Board Review Series

Neuroanatomy

Board Review Series

Neuroanatomy

James D. Fix, Ph.D.

Professor of Anatomy
Department of Anatomy
Marshall University
School of Medicine
Huntington, West Virginia

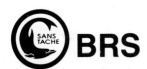

BRS

Board Review Series from Williams & Wilkins
Baltimore, Hong Kong, London, Sydney

Harwal Publishing Company, Malvern, Pennsylvania

**Williams
& Wilkins**

Managing Editor: Susan E. Kelly
Project Editors: Michael N. Samsot, Judd L. Howard
Illustration: Lydia V. Kibiuk
Production Supervisor: Laurie Forsyth

Library of Congress Cataloging-in-Publication Data

Fix, James D.
  Neuroanatomy/James D. Fix.
     p.   cm.—(Board review series)
  Includes bibliographical references and index.
  ISBN 0-683-03250-X
  1. Neuroanatomy—Examinations, questions, etc.   2. Neuroanatomy—
Outlines, syllabi, etc.   I. Title.   II. Series.
  [DNLM: 1. Neuroanatomy—examination questions. 2. Neuroanatomy—
outlines. WL 18 F566n]
QM451.F59   1992
611.8'076—dc20
DNLM/DLC
for Library of Congress   91-30099
                                                                         CIP

10 9 8 7 6 5 4 3 2 1

Dedication

To Ilse, for her constant support and
understanding

Contents

Preface

Designed as a concise review of human neuroanatomy, this book is intended primarily for medical and dental students preparing for the National Board Comprehensive Part I Examination as well as other examinations. It presents the essentials of human neuroanatomy in a concise, tightly outlined, well-illustrated format. There are over 500 National Board-type questions with complete answers and explanations included at the end of each chapter and in a Comprehensive Examination at the end of the book.

Organization

The content has been carefully selected and organized to minimize the time required to review neuroanatomy. The text is hierarchically structured to indicate clearly its relative importance. The illustrations, which play a particularly important role in the understanding of this subject, are used to augment and clarify the outline.

Neurohistology, neuroembryology, and neurotransmitters are discussed in separate chapters. The chapter on neurotransmitters covers recent information on the neurochemical coding of neural circuits.

Features

Questions have been developed to reflect the guidelines set forth beginning in 1991 by the National Board of Medical Examiners. Clinical relevance has been integrated wherever possible both in the text and in the questions and explanations.

A Comprehensive Examination at the end of the book serves as a practice exam and self-assessment tool to help students diagnose weaknesses prior to beginning a review of the subject. It also serves as a self-examination upon completion of the book prior to examination. State-of-the-art magnetic resonance images have been included.

Approximately 115 illustrations have been carefully developed to enhance understanding of neuroanatomy.

To the Student

TRY TO CUSTOMIZE YOUR REVIEW, TAILORING IT TO YOUR OWN LEARNING STYLE. You may be a reader, a scanner, a self-tester, or a visual memorizer.

If you feel relatively confident, take the Comprehensive Examination first. It is composed of 117 questions, several with illustrations. All questions are written covering material in the chapters. Additional information is included in the explanations.

For each chapter that you feel you remember the material, start by taking the review test at the end of the chapter. After taking the test, you may decide that you don't need to review the material in that chapter.

If you decide to review a chapter, remember that each chapter is arranged in separate sections by subject. Each section contains a few statements, and most statements contain an emphasized word or phrase that highlights the most important point of that statement. By scanning the emphasized words and phrases, you can use this book as a trigger to recall and review material you have previously studied.

Chapter 13, "Cranial Nerves," is pivotal. It spawns more neuroanatomy National Board questions than any other single topic in the book.

Study the illustrations carefully and read the legends. Numerous National Board questions come from this source. Pay particular attention to the illustrations that show neuroanatomic pathways (e.g., the pyramidal tracts) or the visual pathways. The thalamic nuclei and their connections can easily be relearned by studying Figure 16.1. Study the simplified block (flow) diagrams of the hypothalamus, limbic, and striatal connections.

If you answered a question incorrectly, take the time to read the explanation. Many confusing issues of neuroanatomy are settled in the explanations to the questions; for example, the difference between stria medullaris and stria terminalis or the important difference between a lower motor neuron and an upper motor neuron.

I wish you success.

James D. Fix

Acknowledgments

The author wishes to thank his students, colleagues, and members of the staff of Williams & Wilkins for their valuable comments, suggestions, and help. I especially would like to thank Susan E. Kelly, Managing Editor, for her perceptive editorial suggestions that have made this a better presentation. I thank Lydia V. Kibiuk for her fine illustrations.

I thank Dr. Malcolm B. Carpenter, Uniformed Services University, who kindly provided me with some of the original artwork used in the sixth edition of *Human Neuroanatomy*, Williams & Wilkins. I thank Dr. Stephen E. Fish, Marshall University, who offered valuable suggestions and criticism during the entire preparation of this book. I wish to thank the class of 1994, Marshall University School of Medicine, for their invaluable comments and help.

I also thank Mr. Mohamad Haleem, Curator of the Yakovlev Collection of the Armed Forces Institute of Pathology, Washington, DC, who provided me with the three myelin-stained sections used in Chapter 1. Thanks go to Dr. Emanuel Kanal, Pittsburgh NMR Institute, who provided me with three MRI images used in Chapter 24.

1

Gross Anatomy
of the Brain

I. Introduction—The Brain

—is that part of the central nervous system (CNS) that lies within the cranial vault, the **encephalon**. Its hemispheric surface is convoluted (i.e., gyrencephalic) and has **gyri** and **sulci**.

—consists of the **cerebrum** (cerebral hemispheres and the diencephalon*); the **brainstem** (midbrain, pons, and medulla); and the **cerebellum**.

—weighs 350 g in the newborn and 1400 g in the adult.

—is covered by three connective tissue membranes, the **meninges**.

—is surrounded by **cerebrospinal fluid (CSF),** which supports it and protects it from trauma.

II. Divisions of the Brain

—the brain is classified into six postembryonic divisions: **telencephalon, diencephalon, mesencephalon, pons, medulla oblongata, and cerebellum.**

A. Telencephalon

—consists of the **cerebral hemispheres** (which comprise both cerebral cortex and white matter) and the **basal ganglia**. The cerebral hemispheres contain the **lateral ventricles**.

1. Cerebral hemispheres (Figures 1.1–1.5)

—are separated by the longitudinal cerebral fissure and the falx cerebri.

—are interconnected by the corpus callosum.

—consist of six lobes and the olfactory structures:

a. Frontal lobe (see Figures 1.3 and 1.4)

—extends from the central sulcus to the frontal pole.

—lies above the lateral sulcus and anterior to the central sulcus.

—contains the following gyri:

(1) Precentral gyrus

—consists of the motor area (area 4).

---

*Some authorities classify the diencephalon as part of the brainstem, not as part of the cerebrum.

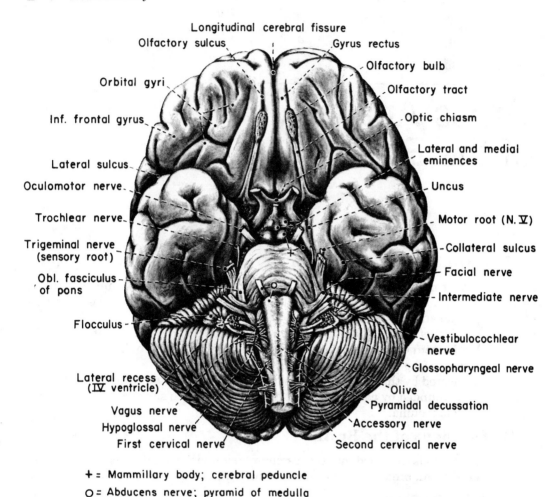

Longitudinal cerebral fissure
Olfactory sulcus
Gyrus rectus
Olfactory bulb
Orbital gyri
Olfactory tract
Inf. frontal gyrus
Optic chiasm
Lateral and medial
eminences
Lateral sulcus
Oculomotor nerve
Uncus
Trochlear nerve
Motor root (N. Ⅴ)
Trigeminal nerve
(sensory root)
Collateral sulcus
Obl. fasciculus
of pons
Facial nerve
Flocculus
Intermediate nerve
Vestibulocochlear
nerve
Lateral recess
(Ⅳ ventricle)
Glossopharyngeal nerve
Olive
Vagus nerve
Pyramidal decussation
Hypoglossal nerve
Accessory nerve
First cervical nerve
Second cervical nerve

\+ = Mammillary body; cerebral peduncle

O = Abducens nerve; pyramid of medulla

Figure 1.1. Base of the brain with the attached cranial nerves. (Reprinted with permission from Truex RC and Kellner CE: *Detailed Atlas of the Head and Neck.* New York, Oxford University Press, 1958, p 34.)

(2) Superior frontal gyrus
–contains the supplementary motor cortex on the medial surface (area 6).

(3) Middle frontal gyrus
–contains the frontal eye field (area 8).

(4) Inferior frontal gyrus
–contains Broca's speech area in the dominant hemisphere (areas 44 and 45).

(5) Gyrus rectus and orbital gyri
–are separated by the olfactory sulcus.

(6) Anterior paracentral lobule
–is found on the medial surface between the superior frontal gyrus (paracentral sulcus) and the central sulcus.
–represents a continuation of the precentral gyrus on the medial hemispheric surface.

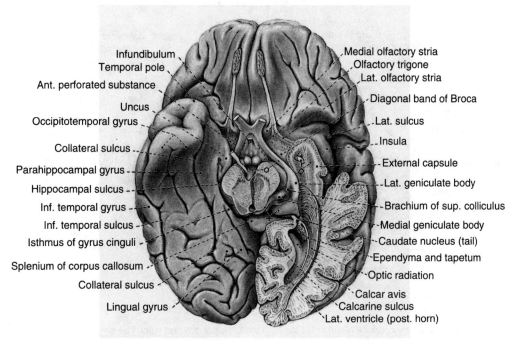

Infundibulum
Temporal pole
Ant. perforated substance
Uncus
Occipitotemporal gyrus
Collateral sulcus
Parahippocampal gyrus
Hippocampal sulcus
Inf. temporal gyrus
Inf. temporal sulcus
Isthmus of gyrus cinguli
Splenium of corpus callosum
Collateral sulcus
Lingual gyrus

Medial olfactory stria
Olfactory trigone
Lat. olfactory stria
Diagonal band of Broca
Lat. sulcus
Insula
External capsule
Lat. geniculate body
Brachium of sup. colliculus
Medial geniculate body
Caudate nucleus (tail)
Ependyma and tapetum
Optic radiation
Calcar avis
Calcarine sulcus
Lat. ventricle (post. horn)

0 = Post. perforated substance; optic tract

◊ = Ant. commissure; lenticular nucleus

+ = Pulvinar of thalamus; brachium of inf. colliculus

Figure 1.2. Inferior surface of the brain showing principal gyri and sulci. The left hemisphere has been dissected to show the visual pathways and relation of the optic radiation to the lateral ventricle. (Reprinted with permission from Truex RC and Kellner CE: *Detailed Atlas of the Head and Neck.* New York, Oxford University Press, 1958, p 46.)

b. Parietal lobe (see Figures 1.3–1.5)

—extends from the central sulcus to the occipital lobe and lies superior to the temporal lobe.

—contains the following lobules and gyri:

(1) Postcentral gyrus

—is the primary sensory area of the cerebral cortex (areas 3, 1, and 2).

(2) Superior parietal lobule

—comprises association areas involved in somatosensory functions (areas 5 and 7).

(3) Inferior parietal lobule

(a) Supramarginal gyrus

—interrelates somatosensory, auditory, and visual input (area 40).

(b) Angular gyrus

—receives visual impulses (area 39).

(4) Precuneus

—is located between the paracentral lobule and the cuneus.

(5) Posterior paracentral lobule

—is located on the medial surface between the central sulcus and the precuneus.

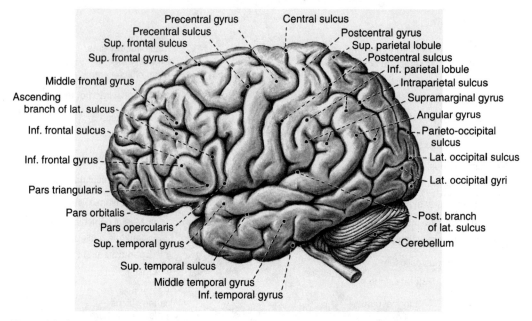

Figure 1.3. Lateral convex surface of the brain showing the principal gyri and sulci. The central sulcus separates the primary motor cortex (precentral gyrus) from the primary somatosensory cortex (postcentral gyrus). (Reprinted with permission from Truex RC and Kellner CE: *Detailed Atlas of the Head and Neck.* New York, Oxford University Press, 1958, p 47.)

—represents a continuation of the postcentral gyrus on the medial hemispheric surface.

c. Temporal lobe (see Figures 1.2–1.4)

—extends from the temporal pole to the occipital lobe, lying below the lateral sulcus.

—extends from the lateral sulcus to the collateral sulcus.

—contains the following gyri:

(1) Transverse temporal gyri of Heschl

—lie buried within the lateral sulcus.

—extend from the superior temporal gyrus toward the medial geniculate body (Figure 1.6).

—are the primary auditory areas of the cerebral cortex (areas 41 and 42).

(2) Superior temporal gyrus

—is associated with auditory functions.

—contains **Wernicke's speech area** in the dominant hemisphere (area 22).

—contains the planum temporale on its superior hidden surface.

(3) Middle temporal gyrus

(4) Inferior temporal gyrus

(5) Lateral occipitotemporal gyrus (fusiform gyrus)

—lies between the inferior temporal sulcus and the collateral sulcus.

d. Occipital lobe (see Figures 1.3–1.5)

—lies posterior to a line connecting the parieto-occipital sulcus and the preoccipital notch.

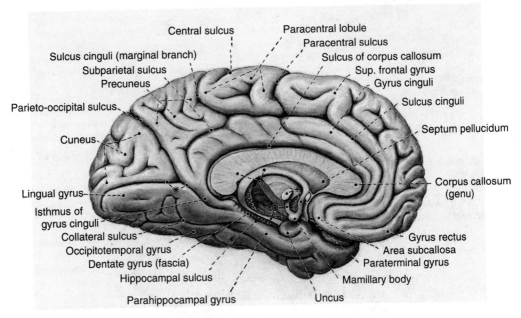

* = Calcarine fissure

◊ = Splenium of corpus callosum; body of fornix

+ = Interthalamic connection; ant. column of fornix

0 = Fimbria of hippocampus; mamillothalamic tract

Figure 1.4. Medial surface of the brain showing the principal gyri and sulci. Parts of the thalamus and hypothalamus have been removed to show the fimbria and anterior column of the fornix and the mamillothalamic tract. (Reprinted with permission from Truex RC and Kellner CE: *Detailed Atlas of the Head and Neck.* New York, Oxford University Press, 1958, p 49.)

—contains two structures:

(1) Cuneus

—lies between the parieto-occipital sulcus and the calcarine sulcus.

—contains the visual cortex (areas 17, 18, and 19).

(2) Lingual gyrus (medial occipitotemporal gyrus)

—lies below the calcarine sulcus.

—contains the visual cortex (areas 17, 18, and 19).

e. Insular lobe (insula) [Figures 1.8 and 1.9; see Figure 1.2]

—lies buried within the lateral sulcus.

—has short and long gyri.

f. Limbic lobe (see Figures 1.4 and 23.1*B*)

—is a C-**shaped structure** of the medial hemispheric surface that encircles the corpus callosum and the lateral aspect of the midbrain.

—includes the following structures:

(1) Paraterminal gyrus and subcallosal area

—is located anterior to the lamina terminalis and ventral to the rostrum of the corpus callosum.

(2) Cingulate gyrus

—lies directly above the corpus callosum.

—merges with the parahippocampal gyrus at the isthmus.

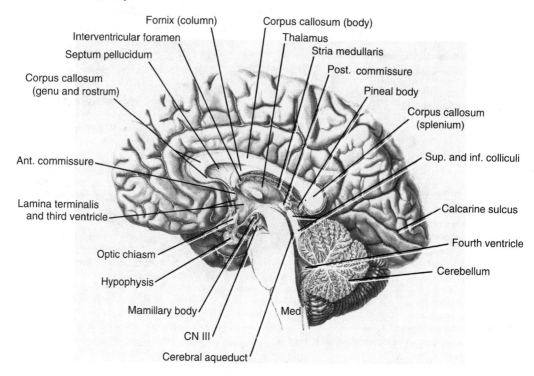

Figure 1.5. Midsagittal section of the brain and brainstem showing the structures surrounding the third and fourth ventricles. The brainstem includes the midbrain (*M*), pons (*P*), and medulla oblongata (*Med*). (Reprinted with permission from Wolf-Heidegger G: *Atlas der systematischen Anatomie des Menschen*, vol III, 3rd ed. Basel, S Karger AG, 1972.)

(3) Parahippocampal gyrus[*]
    —lies between the hippocampal and collateral sulci and terminates in the **uncus**.
(4) Hippocampal formation (see Figures 1.2 and 1.4)
    —lies between the choroidal and hippocampal fissures.
    —is jelly-rolled into the parahippocampal gyrus.
    —is connected to the hypothalamus and septal area via the **fornix** (see Figure 1.4).
    —includes the following three structures:
    (a) Dentate gyrus
    (b) Hippocampus
    (c) Subiculum

g. Olfactory structures (see Figure 1.2)
    —are found on the orbital surface of the brain and include:
    (1) Olfactory bulb and tract
        —are an outpouching of the telencephalon.
    (2) Olfactory bulb
        —receives the olfactory nerve (CN I).
    (3) Olfactory trigone and striae
    (4) Anterior perforated substance
        —is created by penetrating striate arteries.

---

[*]Some authorities include the parahippocampal gyrus as a temporal lobe structure.

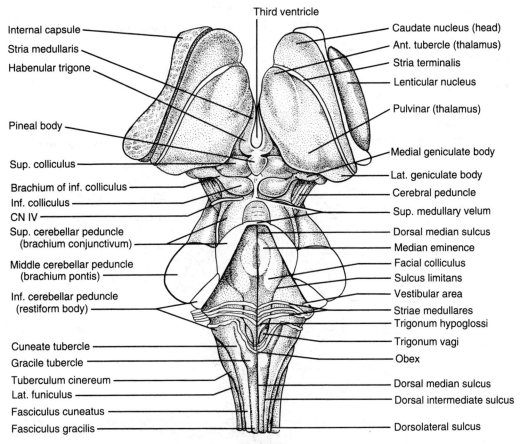

Figure 1.6. Surface anatomy of the brainstem and relationships of the attached cranial nerves. The dorsal surface with the cerebellum removed to show the three cerebellar peduncles and the floor of the fourth ventricle (rhomboid fossa). [Reprinted with permission from Truex RC and Carpenter MB: *Human Neuroanatomy*. Baltimore, Williams & Wilkins, 1969, p 31.]

(5) **Diagonal band of Broca**
–interconnects the amygdaloid nucleus and the septal area.

2. **Basal ganglia** (Figures 1.10 and 1.11; see Figures 1.6–1.9 and 21.1)
–are the subcortical nuclei of the telencephalon and include the following structures:

a. **Caudate nucleus**

b. **Putamen**

c. **Globus pallidus**

d. **Amygdaloid nuclear complex (amygdala)**

3. **Lateral ventricles** (see Figures 1.8–1.11 and 2.4)
–are ependyma-lined cavities of the cerebral hemispheres.
–contain **CSF and choroid plexus**.
–communicate with the third ventricle via the two interventricular foramina of Monro (see Figure 2.3).
–are separated from each other by the septa pellucida.

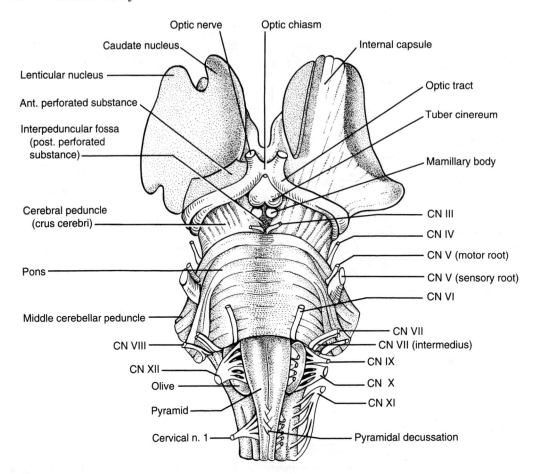

Figure 1.7. Surface anatomy of the brainstem and relationships of the attached cranial nerves; ventral surface. (Reprinted with permission from Truex RC and Carpenter MB: *Human Neuroanatomy*. Baltimore, Williams & Wilkins, 1969, p 31.

4. Cerebral cortex
—consists of a thin layer or mantle of gray substance.
—covers the surface of each cerebral hemisphere.
—is folded into gyri that are separated by sulci.

5. White matter
—includes the cerebral commissures and the internal capsule.

a. Cerebral commissures (see Figures 1.4 and 1.5)
—interconnect the cerebral hemispheres and include:

(1) Corpus callosum
—is the largest commissure of the brain.
—has four parts:
(a) Rostrum
(b) Genu
(c) Body
(d) Splenium

(2) Anterior commissure
—is located in the midsagittal section between the lamina terminalis and the column of the fornix.

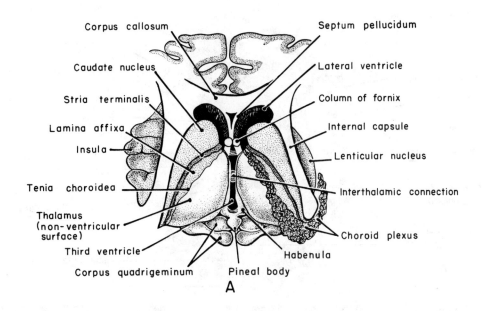

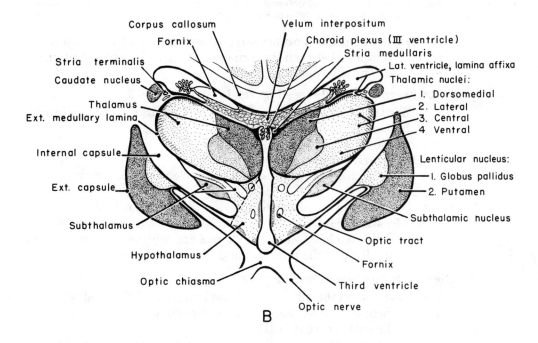

Figure 1.8. (*A*) Dorsal aspect of the diencephalon. The stria terminalis lies between the caudate nucleus and the thalamus. The stria medullaris thalami passes into the habenula. (*B*) Coronal section through the diencephalon showing the boundaries of the thalamus, hypothalamus, and the subthalamus. (Reprinted with permission from Truex RC and Carpenter MB: *Human Neuroanatomy.* Baltimore, Williams & Wilkins, 1969, p 42.)

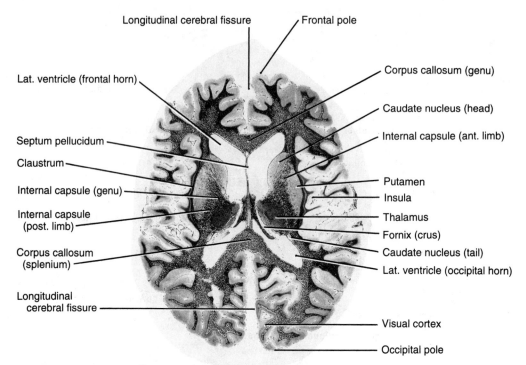

Figure 1.9. Horizontal (axial) section through the brain at the level of the genu and splenium of the corpus callosum. The boundaries of the internal capsule are well delineated. (Published with permission from the Yakovlev Collection. Washington, D.C., The Armed Forces Institute of Pathology.)

(3) Hippocampal commissure (commissure of the fornix)
   –is located between the fornices and ventral to the splenium of the corpus callosum.

b. Internal capsule (see Figures 1.8–1.11 and 16.3)
   –consists of the white matter located between the basal ganglia and the thalamus.
   –has three parts:
(1) Anterior limb
   –is located between the caudate nucleus and putamen.
(2) Genu
   –is located between the anterior and posterior limbs.
(3) Posterior limb
   –is located between the thalamus and lentiform nucleus (which is made up of the putamen and the globus pallidus).

B. Diencephalon (see Figures 1.5–1.8)
   –is located between the telencephalon and mesencephalon and between the interventricular foramen and the posterior commissure.
   –receives the optic nerve (CN II).
   –consists of the epithalamus, thalamus, hypothalamus, subthalamus, and the third ventricle and associated structures.

1. Epithalamus (see Figures 1.5 and 1.6)

a. Pineal body (epiphysis cerebri)

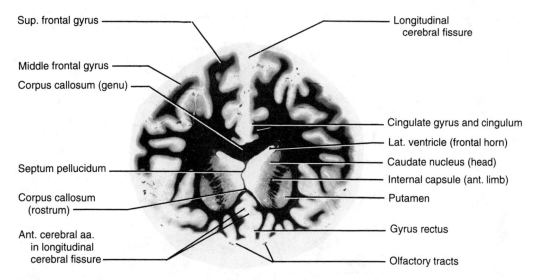

Sup. frontal gyrus

Middle frontal gyrus

Corpus callosum (genu)

Septum pellucidum

Corpus callosum (rostrum)

Ant. cerebral aa. in longitudinal cerebral fissure

Longitudinal cerebral fissure

Cingulate gyrus and cingulum

Lat. ventricle (frontal horn)

Caudate nucleus (head)

Internal capsule (ant. limb)

Putamen

Gyrus rectus

Olfactory tracts

Figure 1.10. Coronal (frontal) section through the striatum (caudate nucleus and putamen) at the level of the rostrum of the corpus callosum. The anterior limb of the internal capsule lies between the caudate nucleus and the putamen. (Published with permission from the Yakovlev Collection. Washington, D.C., The Armed Forces Institute of Pathology.)

  b. Habenular trigone

  c. Medullary stria of the thalamus

  d. Posterior commissure

  e. Tela choroidea and choroid plexus of the third ventricle

2. **Thalamus** (see Figures 1.6 and 1.8)

 −is separated from the hypothalamus by the **hypothalamic sulcus.**
 −consists of the following surface structures:

  a. Pulvinar

  b. Metathalamus
   (1) Medial geniculate body (auditory system)
   (2) Lateral geniculate body (visual system)

  c. Anterior tubercle

  d. Interthalamic adhesion (massa intermedia)

3. **Hypothalamus** (see Figures 1.1, 1.2, 1.6, and 1.8*B*)

  a. Optic chiasm

  b. Mamillary body

  c. Infundibulum

  d. Tuber cinereum

4. **Subthalamus (ventral thalamus)** [see Figure 1.8*B*]

 −lies ventral to the thalamus and lateral to the hypothalamus.
 −is not visible on midsagittal sections through the third ventricle.
 −consists of:

  a. Subthalamic nucleus

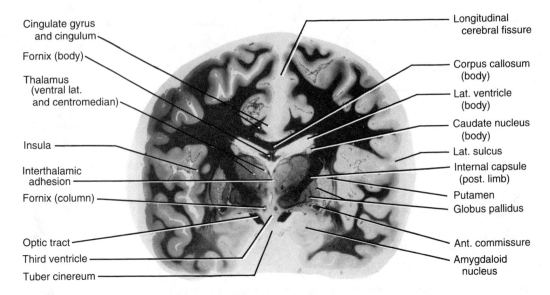

Cingulate gyrus and cingulum

Fornix (body)

Thalamus (ventral lat. and centromedian)

Insula

Interthalamic adhesion

Fornix (column)

Optic tract

Third ventricle

Tuber cinereum

Longitudinal cerebral fissure

Corpus callosum (body)

Lat. ventricle (body)

Caudate nucleus (body)

Lat. sulcus

Internal capsule (post. limb)

Putamen

Globus pallidus

Ant. commissure

Amygdaloid nucleus

Figure 1.11. Coronal (frontal) section through the midthalamus at the level of the ventral lateral nucleus, the interthalamic adhesion, and the tuber cinereum. The posterior limb of the internal capsule lies between the thalamus and the lentiform nucleus (putamen and globus pallidus). The amygdaloid nucleus underlies the uncus of the parahippocampal gyrus. (Published with permission from the Yakovlev Collection. Washington, D.C., The Armed Forces Institute of Pathology.)

   b. Zona incerta and fields of Forel (see Figure 21.3)

 5. Third ventricle and associated structures (see Figures 1.5 and 2.4)

   a. Lamina terminalis

   b. Tela choroidea

   c. Choroid plexus

   d. Interventricular foramen

   e. Optic recess

   f. Infundibular recess

   g. Suprapineal recess

   h. Pineal recess

C. Mesencephalon (midbrain) [see Figure 1.6]

   −is located between the diencephalon and the pons.

   −extends from the posterior commissure to the frenulum of the superior medullary velum.

   −contains the **cerebral aqueduct,** which interconnects the third and fourth ventricles.

   1. Ventral surface

   a. Cerebral peduncle

   b. Interpeduncular fossa

   (1) Oculomotor nerve (CN III)

   (2) Posterior perforated substance

   −is created by penetrating branches of the posterior cerebral and posterior communicating arteries.

    2. Dorsal surface

      a. Superior colliculus

      b. Brachium of the superior colliculus

      c. Inferior colliculus

      d. Brachium of the inferior colliculus

      e. Trochlear nerve (CN IV)

           –is the only cranial nerve to exit the brainstem from the dorsal aspect.

D. Pons (see Figures 1.1 and 1.7)

    –is located between the midbrain and the medulla.

    –extends from the inferior pontine sulcus to the superior pontine sulcus.

    1. Ventral surface

      a. Base of the pons

      b. Cranial nerves

         (1) Trigeminal nerve (CN V)

         (2) Abducent nerve (CN VI)

         (3) Facial nerve (CN VII)

         (4) Vestibulocochlear nerve (CN VIII)

    2. Dorsal surface (rhomboid fossa)

         (1) Locus ceruleus

         (2) Facial colliculus

         (3) Sulcus limitans

         (4) Striae medullares of the rhomboid fossa

            –divide the rhomboid fossa into the superior pontine portion and the inferior medullary portion.

E. Medulla oblongata (myelencephalon) [see Figures 1.1 and 1.7]

    –is located between the pons and the spinal cord.

    –extends from the first cervical nerve (C1) to the inferior pontine sulcus (also called the pontobulbar sulcus).

    1. Ventral surface

      a. Pyramid

      b. Olive

      c. Cranial nerves

         (1) Glossopharyngeal nerve (CN IX)

         (2) Vagal nerve (CN X)

         (3) Accessory nerve (CN XI)

         (4) Hypoglossal nerve (CN XII)

    2. Dorsal surface

      a. Gracile tubercle

      b. Cuneate tubercle

      c. Rhomboid fossa

         (1) Striae medullares of the rhomboid fossa

         (2) Vagal trigone

(3) **Hypoglossal trigone**

(4) **Sulcus limitans**

(5) **Area postrema**

F. **Cerebellum** (see Figures 1.1 and 1.5)

   –is located in the posterior cranial fossa.

   –is attached to the brainstem by three cerebellar peduncles.

   –forms the roof of the fourth ventricle.

   –is separated from the occipital and temporal lobes by the **tentorium cerebelli**.

   –consists of **folia** and **fissures** on its surface.

   –contains the following surface structures:

1. **Hemispheres**

   –are made up of two lateral lobes.

2. **Vermis**

   –is a midline structure.

3. **Flocculus and vermal nodulus**

   –form the flocculonodular lobule.

4. **Tonsil**

   –is a rounded lobule on the inferior surface of each cerebellar hemisphere.

5. **Superior cerebellar peduncle** (see Figure 1.6)

   –connects the cerebellum to the pons and midbrain.

6. **Middle cerebellar peduncle** (see Figure 1.6)

   –connects the cerebellum to the pons.

7. **Inferior cerebellar peduncle** (see Figure 1.6)

   –connects the cerebellum to the medulla.

8. **Anterior lobe**

   –lies anterior to the primary fissure.

9. **Posterior lobe**

   –is located between the primary and posterolateral fissures.

10. **Flocculonodular lobe**

   –lies posterior to the posterolateral fissure.

Review Test

Directions: Each of the numbered items or incomplete statements in this section is followed by answers or by completions of the statement. Select the **one** lettered answer or completion that is **best** in each case.

1. The medulla includes all of the following structures EXCEPT the

(A) cuneate tubercle.
(B) olive.
(C) vagal trigone.
(D) facial colliculus.
(E) glossopharyngeal nerve.

2. The fourth cranial nerve emerges from the

(A) interpeduncular fossa.
(B) superior pontine sulcus.
(C) dorsal surface of the midbrain.
(D) lateral aspect of the pons.
(E) cerebellopontine angle.

3. Which of the following structures separates the anterior cerebellar lobe from the posterior cerebellar lobe?

(A) Sulcus limitans
(B) Horizontal fissure
(C) Primary fissure
(D) Posterolateral fissure
(E) Prepyramidal fissure

4. The limbic lobe includes all of the following structures EXCEPT the

(A) cingulate gyrus.
(B) paraterminal gyrus.
(C) parahippocampal gyrus.
(D) dentate gyrus.
(E) lingual gyrus.

5. All of the following statements concerning the hippocampal formation are correct EXCEPT

(A) it gives rise to the fornix.
(B) it includes the subiculum.
(C) it includes the dentate gyrus.
(D) it includes the posterior commissure.
(E) it lies between the hippocampal and choroidal fissures.

6. All of the following statements concerning the central sulcus are correct EXCEPT

(A) it separates the frontal lobe from the parietal lobe.
(B) it separates the motor cortex from the sensory cortex.
(C) it extends into the paracentral lobule.
(D) it is located on the lateral convex surface of the hemisphere.
(E) it joins the lateral sulcus.

7. The basal ganglia include all of the following structures EXCEPT the

(A) caudate nucleus.
(B) putamen.
(C) thalamus.
(D) globus pallidus.
(E) amygdaloid nucleus.

8. The telencephalon includes all of the following structures EXCEPT the

(A) thalamus.
(B) cerebral hemispheres.
(C) globus pallidus.
(D) caudate nucleus.
(E) internal capsule.

9. The mesencephalon includes all of the following structures EXCEPT the

(A) cerebral peduncle.
(B) cerebral aqueduct.
(C) inferior colliculus.
(D) pineal body.
(E) oculomotor nerve.

10. Which of the following areas is not included in the frontal lobe?

(A) Wernicke's speech area
(B) The motor strip (area 4)
(C) The precentral gyrus
(D) Broca's speech area
(E) The center controlling eye movements

11. All of the following statements concerning the cerebellum are correct EXCEPT it

(A) is found in the posterior cranial fossa.
(B) is part of the brainstem.
(C) is separated from the occipital lobes by the tentorium cerebelli.
(D) has three lobes.
(E) has a tonsil.

12. The parietal lobe contains all of the following structures EXCEPT the

(A) angular gyrus.
(B) sensory strip (areas 3, 1, and 2).
(C) supramarginal gyrus.
(D) primary auditory cortex.
(E) precuneus.

Answers and Explanations

1–D. The facial colliculus is located in the pontine half of the rhomboid fossa and overlies the internal genu of the facial nerve and the abducent nucleus. The facial colliculus is a structure of the pontine tegmentum.

2–C. The fourth cranial nerve (trochlear nerve) emerges from the dorsal surface of the midbrain, just caudal to the inferior colliculus.

3–C. The primary fissure separates the anterior from the posterior cerebellar lobe.

4–E. The lingual gyrus lies below the calcarine fissure in the occipital lobe. It contains primary visual cortex and is not part of the limbic lobe.

5–D. The posterior commissure interconnects the pretectal nuclei of the midbrain and serves the pupillary light reflex.

6–E. The central sulcus is an important cerebral landmark. It separates the frontal lobe from the parietal lobe, and it separates motor cortex from sensory cortex. It extends into the paracentral lobule on the medial surface, dividing it into anterior and posterior parts. It rarely joins the lateral sulcus.

7–C. The thalamus is the largest part of the diencephalon; it is not a basal ganglion.

8–A. The telencephalon contains the cerebral hemispheres, which contain the cerebral cortex and white matter, the basal ganglia (caudate nucleus, putamen, globus pallidus, and amygdaloid nucleus), and the lateral ventricles. The thalamus is a part of the diencephalon.

9–D. The mesencephalon (or midbrain) includes the cerebral peduncles, the superior and inferior colliculi, the oculomotor nerves, and the cerebral aqueduct. The pineal body (epiphysis cerebri) is a part of the epithalamus.

10–A. The frontal lobe includes the motor strip, which is the precentral gyrus (area 4), and Broca's speech area in the dominant hemisphere (areas 44 and 45). The frontal eye field (area 8) lies in the middle frontal gyrus. Wernicke's speech area (area 22) lies in the posterior part of the superior temporal gyrus of the temporal lobe.

11–B. The cerebellum is found below the tentorium cerebelli in the posterior cranial fossa. It has three lobes: an anterior, a posterior, and a flocculonodular lobe. It has a tonsil that rests on the foramen magnum. It is not a part of the brainstem. The brainstem includes the midbrain, pons, and medulla.

12–D. The parietal lobe contains the sensory strip, which is the postcentral gyrus (areas 3, 1, and 2), the supramarginal, and the angular gyri. The precuneus (area 7) lies on the medial aspect of the parietal lobe. Primary auditory cortex (areas 41 and 42) is found in Heschl's gyrus in the temporal lobe.

2

Meninges and Cerebrospinal Fluid

I. Meninges (Figure 2.1)

—are three connective tissue membranes that invest the spinal cord and brain.
—consist of the **pia mater** and the **arachnoid** (together known as the lepto-meninges) and the **dura mater** (pachymeninx).

A. Pia mater

—is a delicate, highly vascular layer of connective tissue.
—closely covers the surface of the brain and spinal cord.
—is connected to the arachnoid by trabeculae.

1. Denticulate ligaments (see Figure 2.1)

—consist of two lateral flattened bands of pial tissue.
—attach to the spinal dura mater with 21 teeth.

2. Filum terminale (Figure 2.2)

—consists of a nonneural band of tissue that is a condensation of the pia mater.
—extends from the conus medullaris to the end of the dural sac and fuses with it.

B. Arachnoid

—is a delicate, nonvascular connective tissue membrane located between the dura mater and the pia mater.

1. Arachnoid granulations or arachnoid villi

—enter the venous dural sinuses and permit the one-way flow of cere-brospinal fluid (**CSF**) from the subarachnoid space into the venous cir-culation.
—are found in large numbers along the **superior sagittal sinus** but are associated with all dural sinuses.

2. Subarachnoid space (see p 20)

C. Dura mater

—is the outer layer of the meninges and consists of dense connective tissue.

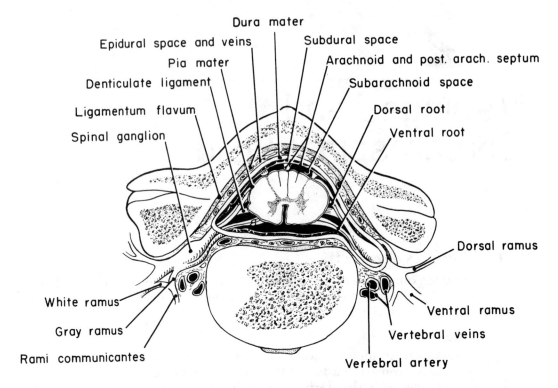

Figure 2.1. Cross section of the spinal cord and its meningeal investments. The subarachnoid, subdural, and epidural spaces are visible. The anterior and posterior longitudinal ligaments are seen but are not labeled. (Reprinted with permission from Carpenter MB and Sutin J: *Human Neuroanatomy,* 8th ed. Baltimore, Williams & Wilkins, 1983, p 9.)

—the supratentorial dura is innervated by the trigeminal nerve; the posterior fossa is innervated by the vagal and upper spinal nerves.
—forms three major reflections and the walls of the dural venous sinuses:

1. **Falx cerebri**
   —lies between the cerebral hemispheres in the longitudinal cerebral fissure.
   —contains the superior and inferior sagittal sinuses between its two layers.

2. **Tentorium cerebelli** (Figure 2.3)
   —separates the posterior cranial fossa from the middle cranial fossa.
   —separates the temporal and occipital lobes from the cerebellum and infratentorial brainstem.
   —contains the **tentorial incisure,** or notch, through which the brainstem passes.

3. **Diaphragma sellae**
   —forms the roof of the **hypophyseal fossa**.
   —contains an aperture through which the **hypophyseal stalk** (infundibulum) passes.

4. **Dural sinuses** (see Figure 2.3)
   —are endothelium-lined, valveless venous blood channels.

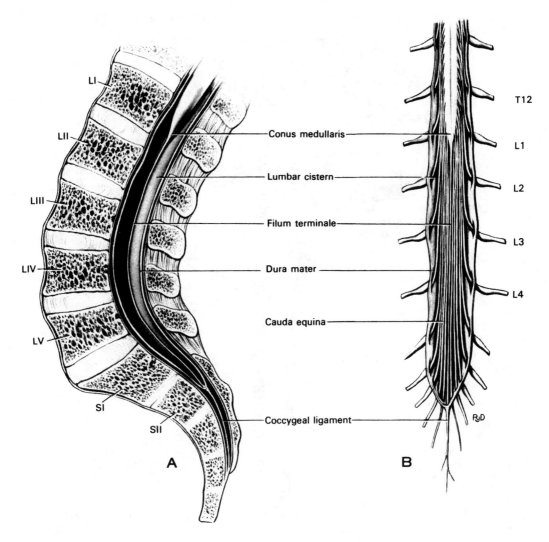

Figure 2.2. Diagrammatic drawings of the caudal part of the spinal cord and lumbar cistern. (*A*) Longitudinal section through the caudal vertebral column and canal showing the conus medullaris and the lumbar cistern. Lumbar puncture is made between the spinous processes of *L3* and *L4* (or *L4* and *L5*). (*B*) Dorsal view of the cauda equina and the spinal nerves. The adult spinal cord terminates at the *L1–L2* interspace. (Reprinted with permission from Carpenter MB and Sutin J: *Human Neuroanatomy,* 8th ed. Baltimore, Williams & Wilkins, 1983, p 8.)

D. Meningeal spaces (see Figures 2.1–2.3)

1. Spinal epidural space

–is located between the dura and the vertebral periosteum.

–contains loose areolar tissue, venous plexuses, and lymphatics.

–may be injected with a local anesthetic to produce a paravertebral nerve block.

2. Cranial epidural space

–is a *potential* space between the periosteal and meningeal layers of the dura.

–contains the meningeal arteries and veins.

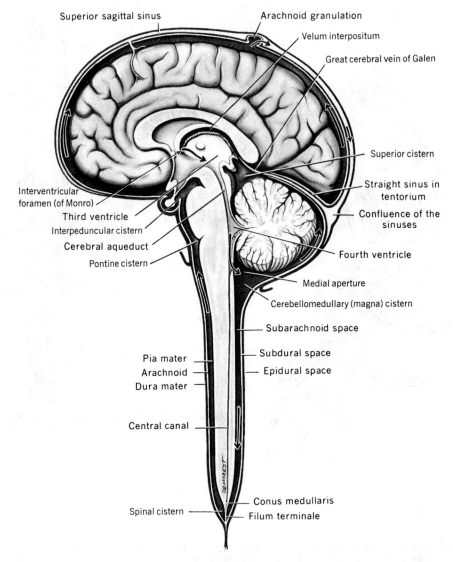

Superior sagittal sinus

Arachnoid granulation

Velum interpositum

Great cerebral vein of Galen

Superior cistern

Straight sinus in tentorium

Confluence of the sinuses

Fourth ventricle

Medial aperture

Cerebellomedullary (magna) cistern

Subarachnoid space

Subdural space

Epidural space

Interventricular foramen (of Monro)

Third ventricle

Interpeduncular cistern

Cerebral aqueduct

Pontine cistern

Pia mater

Arachnoid

Dura mater

Central canal

Spinal cistern

Conus medullaris

Filum terminale

Figure 2.3. The subarachnoid spaces and cisterns of the brain and spinal cord. Cerebrospinal fluid is produced in the choroid plexuses of the ventricles, exits the fourth ventricle, circulates in the subarachnoid space, and enters the superior sagittal sinus via the arachnoid granulations. (Reprinted with permission from Noback CR, Strominger NL, and Demarest RJ: *The Human Nervous System,* 4th ed. Malvern, Pa, Lea & Febiger, 1991, p 68.)

3. Subdural space

–is a *potential* space between the dura and the arachnoid.

–intracranially transmits the superior cerebral veins to the venous lacunae of the superior sagittal sinus.

–laceration of these "bridging veins" results in **subdural hemorrhage** (hematoma).

4. Subarachnoid space

–is located between the pia mater and the arachnoid.

–contains **CSF**.

–surrounds the entire brain and spinal cord.

–extends, in the adult, below the conus medullaris to the level of the second sacral vertebra, the **lumbar cistern** (see Figure 2.2A).

5. **Subarachnoid cisterns** (see Figure 2.3)

–are dilatations of the subarachnoid space, which contains CSF.
–are named after the structures over which they lie (e.g., the pontine, chiasmatic, and interpeduncular cisterns).

a. **Cerebellopontine angle cistern**

–receives CSF from the fourth ventricle via the lateral foramina of Luschka.
–contains the facial nerve (**CN VII**) and the vestibulocochlear nerve (**CN VIII**).

b. **Cerebellomedullary cistern (cisterna magna)**

–is located in the midline between the cerebellum and and the medulla.
–receives CSF from the fourth ventricle via the median foramen of Magendie.
–can be tapped for CSF (suboccipital tap).

E. **Meningiomas**

–are benign, slow-growing, well-demarcated tumors that arise from meningotheal arachnoid cells.
–comprise 20% of primary intracranial tumors and 25% of spinal tumors.
–are found most frequently in the anterior cranial fossa (parasagittal 25%, convexity 20%, and basal 40%).
–are histologically characterized by a whorling pattern and calcified **psammoma bodies**.
–enlarge slowly and create a cavity in the adjacent brain.
–occur in adults between the ages of 20 and 60 years; occur most often in women (60%).

II. Ventricles (Figure 2.4.; see Figure 2.3)

–are lined with ependyma and contain CSF.
–contain choroid plexus, which produces CSF at a rate of 500 ml/day.
–communicate with the subarachnoid space via three foramina in the fourth ventricle.
–consist of four fluid-filled communicating cavities within the brain.

A. **Lateral ventricles**

–are the two ventricles located within the cerebral hemispheres.
–communicate with the third ventricle via the **interventricular foramina of Monro**.
–consist of five parts:

1. **Frontal (anterior) horn**

–is located in the frontal lobe; its lateral wall is formed by the head of the caudate nucleus.
–lacks choroid plexus.

2. **Body**

–is located in the medial portion of the frontal and parietal lobes.
–has choroid plexus.

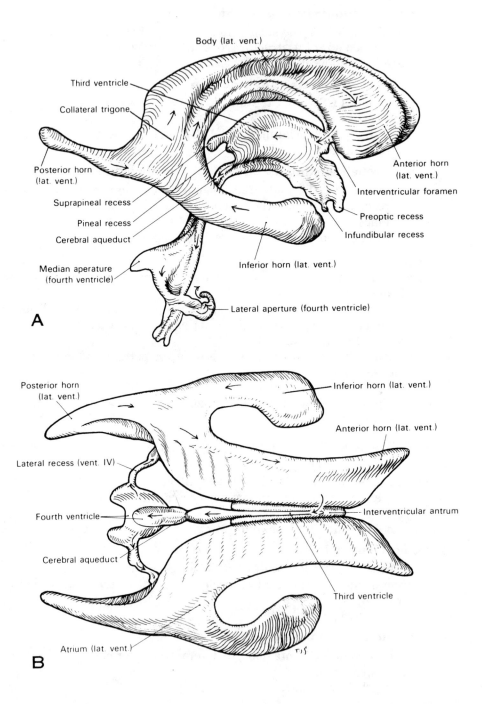

Figure 2.4. The ventricle system of the brain. (*A*) Lateral aspect. (*B*) Dorsal aspect. (Reprinted with permission from Carpenter MB and Sutin J: *Human Neuroanatomy,* 8th ed. Baltimore, Williams & Wilkins, 1983, p 44.)

—communicates via the interventricular foramen of Monro with the third ventricle.

3. Temporal (inferior) horn

—is located in the medial part of the temporal lobe.
—has choroid plexus.

4. Occipital (posterior) horn (see Figure 1.2)

—is located in the parietal and occipital lobes.
—lacks choroid plexus.

5. Trigone (atrium)

—is found at the junction of the body, occipital horn, and temporal horn of the lateral ventricle.
—contains the **glomus,** a large tuft of choroid plexus, which is calcified in adults and is visible on x-ray and CT.

B. Third ventricle (see Figures 1.5, 2.3, and 2.4)

—is a slit-like, vertical midline cavity of the diencephalon.
—communicates with the lateral ventricles via the interventricular foramina of Monro and with the fourth ventricle via the cerebral aqueduct.
—contains a pair of choroid plexuses in its roof.

C. Fourth ventricle (see Figures 1.5, 2.3, and 2.4)

—lies between the cerebellum and the brainstem.
—contains a pair of choroid plexuses in its caudal roof.
—expresses CSF into the subarachnoid space via the two lateral foramina of Luschka and the single medial foramen of Magendie.

D. Cerebral aqueduct (aqueduct of Sylvius)

—lies in the midbrain.
—connects the third ventricle with the fourth ventricle.
—lacks choroid plexus.
—blockage leads to hydrocephalus (aqueductal stenosis).

III. Cerebrospinal Fluid

—is a clear, colorless, acellular fluid found in the subarachnoid space and in the ventricles.

A. Formation—CSF

—is produced by the **choroid plexus** at a rate of 500 ml/day; total CSF volume equals 140 ml (see Figures 1.5, 1.7, and 2.3).

B. Function—CSF

—supports and cushions the central nervous system (CNS) against concussive injury.
—transports hormones and hormone-releasing factors.
—removes metabolic waste products through absorption; the sites of greatest absorption are the **arachnoid villi** (see Figure 2.3).

C. Circulation—CSF (see Figure 2.3)

—flows from the ventricles via the three foramina of the fourth ventricle into the subarachnoid space and over the convexity of the hemisphere to the superior sagittal sinus, where it enters the venous circulation.

D. Composition—CSF

—contains no more than 5 lymphocytes/ml and usually is sterile (gram negative).

—other **normal values** are:

—**pH:** 7.35

—**specific gravity:** 1.007

—**glucose:** 65 mg/dl

—**total protein:** 15–50 mg/dl in the lumbar cistern.

E. Normal pressure—CSF

—is 50–200 mm of water in the lumbar subarachnoid space, when the patient is in a lateral recumbent position.

IV. Circumventricular Organs

—are chemosensitive zones that monitor the varying concentrations of circulating hormones in blood and CSF.

—are located in the periphery of the third ventricle; the **area postrema** is found in the floor of the fourth ventricle.

—are highly vascularized with fenestrated capillaries and no blood–brain barrier (the subcommissural organ is an exception).

—include the following structures:

A. Organum vasculosum of the lamina terminalis

—is considered to be a vascular outlet for luteinizing hormone-releasing hormone and somatostatin.

B. Median eminence of the tuber cinereum (see Figure 1.1)

—contains neurons that elaborate releasing and inhibiting hormones into the hypophyseal portal system.

C. Subfornical organ

—is located on the inferior surface of the fornix at the level of the interventricular foramen of Monro.

—contains neurons that project to the supraoptic nuclei and the organum vasculosum.

—is a central receptor site for angiotensin II.

D. Subcommissural organ

—is located below the posterior commissure at the junction of the third ventricle and the cerebral aqueduct.

—is composed of specialized ependymal cells, glial elements, and a capillary bed containing nonfenestrated endothelial cells.

E. Pineal body (see Figures 1.5 and 1.6A)

—contains **calcareous granules, brain sand** or acervulus, which are seen on x-ray and CT; calcification occurs after 16 years of age.

—contains **pinealocytes** (epiphyseal cells) and is highly vascular with fenestrated capillaries.

—is derived from the diencephalon.

—is innervated solely via postganglionic fibers from the superior cervical ganglion of the autonomic nervous system.

—synthesizes serotonin and melatonin.

–clinical observation suggests an **antigonadotrophic function**.

–**pinealomas** may result in dorsal midbrain syndrome (see Figure 14.3*A*).

F. Area postrema

–consists of two small subependymal oval areas on either side of the fourth ventricle rostral to the obex.

–contains modified neurons and astrocyte-like cells surrounded by fenestrated capillaries.

–is considered to be a chemoreceptor zone that triggers vomiting in response to circulating emetic substances.

–plays a role in food intake and cardiovascular regulation.

Review Test

Directions: Each of the numbered items or incomplete statements in this section is followed by answers or by completions of the statement. Select the **one** lettered answer or completion that is **best** in each case.

1. Which of the following is only a potential space?

(A) Subarachnoid space
(B) Subarachnoid cistern
(C) Spinal epidural space
(D) Cerebral aqueduct
(E) Cranial epidural space

2. The cranial dura is innervated by the

(A) ophthalmic nerve.
(B) facial nerve.
(C) intermediate nerve.
(D) glossopharyngeal nerve.
(E) major petrosal nerve.

3. The calcified glomus of the choroid plexus is visible on x-ray and CT. It is seen in the

(A) frontal horn.
(B) third ventricle.
(C) occipital horn.
(D) trigone.
(E) fourth ventricle.

4. The caudate nucleus is a boundary of all of the following structures EXCEPT the

(A) frontal horn.
(B) body of the lateral ventricle.
(C) occipital horn.
(D) trigone.
(E) temporal horn.

5. All of the following statements concerning the pia mater are correct EXCEPT it

(A) is a delicate, highly vascular layer of connective tissue.
(B) gives rise to the denticulate ligaments.
(C) extends into the sulci and fissures.
(D) is connected to the arachnoid by trabeculae.
(E) is a boundary of the epidural space of the vertebral canal.

6. All of the following statements concerning the arachnoid granulations are correct EXCEPT they

(A) are found along the superior sagittal sinus.
(B) project into the dural venous sinuses.
(C) play a role in the absorption of CSF.
(D) produce CSF.
(E) consist of arachnoid villi.

7. All of the following statements concerning the dura mater are correct EXCEPT it

(A) forms the periosteum of the vertebral canal.
(B) forms the walls of the venous sinuses.
(C) forms the roof of the pituitary fossa.
(D) is innervated by two cranial nerves.
(E) is continuous with the sclera of the eyeball.

8. Which of the following statements concerning the spinal epidural space is true?

(A) It contains the denticulate ligaments.
(B) It contains CSF.
(C) It contains the dorsal root ganglia.
(D) It may be injected with an anesthetic to produce a paravertebral nerve block.
(E) It contains the cauda equina.

9. All of the following statements concerning the cranial epidural space are correct EXCEPT

(A) it contains a branch of the facial artery.
(B) it contains meningeal veins.
(C) it usually is associated with arterial hemorrhage.
(D) it is bounded by two layers of dura.
(E) it is normally a potential space.

10. All of the following statements concerning the subarachnoid space are correct EXCEPT it

(A) communicates via the foramina of Luschka with the fourth ventricle.
(B) is found between the arachnoid and the pia mater.
(C) extends, in the adult, from the conus medullaris to S2.
(D) is lined with ependymal cells.
(E) communicates via the median foramen of Magendie with the fourth ventricle.

11. All of the following statements concerning meningiomas are correct EXCEPT they

(A) are derived from arachnoid cells.
(B) are characterized by cellular whorls and psammoma bodies.
(C) are more frequent in males.
(D) are benign, slow growing, and well-circumscribed tumors.
(E) comprise approximately 20% of primary intracranial tumors.

Answers and Explanations

1–E. The cranial epidural space and the subdural space are normally potential spaces. Hemorrhage of a meningeal artery creates an epidural space between the periosteal and meningeal layers of the dura (epidural hematoma). Laceration of the superior cerebral veins ("bridging veins") as they enter the superior sagittal sinus creates a subdural space between the dura and the arachnoid (subdural hematoma).

2–A. The cranial dura is innervated by the trigeminal nerve (CN V), the meningeal (recurrent) branches of the vagal nerve (CN X), and the upper spinal nerves (C1 and C2), via the hypoglossal nerve (CN XII).

3–D. The calcified glomus is found in the trigone of the lateral ventricle. It, as well as the calcified pineal gland, can be seen on x-ray and CT (but not on MRI).

4–C. The caudate nucleus forms the lateral wall of the frontal horn, body, trigone of the lateral ventricle, and the roof of the temporal horn. It does not extend into the occipital horn.

5–E. The pia mater is a delicate, highly vascular layer of connective tissue, which gives rise to the denticulate ligaments. It extends into the sulci and fissures of the brain and spinal cord and is connected via trabeculae to the arachnoid membrane. The spinal epidural space lies between the dura and the periosteum of the vertebrae; it contains loose areolar tissue and a venous plexus.

6–D. Arachnoid granulations are tufts of pia–arachnoid tissue that extend into the venous lacunae or directly into the venous dural sinuses. Microscopically, they are arachnoid villi and are prominent along the superior sagittal sinus. They play a major role in the absorption of CSF.

7–A. The dura mater forms the walls of the venous sinuses and the diaphragma sellae, which forms the roof of the hypophyseal fossa. The dura of the anterior and middle cranial fossae is innervated by the ophthalmic and maxillary divisions of the trigeminal nerve (CN V). The infratentorial dura of the posterior cranial fossa is innervated by the vagal nerve (CN X) and the meningeal branches of the upper cervical spinal nerves. The spinal dura consists of one layer, the meningeal dura; it does not form the periosteum of the vertebrae. The dura is continuous with the sclera; it forms the outer connective tissue layer of the optic nerve (CN II).

8–D. The spinal epidural space contains loose areolar tissue, venous plexuses, and lymphatics. It may be injected with an anesthetic to produce a paravertebral nerve block. The denticulate ligaments are subdural pial structures that extend from the surface of the spinal cord and attach to the internal surface of the dura. The dorsal root ganglia are located within the intervertebral foramina. CSF and the cauda equina are found in the subarachnoid space.

9–A. The cranial epidural space is actually a potential intradural space that is created only after trauma and hemorrhage. Epidural hematomas are arterial hemorrhages. The cranial epidural space lies between the periosteal and meningeal dural layers. Meningeal arteries and veins are found in this space.

10–D. The subarachnoid space is found between the arachnoid and the pia. It extends in the adult from the conus medullaris to S2. The subarachnoid space is lined with leptomeningeal (mesothelial) cells. The subarachnoid space communicates via the foramina of Luschka and the median foramen of Magendie with the fourth ventricle. Ependymal cells line the ventricles.

11–C. Meningiomas occur more frequently in women (60%) than in men.

3

Blood Supply of the Central Nervous System

I. Arteries of the Spinal Cord

—arise from the vertebral and segmental arteries.

A. Vertebral artery (Figure 3.1)

—is a branch of the subclavian artery.

—gives rise to the anterior spinal artery and may give rise to the posterior spinal artery.

1. Anterior spinal artery

—supplies the anterior two-thirds of the spinal cord, including the anterior and lateral horns.

—supplies the pyramids, medial lemniscus, and intra-axial fibers of cranial nerve XII in the medulla.

2. Posterior spinal arteries

—supply the posterior one-third of the spinal cord, including the posterior horns and columns.

—supply the gracile and cuneate fasciculi and nuclei in the medulla.

B. Segmental arteries

—give rise to the medullary arteries, which supply the anterior and posterior spinal arteries.

—provide the main blood supply to the spinal cord at thoracic and lumbar levels.

—the second lumbar artery gives rise to a large anterior medullary artery, the **artery of Adamkiewicz**.

II. Venous Drainage of the Spinal Cord

—follows, in general, the arterial pattern.

—passes from spinal veins within the subarachnoid space to the epidural internal venous plexus before draining into intracranial, cervical, thoracic, intercostal, or abdominal veins.

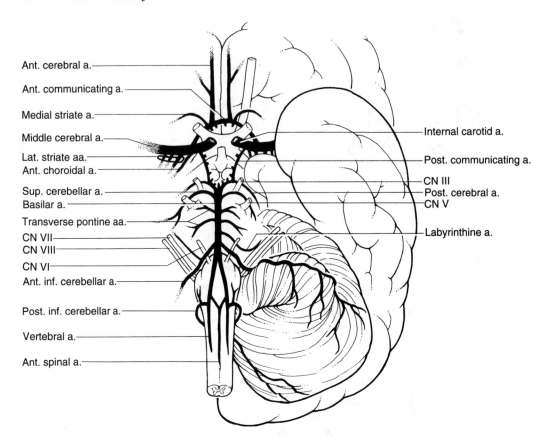

Figure 3.1. Arteries of the base of the brain and brainstem, including the arterial circle of Willis. The medial and lateral striate arteries and the anterior choroidal artery supply the basal ganglia and internal capsule.

—is conducted by valveless veins that permit bidirectional flow, depending on the existing pressure gradients.
—is a pathway for transmission of infectious agents and tumor cells.

III. Arteries of the Brain (Figures 3.2–3.5; see Figure 3.1)

—supply 15% of cardiac output to the brain.
—provide the brain with 20% of the oxygen used by the body.
—normal bloodflow is 50 ml/100 g of brain tissue/minute.
—consist of two pairs of vessels, the **internal carotid arteries** and the **vertebral arteries,** and their divisions. At the junction between the medulla and the pons, the two vertebral arteries fuse to form the **basilar artery**.

A. Internal carotid artery

—enters the cranium via the carotid canal of the temporal bone.
—lies within the cavernous sinus as a carotid siphon.
—supplies tributaries to the dura, hypophysis, tympanic cavity, and trigeminal ganglion.
—gives direct branches to the optic nerve, optic chiasm, hypothalamus, and genu of the internal capsule.
—gives off the following branches:

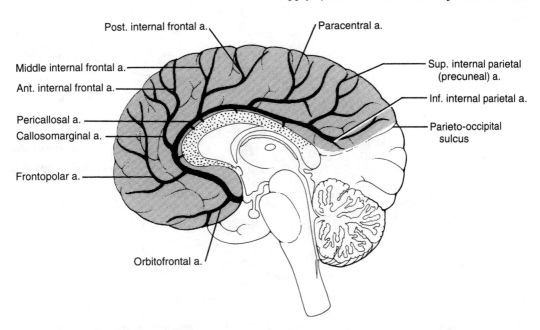

Figure 3.2. Cortical branches of the anterior cerebral artery on the medial hemispheric surface. The temporal pole is supplied by the middle cerebral artery; the occipital lobe is supplied by the posterior cerebral artery.

1. Ophthalmic artery
   —enters the orbit via the optic canal with the optic nerve.

2. Central artery of the retina
   —is a branch of the **ophthalmic artery**.
   —provides the only blood supply to the inner five layers of the retina.
   —is an end artery; its **occlusion results in blindness**.

3. Posterior communicating artery
   —arises from the carotid siphon and joins the posterior cerebral artery.
   —supplies the optic chiasm and tract, hypothalamus, subthalamus, and the anterior half of the ventral portion of the thalamus.

4. Anterior choroidal artery (see Figures 3.1 and 3.5)
   —arises from the internal carotid artery.
   —supplies the choroid plexus of the temporal horn of the lateral ventricle, hippocampus, amygdala, optic tract, lateral geniculate body, globus pallidus, and the ventral part of the posterior limb of the internal capsule.
   —supplies the proximal portion of optic radiations as they leave the lateral geniculate body to form Meyer's loop.

5. Anterior cerebral artery (see Figure 3.2)
   —originates at the terminal bifurcation of the internal carotid artery.
   —gives direct branches to the optic chiasm.
   —supplies the medial surface of the frontal and parietal lobes and corpus callosum.
   —supplies part of the caudate nucleus and putamen and the anterior limb of the internal capsule via the **medial striate artery** (Heubner).

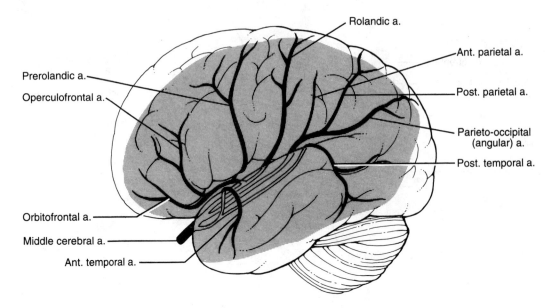

Figure 3.3. Cortical branches of the middle cerebral artery. The *unshaded* area represents the terminal territories of the anterior and posterior cerebral arteries.

—supplies the leg and foot area of the motor and sensory cortices (paracentral lobule) [see Figure 23.1].

6. Anterior communicating artery

—connects the two anterior cerebral arteries.

7. Middle cerebral artery (see Figures 3.3 and 3.5)

—begins at the bifurcation of the internal carotid artery.
—supplies the lateral convexity of the hemisphere and underlying insula.
—supplies the trunk, arm, and face areas of the motor and sensory cortices.
—supplies Broca's and Wernicke's speech areas.
—supplies the caudate nucleus, putamen, globus pallidus, and anterior and posterior limbs of the internal capsule via the **lateral striate arteries**.

B. Vertebral artery (see Figure 3.1)

—is a branch of the subclavian artery.
—joins its opposite partner to form the basilar artery.
—gives rise to:

1. Anterior spinal artery

2. Posterior spinal artery

—is occasionally a branch of the vertebral artery.

3. Posterior inferior cerebellar artery

—gives rise to the posterior spinal artery.
—supplies the dorsolateral zone of the medulla.
—supplies the inferior surface of the cerebellum and the choroid plexus of the fourth ventricle.
—supplies the medial and inferior vestibular nuclei, inferior cerebellar peduncle, nucleus ambiguus, intra-axial fibers of CN IX and CN X, spinothalamic tract, and spinal trigeminal nucleus and tract.

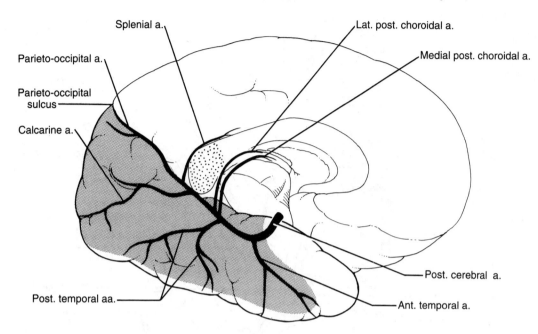

Splenial a.

Lat. post. choroidal a.

Parieto-occipital a.

Medial post. choroidal a.

Parieto-occipital sulcus

Calcarine a.

Post. cerebral a.

Post. temporal aa.

Ant. temporal a.

Figure 3.4. Cortical branches of the posterior cerebral artery seen from the ventral and medial surface. The splenium of the corpus callosum is supplied by the callosal branch of the posterior cerebral artery.

C. Basilar artery (see Figure 3.1)

–is formed by the two vertebral arteries.
–gives rise to:

1. Pontine arteries

–include penetrating and short circumferential branches.
–supply corticospinal tracts and the intra-axial exiting fibers of the abducent nerve (CN VI).

2. Labyrinthine artery

–arises, in 15% of the population, from the basilar artery.
–perfuses the cochlea and the vestibular apparatus.

3. Anterior inferior cerebellar artery

–supplies the inferior surface of the cerebellum.
–supplies the facial nucleus and intra-axial fibers, spinal trigeminal nucleus and tract, vestibular nuclei, cochlear nuclei, intra-axial fibers of the vestibulocochlear nerve, spinothalamic tract, and inferior and middle cerebellar peduncles.
–gives rise to the labyrinthine artery in 85% of the population.

4. Superior cerebellar artery

–supplies the superior surface of the cerebellum and the cerebellar nuclei (dentate nucleus).
–supplies the rostral and lateral pons, including the superior cerebellar peduncle and spinothalamic tract.

5. Posterior cerebral artery (see Figure 3.4)

–is formed by bifurcation of the basilar artery.
–provides the major blood supply to the midbrain.

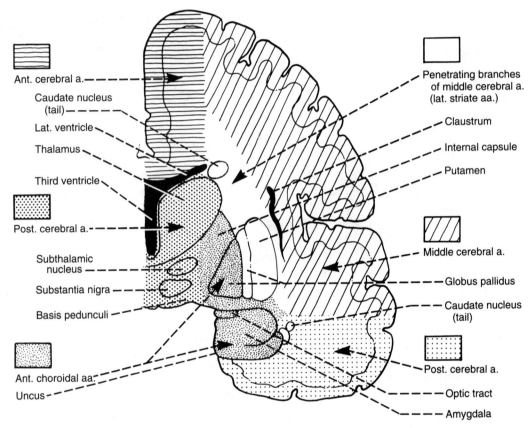

Figure 3.5. Schematic drawing of a coronal (frontal) section through the cerebral hemisphere at the level of the internal capsule and thalamus showing the major vascular territories.

–supplies the posterior half of the thalamus and the medial and lateral geniculate bodies.

–supplies the occipital lobe, visual cortex, and inferior surface of the temporal lobe.

–gives rise to the lateral and medial **posterior choroidal arteries,** which supply the dorsal thalamus, pineal body, and the choroid plexus of the third and lateral ventricles.

IV. Arterial Circle of Willis (see Figure 3.1)

–is formed by the anterior communicating, anterior cerebral, internal carotid, posterior communicating, and posterior cerebral arteries.

–gives off penetrating arteries to supply the ventral diencephalon (hypothalamus, subthalamus, and thalamus) and the midbrain.

V. Meningeal Arteries

–supply the intracranial dura.

–usually arise from branches of the external carotid artery.

A. Anterior meningeal arteries

–arise from the anterior and posterior ethmoidal arteries.

–supply the dura of the anterior cranial fossa.

B. Middle meningeal artery

–is a branch of the **maxillary artery**.

–enters the cranium via the **foramen spinosum**.

–lies between the periosteal and meningeal dura, below the temporal and parietal bones.

–supplies most of the dura and almost its entire calvarial portion.

–laceration results in **epidural hemorrhage** (hematoma).

C. Posterior meningeal arteries

–are branches of the ascending pharyngeal, vertebral, and occipital arteries.

–supply the dura of the posterior cranial fossa.

VI. Veins of the Brain

A. Superficial cerebral veins

–are devoid of valves and lie along surface sulci.

–arise from the cortex and subcortical medullary substance and terminate in the dural sinuses.

–lie superficial to arteries and are considered meningeal veins.

–include the following:

1. Superior cerebral veins

–drain into the superior sagittal sinus ("bridging veins").

–laceration results in **subdural hemorrhage** (hematoma).

2. Middle cerebral vein

–overlies the lateral sulcus and drains into the cavernous sinus.

–communicates with the transverse sinus.

3. Inferior cerebral veins

–drain the inferior lateral and basal surface of the hemisphere.

4. Medial cerebral veins

–drain the medial surface of the hemisphere, including the corpus callosum, into the inferior sagittal sinus.

5. Basal (Rosenthal's) vein*

–drains the orbital surface of the frontal lobe, insula, and corpus striatum (the caudate nucleus, putamen, and globus pallidus).

–encircles the brainstem and drains into the **great vein of Galen**.

B. Deep cerebral veins

–are more consistent in configuration than the superficial veins.

–drain the deep subcortical structures of the cerebral hemispheres: **septal area, thalamus, and basal ganglia**.

1. Internal cerebral veins

–are paired, parallel vessels situated lateral to the midline and on the roof of the third ventricle.

–extend from the interventricular foramina to the superior cistern, where they join the great vein of Galen.

---

*Some authorities consider the basal vein a deep vein because, in addition to cortical areas, it also drains some deep structures.

2. Great cerebral vein of Galen (see Figure 2.3)

—is located below the splenium of the corpus callosum in the transverse cerebral fissure.

—receives two internal cerebral veins, two basal veins, two occipital veins, and the posterior callosal vein.

—joins the inferior sagittal sinus and the straight sinus, which usually drains into the left transverse sinus.

VII. Venous Dural Sinuses

—are endothelium-lined, valveless channels whose walls are formed by two layers of dura mater.

—collect blood from the superficial and deep cerebral veins and the calvarium and represent the major drainage pathway of the cranial cavity.

—receive arachnoid granulations and absorb cerebrospinal fluid (CSF).

A. Superior sagittal sinus (see Figure 2.3)

—extends from the foramen cecum to the internal occipital protuberance and usually terminates in the right transverse sinus.

—communicates with the nasal emissary veins.

—receives superficial cerebral veins, diploic veins, and parietal emissary veins.

—receives arachnoid granulations and drains CSF from the subarachnoid space.

B. Inferior sagittal sinus

—courses in the inferior free edge of the falx cerebri.

—joins the great cerebral vein to form the straight sinus.

C. Straight sinus (see Figure 2.3)

—is formed by the great cerebral vein and the inferior sagittal sinus.

—terminates at the internal occipital protuberance and usually drains into the left transverse sinus.

—drains the superior surface of the cerebellum.

D. Left and right transverse sinuses

—originate at the confluence of the sinuses and course anterolaterally along the edge of the tentorium cerebelli to become the sigmoid sinus.

—receive venous blood from the temporal and occipital lobes.

E. Confluence of the sinuses (see Figure 2.3)

—lies at the internal occipital protuberance.

—is formed by the union of the superior sagittal, straight, and transverse sinuses.

F. Sigmoid sinus

—is a continuation of the transverse sinus.

—passes inferiorly and medially into the jugular foramen.

G. Sphenoparietal sinus

—lies along the curve of the lesser wing of the sphenoid bone and drains into the cavernous sinus.

H. Superior petrosal sinus

—extends from the cavernous sinus to the sigmoid sinus.

—receives tributaries from the pons, medulla, cerebellum, and inner ear.

I. Inferior petrosal sinus

—passes between the glossopharyngeal and vagal nerves and drains into the jugular bulb.

—receives major venous drainage from the inferior portion of the cerebellum.

—drains the cavernous sinus and clival plexus into the internal jugular vein.

J. Cavernous sinus (see Figure 10.5)

—surrounds the sella turcica and the body of the sphenoid bone.

—contains, *within the sinus,* the internal carotid artery, sympathetic plexus, and abducent nerve (CN VI).

—contains, *within the lateral wall of the sinus,* the oculomotor nerve (CN III), the trochlear nerve (CN IV), the ophthalmic nerve (CN V-1), and the maxillary branches (CN V-2) of the trigeminal nerve.

—receives blood from the superior and the inferior ophthalmic veins.

VIII. Intracranial Hemorrhage

A. Aneurysms

—are circumscribed **dilatations (ectasias) of an artery**.

1. Berry (saccular) aneurysms

—develop at arterial bifurcations.

—90% are found in the **arterial circle of Willis.**

—10% are found in the vertebrobasilar system.

—rupture is the most common cause of nontraumatic **subarachnoid hemorrhage**.

2. Microaneurysms (Charcot-Bouchard aneurysms)

—are found in small arteries, most frequently within the territory of the middle cerebral artery (the lenticulostriate arteries).

—rupture is the most common cause of nontraumatic **intraparenchymal hemorrhage**.

—rupture occurs most frequently in the basal ganglia.

B. Subdural hemorrhage (hematoma)

—results from **rupture of the superior cerebral veins,** the "bridging" veins that drain into the superior sagittal sinus.

C. Epidural hemorrhage (hematoma)

—results from **rupture of the middle meningeal artery,** which lies between the dura and the inner table of the skull.

Review Test

Directions: Each of the numbered items or incomplete statements in this section is followed by answers or by completions of the statement. Select the **one** lettered answer or completion that is **best** in each case.

1. The thalamus, hypothalamus, and subthalamus are perfused by the

(A) anterior choroidal artery.
(B) medial striate artery.
(C) anterior communicating artery.
(D) posterior communicating artery.
(E) anterior cerebral artery.

2. The optic chiasm is supplied by all of the following arteries EXCEPT the

(A) internal carotid artery.
(B) anterior communicating artery.
(C) anterior choroidal artery.
(D) posterior communicating artery.
(E) anterior cerebral artery.

3. The internal capsule is supplied by all of the following arteries EXCEPT the

(A) internal carotid artery.
(B) posterior cerebral artery.
(C) anterior choroidal artery.
(D) anterior cerebral artery.
(E) middle cerebral artery.

4. All of the following statements concerning the internal carotid artery are correct EXCEPT

(A) it enters the skull via the sphenoid bone.
(B) it lies within the cavernous sinus.
(C) it gives off direct branches to the internal capsule.
(D) it gives rise to the anterior choroidal artery.
(E) it gives rise to the posterior communicating artery.

5. All of the following statements concerning the vertebral artery are correct EXCEPT it

(A) may give off a posterior spinal artery.
(B) gives rise to the labyrinthine artery.
(C) is a branch of the subclavian artery.
(D) gives rise to the anterior spinal artery.
(E) gives rise to the posterior inferior cerebellar artery.

6. The cavernous sinus and its lateral wall contain all of the following structures EXCEPT the

(A) carotid siphon.
(B) oculomotor, abducent, and trochlear nerves.
(C) ophthalmic and maxillary nerves.
(D) optic nerve.
(E) postganglionic sympathetic fibers.

7. All of the following statements concerning the ophthalmic artery are correct EXCEPT it

(A) enters the orbit via the superior orbital fissure.
(B) is a branch of the internal carotid artery.
(C) accompanies the optic nerve to the orbit.
(D) supplies the inner layers of the retina.
(E) gives rise to the central artery of the retina.

8. All of the following statements concerning the middle meningeal artery are correct EXCEPT

(A) it is usually a branch of the maxillary artery.
(B) it enters the cranium through the foramen spinosum.
(C) laceration results in epidural hemorrhage.
(D) it supplies most of the dura of the calvarium.
(E) it supplies the dura of the posterior cranial fossa.

Directions: Each group of items in this section consists of lettered options followed by a set of numbered items. For each item, select the **one** lettered option that is most closely associated with it. Each lettered option may be selected once, more than once, or not at all.

Questions 9–13

Match each of the descriptions with the most appropriate artery.

(A) Anterior cerebral artery
(B) Middle cerebral artery
(C) Posterior cerebral artery
(D) Anterior choroidal artery
(E) Anterior communicating artery

9. Is not an artery of the circle of Willis

10. Provides the major blood supply to the midbrain

11. Supplies Broca's speech area

12. Supplies the visual cortex

13. Supplies the foot area of the sensory and motor cortex

Questions 14–18

Match each of the descriptions with the most appropriate artery.

(A) Posterior cerebral artery
(B) Superior cerebellar artery
(C) Anterior inferior cerebellar artery
(D) Posterior inferior cerebellar artery
(E) Anterior spinal artery

14. Usually gives rise to the artery that supplies the inner ear

15. Supplies the facial nucleus and the spinal trigeminal nucleus and tract

16. Is the terminal branch of the basilar artery

17. Supplies the deep cerebellar nuclei

18. Supplies the nucleus ambiguus

Answers and Explanations

1–D. The thalamus, hypothalamus, and subthalamus are irrigated by the posterior communicating artery and the thalamoperforating branches of the posterior cerebral artery.

2–C. The anterior choroidal artery lies outside of the circle of Willis and does not supply the optic chiasm.

3–B. The internal capsule is supplied by the anterior cerebral artery, the internal carotid artery, the anterior choroidal artery, and the middle cerebral artery.

4–A. The internal carotid artery enters the skull via the carotid canal of the temporal bone.

5–B. The vertebral artery, a branch of the subclavian artery, *may* give off a posterior spinal artery and does give off an anterior spinal artery. The posterior spinal artery is most commonly a branch of the posterior inferior cerebellar artery. The anterior inferior cerebellar artery is the first major branch of the basilar artery and usually (in 85% of the population) gives rise to the labyrinthine artery. In the remaining cases, the labyrinthine artery is a branch of the basilar artery. The posterior inferior cerebellar artery is the largest branch of the vertebral artery.

6–D. The cavernous sinus and its lateral wall contain the carotid siphon, the oculomotor, abducent, and trochlear nerves, a sympathetic plexus, and the ophthalmic and maxillary divisions of the trigeminal nerve. The optic nerve and ophthalmic artery reach the orbit via the optic canal.

7–A. The ophthalmic artery is the first major branch of the internal carotid artery. It reaches the orbit with the optic nerve via the optic canal. It gives rise to the central artery of the retina, which perfuses the inner five layers of the retina. The ophthalmic nerve, a division of the trigeminal nerve, enters the orbit with the ophthalmic vein via the superior orbital fissure.

8–E. The middle meningeal artery usually is a branch of the maxillary artery, which enters the cranium via the foramen spinosum and supplies most of the dura of the calvarium. Laceration of this artery leads to epidural hemorrhage (hematoma). The artery and its accompanying dural veins lie between the periosteal and meningeal layers of the dura. The dura of the posterior fossa is supplied by branches of the ascending pharyngeal, vertebral, and occipital arteries (posterior meningeal arteries).

9–D. The anterior choroidal artery is not an artery of the circle of Willis.

10–C. The posterior cerebral artery provides the major blood supply to the midbrain.

11–B. The middle cerebral artery supplies Broca's speech area.

12–C. The posterior cerebral artery supplies the visual cortex of the occipital lobe.

13–A. The anterior cerebral artery supplies the medial surface of the hemisphere, including the motor and sensory areas for the leg and foot.

14–C. The anterior inferior cerebellar artery usually gives rise to the labyrinthine artery, which supplies the structures of the inner ear (i.e., the cochlea and vestibular apparatus).

15–C. The facial nucleus and the spinal trigeminal nucleus and tract are supplied by the anterior inferior cerebellar artery.

16–A. The posterior cerebral artery is the terminal branch of the basilar artery.

17–B. The superior cerebellar artery supplies the superior surface of the cerebellum and the cerebellar nuclei (dentate nucleus).

18–D. The posterior inferior cerebellar artery supplies the dorsolateral medullary field, including the nucleus ambiguus.

4

Development of the Nervous System

I. Overview

A. Central nervous system (CNS)

–begins development in the third week of embryonic development as the **neural plate**.

–the neural plate becomes the **neural tube,** which gives rise to the brain and spinal cord.

B. Peripheral nervous system (PNS)

–consists of spinal, cranial, and visceral nerves and spinal, cranial, and autonomic ganglia.

–is derived from three sources:

1. Neural crest cells

–give rise to peripheral ganglia, Schwann cells, and afferent nerve fibers.

2. Neural tube

–gives rise to all preganglionic autonomic fibers and all fibers that innervate skeletal muscles.

3. Mesoderm

–gives rise to the dura mater and to connective tissue investments of peripheral nerve fibers (endoneurium, perineurium, and epineurium).

II. Development of the Neural Tube (Figures 4.1 and 4.2)

–begins in the third week and is completed in the fourth week.

A. Neural plate

–is a thickened pear-shaped region of embryonic ectoderm, located between the **primitive knot** and the **oropharyngeal membrane**.

B. Neural groove

–forms as the neural plate begins to fold inward.

–is flanked by neural folds, which are parallel.

–deepens as the neural folds begin to close over it.

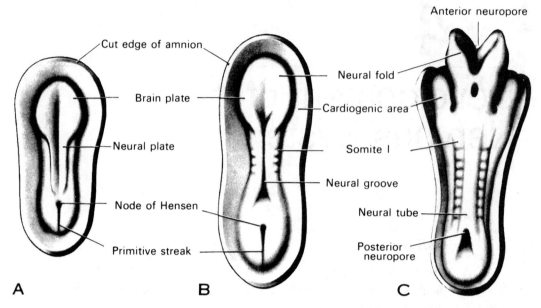

Figure 4.1. Diagrams illustrating the dorsal aspect of the human embryo. (*A*) Late presomite and early neural plate stage. (*B*) Early somite stage and neural groove stage. (*C*) Eight-somite stage and early neural tube stage. The anterior and posterior neuropores provide transitory communication between the neural canal and the amniotic cavity. (Reprinted with permission from Carpenter MB and Sutin J: *Human Neuroanatomy*. Baltimore, Williams & Wilkins, 1983, p 63.)

C. Neural folds
   –fuse in the midline to form the neural tube.
   –are the sites of neural crest cell differentiation.

D. Neural tube
   –forms as the neural folds fuse in the midline and separate from the surface ectoderm.
   –lies between the surface ectoderm and the notochord.
   –gives rise to the CNS:

   1. The **cranial part** becomes the brain.

   2. The **caudal part** becomes the spinal cord.

   3. The **cavity** gives rise to the central canal of the spinal cord and ventricles of the brain.

   4. The **two openings** in the neural tube connect the central canal with the amniotic cavity:

   a. Anterior neuropore
      –closes in the fourth week (day 25) and becomes the **lamina terminalis**.

   b. Posterior neuropore
      –closes in the fourth week (day 27).

III. Neural Crest (see Figure 4.2)
   –gives rise to:

A. Pseudounipolar ganglion cells of the spinal and cranial nerve ganglia

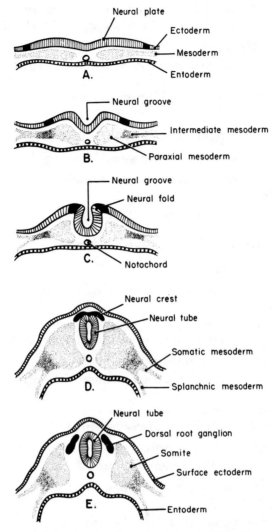

Figure 4.2. Schematic diagrams of transverse sections of embryos at various stages. (*A*) Neural plate stage. (*B*) Early neural groove stage. (*C*) Late neural groove stage. (*D*) Early neural tube and neural crest stage. (*E*) Neural tube and dorsal root ganglion stage. (Reprinted with permission from Truex RC and Carpenter MB: *Human Neuroanatomy.* Baltimore, Williams & Wilkins, 1969, p 91.)

B. Schwann cells (neurolemmal sheath cells that form myelin in the PNS)

C. Multipolar ganglion cells of the autonomic ganglia

D. Leptomeninges (pia–arachnoid cells)

E. Chromaffin cells of the suprarenal medulla

F. Pigment cells (melanocytes)

G. Odontoblasts (dentine-forming cells)

IV. Placodes

—are localized thickenings of the cephalic surface ectoderm.

—give rise to cells that migrate into the underlying mesoderm and develop into the sensory receptive organs of cranial nerves I and VIII.

A. Olfactory placodes

—differentiate into neurosensory cells that give rise to the **olfactory nerve (CN I)**.
—induce formation of the **olfactory bulbs**.

B. Otic placodes

—give rise to the following statoacoustic organs:

1. Organ of Corti and spiral ganglion

2. Cristae ampullares, maculae utriculi and sacculi, and vestibular ganglion

3. Vestibulocochlear nerve (CN VIII)

V. Stages of Neural Tube Development

A. Vesicle development

1. The three primary brain vesicles and associated flexures (Figure 4.3*A* and 4.3*B*)

—development occurs during the fourth week.
—give rise to dilatations of the primary brain vesicles and two curvatures.

a. Prosencephalon (forebrain)

—is associated with the appearance of the **optic vesicles**.
—gives rise to:
(1) Telencephalon (endbrain)
(2) Diencephalon (between-brain)

b. Mesencephalon (midbrain)

—remains as the mesencephalon.

c. Rhombencephalon (hindbrain)

—gives rise to:
(1) Metencephalon (afterbrain)
—forms the pons and the cerebellum.
(2) Myelencephalon (medulla oblongata)

d. Cephalic flexure (midbrain flexure)

—is located between the prosencephalon and the rhombencephalon.

e. Cervical flexure

—is located between the rhombencephalon and the future spinal cord.

2. The five secondary brain vesicles (with four ventricles) [Figure 4.4; see Figure 4.3*C* and 4.3*D*]

—become visible in the sixth week; the brain vesicles are visible as the primordia of the five major brain divisions.

a. Telencephalon

—lateral outpocketings form the **cerebral hemispheres**.
—ventral outpocketings form the **olfactory bulbs**.
—lateral ventricles are visible.

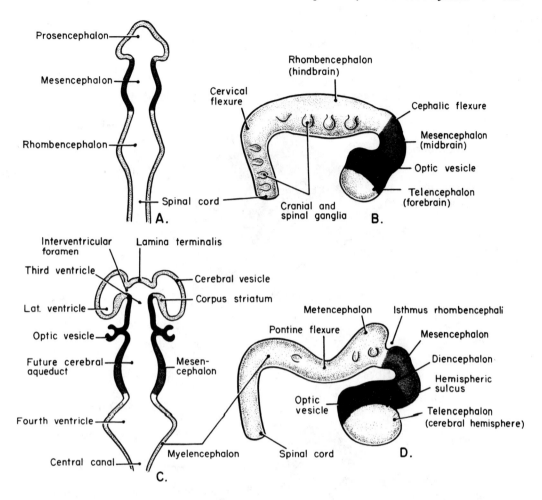

Figure 4.3. Schematic illustrations of the developing brain vesicles and ventricular system. (*A* and *B*) Three-brain vesicle stage of a 4-week old embryo. (*C* and *D*) Five-brain vesicle stage of a 6-week old embryo. (Reprinted with permission from Truex RC and Carpenter MB: *Human Neuroanatomy*. Baltimore, Williams & Wilkins, 1969, p 97.)

b. Diencephalon

–the third ventricle, optic chiasm and optic nerves, infundibulum, and mamillary eminences become visible.

c. Mesencephalon

–contains a large cavity that will become the **cerebral aqueduct**.

d. Metencephalon

–is separated from the mesencephalon by the rhombencephalic isthmus.
–is separated from the myelencephalon by the pontine flexure.
–contains rhombic lips on the dorsal surface, which give rise to the cerebellum.
–becomes the pons and the cerebellum.
–contains the **rostral half of the fourth ventricle**.

e. Myelencephalon (medulla oblongata)

–lies between the pontine and cervical flexures.

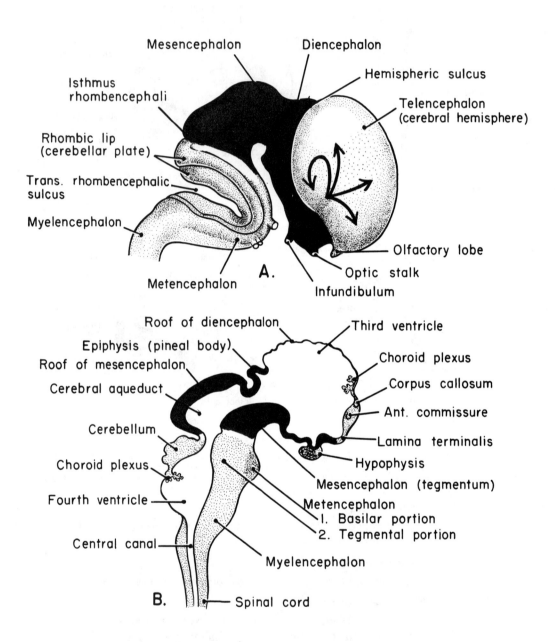

Figure 4.4. Diagrams of the developing brain vesicles and ventricular system. (*A*) Lateral view of the cerebral vesicle and developing brainstem in an 8-week old embryo. *Arrows* indicate directions of growth and expansion of the cerebral hemisphere. (*B*) Midsagittal section through the brainstem of a 12-week old fetus. Note that the corpus callosum and the anterior commissure develop in the lamina terminalis. (Reprinted with permission from Truex RC and Carpenter MB: *Human Neuroanatomy*. Baltimore, Williams & Wilkins, 1969, p 101.)

–becomes the medulla.

–contains the **caudal half of the fourth ventricle**.

B. Histogenesis

1. Cells of the neural tube wall

–are neuroepithelial cells that give rise to:

a. Neuroblasts

–form all neurons found in the CNS.

b. Glioblasts (spongioblasts)

–form supporting cells of the CNS.

(1) Macroglia

(a) Astroglia (astrocytes)

–surround blood capillaries with their vascular feet.

(b) Oligodendroglia (oligodendrocytes)

–produce the myelin of the CNS.

(2) Ependymal cells

(a) Ependymocytes

–line the ventricles and the central canal.

(b) Tanycytes

–are located in the wall of the third ventricle.

(c) Choroid plexus cells

–produce cerebrospinal fluid (**CSF**).

c. Microglia

–are the scavenger cells of the CNS.

–arise from monocytes, not from glioblasts.

–invade the developing nervous system, in the third week, with the developing blood vessels.

2. Layers of the neural tube wall

–are formed within the wall of the primitive neural tube.

a. Neuroepithelial (ventricular) layer

–is the innermost layer.

–is a monocellular layer of ependymal cells that lines the central canal and future brain ventricles.

b. Mantle (intermediate) layer

–is the middle layer.

–consists of neurons and glial cells, the central **gray matter of the spinal cord**.

–contains the developing **alar** and **basal plates**.

c. Marginal layer

–is the outermost layer.

–contains nerve fibers of neuroblasts of the mantle layer and glial cells.

–produces the **white matter of the spinal cord** through the myelination of axons growing into this layer.

VI. Spinal Cord (Medulla Spinalis)

–develops from the neural tube caudal to the fourth pair of somites.

A. Alar and basal plates, sulcus limitans, and roof and floor plates

1. Alar plate
—is a dorsolateral thickening of the mantle layer of the neural tube.
—gives rise to **sensory neuroblasts** of the dorsal horn (general somatic afferent [GSA] and general visceral afferent [GVA] cell regions).
—receives axons, which become the dorsal roots, from the dorsal root ganglion.
—becomes the **dorsal horn** of the spinal cord.

2. Basal plate
—is a ventrolateral thickening of the mantle layer of the neural tube.
—gives rise to the **motor neuroblasts** of the ventral and lateral horns (general somatic efferent [GSE] and general visceral efferent [GVE] cell regions). Axons from motor neuroblasts exit the spinal cord and form the ventral roots.
—becomes the **ventral horn** of the spinal cord.

3. Sulcus limitans
—is a longitudinal groove in the lateral wall of the neural tube that appears during the fourth week.
—separates the alar (sensory) and the basal (motor) plates.
—disappears in the adult spinal cord but is retained in the rhomboid fossa of the brainstem.
—extends from the spinal cord to the rostral midbrain.

4. Roof plate
—is the nonneural roof of the central canal.

5. Floor plate
—is the nonneural floor of the central canal.
—contains the **ventral white commissure**.

B. Myelination
—of the CNS is accomplished by oligodendrocytes.
—of the PNS is accompished by Schwann cells.
—commences in the fourth fetal month.
—is not completed until the end of the second postnatal year (e.g., when corticospinal tracts become myelinated and functional).

C. Positional changes of the spinal cord
—at **birth,** the conus medullaris extends to the level of the third lumbar vertebra (VL3).
—at **8 weeks,** the spinal cord extends the length of the vertebral canal
—in **adults,** the conus medullaris terminates at the VL1–VL2 interspace.
—disparate growth results in formation of the **cauda equina,** consisting of dorsal and ventral roots (L3–Co) that descend below the level of the conus medullaris.

VII. Medulla Oblongata (Myelencephalon) [see Figure 4.4]

—develops from the caudal rhombencephalon.
—contains the medullary pyramids (corticospinal tracts) in its base.

A. Closed (caudal) medulla
—extends from the pyramidal decussation to the obex.
—contains a central canal.

1. Alar plate sensory neuroblasts give rise to:

a. Dorsal column nuclei
   —consist of the nuclei gracilis and cuneatus.

b. Inferior olivary nuclei
   —are cerebellar relay nuclei.

c. Solitary nucleus
   —forms the GVA and special visceral afferent (SVA) columns.

d. Spinal trigeminal nucleus
   —forms the GSA column.

2. Basal plate motor neuroblasts give rise to:

a. Hypoglossal nucleus
   —forms the GSE column.

b. Nucleus ambiguus
   —forms the special visceral efferent (SVE) column (innervates branchiomeric muscles).

c. Dorsal motor nucleus of the vagal nerve
   —forms the GVE column.

B. Open (rostral) medulla (Figure 4.5)
   —extends from the **obex** and the **striae medullares** of the rhomboid fossa (see Figure 1.6A).
   —formation of the pontine flexure causes the lateral walls of the rostral medulla to open like a book and form the rhomboid fossa (the floor of the fourth ventricle).

1. Alar plate
   —lies lateral to the sulcus limitans.
   —its sensory neuroblasts give rise to:

a. Solitary nucleus
   —forms the GVA and SVA columns.

b. Cochlear and vestibular nuclei
   —form the special somatic afferent (SSA) column.

c. Spinal trigeminal nucleus
   —forms the GSA column.

2. Basal plate
   —lies medial to the sulcus limitans.
   —its motor neuroblasts give rise to:

a. Hypoglossal nucleus
   —forms the GSE column.

b. Nucleus ambiguus
   —forms the SVE column.

c. Dorsal motor nucleus of the vagal nerve and the inferior salivatory nucleus of CN IX
   —form the GVE column.

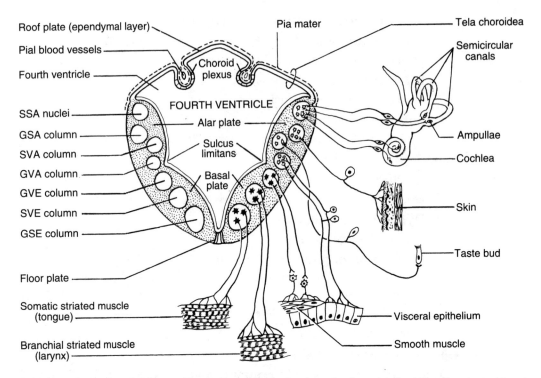

Figure 4.5. Schematized diagram of the brainstem illustrating the cell columns derived from the alar and basal plates. The seven cranial nerve modalities are shown. (Adapted with permission from Patten BM: *Human Embryology,* 3rd ed. New York, The Blakiston Division, McGraw-Hill, 1969, p 298.)

   3. Roof plate
      –forms the caudal roof of the fourth ventricle.
      –is the **tela choroidea,** a monolayer of ependymal cells covered with pia mater.
      –is invaginated by pial vessels to form the choroid plexus of the fourth ventricle.

VIII. Metencephalon (see Figures 4.3 and 4.4)

   –develops from the rostral division of the rhombencephalon.
   –develops between the rhombencephalic isthmus and the pontine flexure.
   –gives rise to the **pons and the cerebellum.**

A. Pons

   1. Alar plate
      –its sensory neuroblasts give rise to:

   a. Solitary nucleus
      –forms the SVA column of CN VII.

   b. Cochlear and vestibular nuclei
      –form the SSA column of CN VIII.

c. Spinal and principal trigeminal nuclei
–form the GSA column of CN V.

d. Pontine nuclei
–consist of cerebellar relay nuclei (pontine gray).

2. Basal plate
–its motor neuroblasts give rise to:

a. Abducent nucleus
–forms the GSE column.

b. Facial and motor trigeminal nuclei
–form the SVE column.

c. Superior salivatory nucleus
–forms the GVE column of CN VII.

3. Base of the pons
–contains pontine nuclei from the alar plate.
–contains corticobulbar, corticospinal, and corticopontine fibers with cell bodies located in the cerebral cortex.
–contains pontocerebellar fibers, which are axons of neurons found in the pontine nuclei.

B. Cerebellum (see Figure 4.4)
–is formed by the rhombic lips, which are the thickened alar plates of the mantle layer.
–the **cerebellar anlage (primordium)** gives rise to:

1. Vermis, by midline growth

2. Cerebellar hemispheres, by lateral growth

3. Three-layered cerebellar cortex and four pairs of cerebellar nuclei, by cell migration from the mantle layer into the marginal layer

4. Folia and fissures, by cortical growth

IX. Mesencephalon (Midbrain) [see Figure 4.4]
–develops from the walls of the mesencephalic vesicle.
–lies between the posterior commissure and the rhombencephalic isthmus.
–contains the **cerebral aqueduct,** which develops from the rhombencephalic cavity.

A. Alar plate
–its neuroblasts form the cell layers of the superior colliculi and the nuclei of the inferior colliculi.

B. Basal plate
–its neuroblasts give rise to:

1. Trochlear and oculomotor nuclei of CN IV and CN III
–form the GSE column.

2. Edinger-Westphal nucleus of CN III
–forms the most rostral cell group of the GVE column.

C. Basis pedunculi

—contains corticobulbar, corticospinal, and corticopontine fibers.
—is derived from the cerebral cortex of the telencephalon.

X. Diencephalon, Optic Structures, and Hypophysis

A. Diencephalon (see Figures 4.3 and 4.4)

—develops from the median part of the prosencephalon, within the walls of the primitive third ventricle.
—extends from the interventricular foramen to the posterior commissure.

1. Epithalamus

—develops from the embryonic roof plate and dorsal parts of the alar plates.
—gives rise to the **pineal body** (epiphysis) and the habenular nuclei.
—gives rise to the habenular and posterior commissures.
—gives rise, from the roof plate and the pia mater, to the tela choroidea and choroid plexus of the third ventricle.

2. Thalamus (dorsal thalamus)

—is an alar plate derivative.
—develops between the epithalamus and the hypothalamus.
—gives rise to the thalamic nuclei.
—gives rise to the **metathalamus,** which includes the lateral geniculate body (relays visual impulses) and the medial geniculate body (relays auditory impulses).

3. Hypothalamus

—develops ventral to the hypothalamic sulcus from the alar plate and floor plate.
—gives rise to the hypothalamic nuclei, including the **mamillary bodies**.
—gives rise to the **neurohypophysis** (Figure 4.6).

4. Subthalamus (ventral thalamus) [Figure 1.8*B*]

—is an alar plate derivative located ventral to the thalamus and lateral to the hypothalamus.
—includes the subthalamic nucleus, zona incerta, and lenticular and thalamic fasciculi (fields of Forel).
—contains subthalamic neuroblasts that migrate into the telencephalon and form the **globus pallidus** (pallidum), a basal ganglion.

B. Optic vesicles, cups, and stalks (see Figures 4.3 and 4.4)

—are derivatives of diencephalic vesicle walls (see Figure 4.4*A*).
—give rise to the retina, optic nerve, optic chiasm, and optic tract.

C. Hypophysis (pituitary gland) [see Figure 4.6]

—is attached by the pituitary stalk to the hypothalamus.

1. Anterior lobe (adenohypophysis)

—develops from **Rathke's pouch,** an ectodermal diverticulum of the primitive mouth cavity (stomodeum). Remnants of Rathke's pouch may give rise to a congenital cystic tumor, a craniopharyngioma.
—includes the pars tuberalis, pars intermedia, and pars distalis.

2. Posterior lobe (neurohypophysis)

—develops from a ventral evagination of the hypothalamus.
—includes the median eminence, infundibular stem, and pars nervosa.

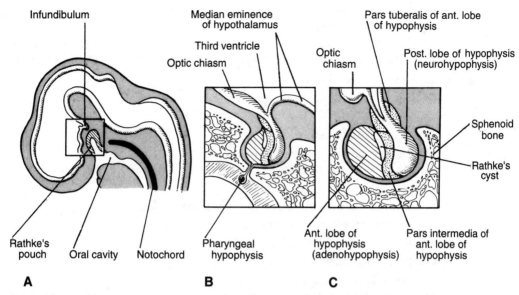

Figure 4.6. Schematic drawings illustrating the development of the hypophysis (pituitary gland). (*A*) Midsagittal section through the 6-week old embryo, showing Rathke's pouch as a dorsal outpocketing of the oral cavity and the infundibulum as a thickening in the floor of the hypothalamus. (*B* and *C*) Development at 11 weeks and 16 weeks, respectively. The anterior lobe, the pars tuberalis, and the pars intermedia are derived from Rathke's pouch. (Adapted with permission from Sadler TW: *Langman's Medical Embryology,* 6th ed. Baltimore, Williams & Wilkins, 1990, p 373.)

XI. Telencephalon

A. Cerebral hemispheres (see Figures 4.3 and 4.4*A*)

–develop as bilateral evaginations of the lateral walls of the prosencephalic vesicle.

–contain the cerebral cortex, cerebral white matter, basal ganglia, and lateral ventricles.

–are interconnected by three commissures: the corpus callosum, anterior commissure, and hippocampal (fornix) commissure.

–continuous hemispheric growth gives rise to frontal, parietal, occipital, and temporal lobes, which overlie the insula and dorsal brainstem.

B. Cerebral cortex (pallium)

–is formed by neuroblasts that migrate in waves from the mantle layer into the marginal layer and give rise to cortical cell layers.

–is classified phylogenetically into:

1. Neocortex (isocortex), a six-layered cortex

–is separated from the paleocortex by the **rhinal sulcus,** a continuation of the collateral sulcus.

2. Paleocortex (allocortex), a three-layered olfactory cortex

3. Archicortex (allocortex), a three-layered hippocampal cortex

C. Corpus striatum

–appears in the fifth week as a bulging striatal eminence in the ventral floor of the lateral telencephalic vesicle.

—gives rise to the **basal ganglia:** the caudate nucleus, putamen, amygdaloid nucleus, and claustrum.

—is divided into the caudate nucleus and the lentiform nucleus by cortico-fugal and corticopetal fibers; these fibers make up the **internal capsule**.

D. Commissures (see Figure 4.4*B*)

—are fiber bundles that interconnect the hemispheres.

—cross the midline via the lamina terminalis.

1. Anterior commissure

—is the first commissure to appear.

—interconnects the olfactory structures and the middle and inferior temporal gyri.

2. Hippocampal commissure (fornical commissure)

—is the second commissure to appear.

—interconnects the two hippocampi.

3. Corpus callosum

—is the third commissure to appear.

—is the largest commissure of the brain and interconnects the corresponding neocortical areas of the two cerebral hemispheres.

E. Gyri and sulci (fissures)

—in the fourth month, no gyri or sulci are present; the brain is smooth or **lissencephalic**.

—at the eighth month, all major gyri and sulci are present; the brain is convoluted or **gyrencephalic**.

XII. Congenital Malformations of the CNS

—result from failure of the neural tube to close or separate from surface ectoderm.

—result from the failure of the vertebral arches to fuse.

A. Spina bifida (Figure 4.7)

—usually occurs in the sacrolumbar region.

—includes the following variations:

1. Spina bifida occulta

—is a defect in the vertebral arches.

—is the least severe variation.

—occurs in 10% of the population.

2. Spina bifida with meningocele

—occurs when the meninges project through a vertebral defect, forming a sac filled with CSF.

—exists with the spinal cord remaining in its normal position.

3. Spina bifida with meningomyelocele

—occurs when the meninges and spinal cord project through a vertebral defect, forming a sac.

4. Spina bifida with myeloschisis

—is the most severe type of spina bifida.

—results in an open neural tube that lies on the surface of the back.

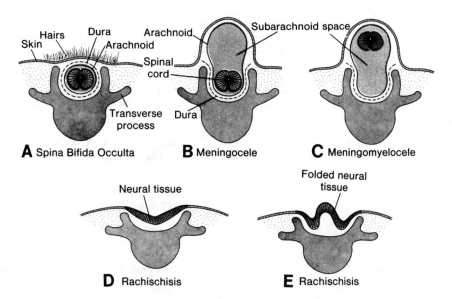

Figure 4.7. Schematic drawings illustrating the various types of spina bifida. (Reprinted with permission from Sadler TW: *Langman's Medical Embryology*, 6th ed. Baltimore, Williams & Wilkins, 1990, p 363.)

B. Ossification defects of the occipital bone

   —are also called **cranium bifidum**.

   —occur once in every 2000 births.

   —include the following variations:

   1. Cranial meningocele

   2. Meningoencephalocele

   3. Meningohydroencephalocele

C. Anencephaly (meroanencephaly)

   —results from failure of the anterior neuropore to close.

   —occurs when the brain fails to develop, a rudimentary brainstem is usually present, and no cranial vault is formed.

   —occurs once in every 1000 births.

D. Arnold-Chiari malformation

   —is a cerebellomedullary malformation in which the caudal vermis, cerebellar tonsils, and medulla herniate through the foramen magnum, resulting in a communicating hydrocephalus.

   —is frequently associated with spina bifida and platybasia, with malformation of the occipitovertebral joint.

   —occurs once in every 1000 births.

E. Dandy-Walker syndrome

   —is a congenital hydrocephalus associated with atresia of the outlet foramina of Luschka and Magendie.

   —is usually associated with dilatation of the fourth ventricle, agenesis of the cerebellar vermis, occipital meningocele, and frequently agenesis of the splenium of the corpus callosum.

Review Test

Directions: Each of the numbered items or incomplete statements in this section is followed by answers or by completions of the statement. Select the **one** lettered answer or completion that is **best** in each case.

1. The anterior and posterior neuropores close during which week of embryonic development?

(A) Second
(B) Third
(C) Fourth
(D) Fifth
(E) Sixth

2. At birth, the conus medullaris is found at which vertebral level?

(A) VT12
(B) VL1
(C) VL3
(D) VS1
(E) VS4

3. The telencephalon gives rise to all of the following structures EXCEPT the

(A) caudate nucleus.
(B) putamen.
(C) globus pallidus.
(D) claustrum.
(E) amygdala

4. Failure of the anterior neuropore to close results in

(A) hydrocephalus.
(B) anencephaly.
(C) mongolism.
(D) craniosynostosis.
(E) meningoencephalocele.

5. The diencephalon gives rise to all of the following structures EXCEPT the

(A) mamillary bodies.
(B) pineal body.
(C) subthalamic nucleus.
(D) adenohypophysis.
(E) neurohypophysis.

6. Caudal herniation of the cerebellar tonsils and medulla through the foramen magnum is called

(A) Dandy-Walker syndrome.
(B) Down's syndrome.
(C) Arnold-Chiari syndrome.
(D) cranium bifidum.
(E) myeloschisis.

7. The alar plate gives rise to all of the following structures EXCEPT the

(A) dentate nucleus.
(B) inferior olivary nucleus.
(C) nucleus gracilis.
(D) nucleus ambiguus.
(E) cerebellar cortex.

8. All of the following statements concerning myelination are correct EXCEPT

(A) it is accomplished by neural crest cells.
(B) it is accomplished by Schwann cells in the PNS.
(C) it is accomplished by oligodendrocytes in the CNS.
(D) it commences in the fourth fetal month.
(E) it is completed by birth.

9. All of the following statements concerning spina bifida are correct EXCEPT

(A) spina bifida results from failure of vertebral arches to fuse.
(B) spina bifida is frequently associated with Arnold-Chiari malformation.
(C) spina bifida usually occurs in the cervicothoracic region.
(D) spina bifida occulta is the least severe variation.
(E) spina bifida with myeloschisis is the most severe variation.

10. The flexure that develops between the metencephalon and the myelencephalon is called the

(A) cephalic flexure.
(B) mesencephalic flexure.
(C) pontine flexure.
(D) cerebellar flexure.
(E) cervical flexure.

11. All of the following statements concerning the neural tube are correct EXCEPT it

(A) lies between the surface ectoderm and the notochord.
(B) is completely closed by the sixth week.
(C) contains the neural crest.
(D) gives rise to the CNS.
(E) gives rise to myelin-producing cells.

12. Which of the following statements best describes the sulcus limitans?

(A) It is found in the interpeduncular fossa.
(B) It is located between the alar and basal plates.
(C) It separates the medulla from the pons.
(D) It separates the hypothalamus from the thalamus.
(E) It separates the neocortex from the allocortex.

13. The cerebellum develops from all of the following structures EXCEPT the

(A) rhombencephalon.
(B) metencephalon.
(C) rhombic lips.
(D) alar plates.
(E) myelencephalon.

14. The neural crest gives rise to all of the following cells EXCEPT

(A) odontoblasts.
(B) oligodendrocytes.
(C) cells of enteric ganglia.
(D) Schwann cells.
(E) chromaffin cells.

Answers and Explanations

1–C. The anterior and posterior neuropores close during the fourth week of embryonic development: the anterior on day 25, the posterior on day 27. Failure of the anterior neuropore to close results in anencephaly; failure of the posterior neuropore to close results in myeloschisis.

2–C. At birth, the conus medullaris extends to VL3, and in the adult it extends to the VL1–VL2 interspace. At 8 weeks, the spinal cord extends the entire length of the vertebral canal.

3–C. The globus pallidus develops from the diencephalon. Globus pallidus cells migrate into the telencephalon.

4–B. Failure of the anterior neuropore to close results in anencephaly. The brain fails to develop; no cranial vault is formed.

5–D. The adenohypophysis (pars distalis, pars tuberalis, and pars intermedia) develops from Rathke's pouch, an ectodermal diverticulum of the stomodeum. The neurohypophysis develops from the infundibulum of the hypothalamus.

6–C. Arnold-Chiari syndrome is a cerebellomedullary malformation in which the inferior vermis and medulla herniate through the foramen magnum, resulting in communicating hydrocephalus. Arnold-Chiari syndrome is frequently associated with spina bifida.

7–D. The alar plate of the mantle layer gives rise to sensory relay nuclei and the cerebellum. The nucleus ambiguus, a SVE nucleus, is derived from the basal motor plate.

8–E. Myelination is not complete at birth. The corticospinal tracts are not completely myelinated until the end of the second postnatal year.

9–C. Spina bifida usually occurs in the lumbosacral region.

10–C. The pontine flexure develops between the metencephalon (pons) and the myelencephalon (medulla). The pontine flexure results in lateral expansion of the walls of the metencephalon and myelencephalon, stretching of the roof of the fourth ventricle, and widening of the floor of the fourth ventricle (rhomboid fossa).

11–C. The neural tube, which lies between the surface ectoderm and the notochord, gives rise to the brain and spinal cord. Closure is already complete in the fifth week. The neural crest lies between the neural tube and the surface ectoderm. The neural tube gives rise to oligodendrocytes, which produce the myelin of the CNS.

12–B. The sulcus limitans separates the sensory alar and motor basal plates. It is found in the developing spinal cord and on the surface of the adult rhomboid fossa of the fourth ventricle. The bulbopontine sulcus separates the medulla from the pons. The hypothalamic sulcus separates the thalamus from the hypothalamus. The rhinal sulcus separates the neocortex from the allocortex.

13–E. The cerebellum arises from the alar plates of the rhombencephalon, which form the rhombic lips. The metencephalon, a division of the rhombencephalon, includes the pons and the cerebellum. The myelencephalon develops from the rhombencephalon and becomes the medulla oblongata.

14–B. The neural crest gives rise to dorsal root ganglion cells, the cells of autonomic and enteric ganglia, Schwann cells, satellite cells, and chromaffin cells of the suprarenal medulla. The neural crest also gives rise to pigment cells (melanocytes), odontoblasts, meninges, and mesenchyme of the branchial arches. Oligodendrocytes arise from the glioblasts of the neural tube.

5

Neurohistology

I. Overview—Nervous Tissue

—develops from ectoderm (the neural tube and neural crest).
—consists of neurons and glial cells.

II. Neurons

—constitute the genetic, anatomic, trophic, and functional units of the nervous system (known as the neuron doctrine).
—have lost the capacity to undergo cell division.
—have the capacity to *receive* impulses from receptor organs or other neurons.
—have the capacity to *transmit* impulses to other neurons or effector organs.
—consist of the **cell body** and its processes, **dendrites,** and a single **axon.**

A. Classification of neurons (Figure 5.1)

—is according to **number of processes** (unipolar, bipolar, or multipolar), **axonal length, function,** and **neurotransmitter.**

1. Processes

a. Unipolar or pseudounipolar neurons

—are sensory neurons located in the dorsal root and cranial nerve ganglia and in the mesencephalic nucleus of the trigeminal nerve (CN V) of the brainstem.

b. Bipolar neurons

—are located in the vestibular and cochlear ganglia of the vestibulocochlear nerve (CN VIII), the retina, and the olfactory epithelium (CN I).

c. Multipolar neurons

—possess one axon and more than one dendrite.
—are the largest population of nerve cells in the nervous system.
—include motor neurons, interneurons, pyramidal cells of the cerebral cortex, and Purkinje cells of the cerebellar cortex.

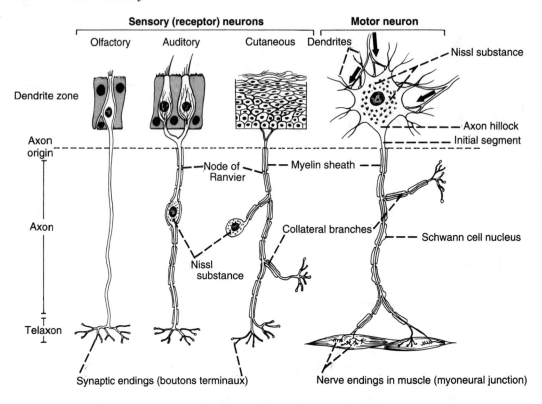

Figure 5.1. Types of nerve cells. Olfactory neurons are bipolar and unmyelinated. Auditory neurons are bipolar and are myelinated. Dorsal root ganglion cells (cutaneous) are pseudounipolar and myelinated. Motor neurons are multipolar and myelinated. *Arrows* indicate input via axons of other neurons. Nerve cells are characterized by the presence of Nissl substance, rough endoplasmic reticulum. (Modified with permission from Carpenter MB and Sutin J: *Human Neuroanatomy*. Baltimore, Williams & Wilkins, 1983, p 92.)

2. Axonal length

a. Golgi type I neurons

–have long axons (e.g., giant pyramidal cells of Betz of the motor cortex).

b. Golgi type II neurons

–have short axons (e.g., interneurons).

3. Function

a. Motor neurons

–conduct impulses to muscles, glands, and blood vessels (e.g., ventral horn cells).

b. Sensory neurons

–receive stimuli from the external and internal environment (e.g., dorsal root ganglion cells).

c. Interneurons

–are intercalated or internuncial neurons that interconnect motor or sensory neurons.

4. Neurotransmitter (cholinergic neurons)

−elaborate acetylcholine as a neurotransmitter (e.g., ventral horn motor neurons).

B. Nerve cell body

−is also called the **soma** or **perikaryon**.

−contains the organelles found in other cells, including a large nucleus and a prominent nucleolus.

−has receptor molecules on its plasmalemmal surface that confer sensitivity to various neurotransmitters.

−incorporates or gives rise to the following structures:

1. Nissl substance

−is characteristic of nerve cells and consists of rosettes of polysomes and rough endoplasmic reticulum.

−plays a role in **protein synthesis**.

−is abundant throughout cytoplasm and dendrites but is *not* found in the axon hillock or in the axon.

2. Lysosomes

−are membrane-bound dense bodies that contain hydrolytic enzymes and are involved in the process of **intracellular digestion**.

−a genetic defect in the synthesis of lysosomal enzymes results in a storage disease (e.g., Tay-Sachs disease [GM_2 gangliosidosis]).

3. Filamentous protein structures

−form an internal supportive network, the **cytoskeleton,** consisting of:

a. Microtubules (25 nm in diameter)

−are found in the cell body, dendrites, and axons.

−play a role in the **development and maintenance of cell shape**.

−play a role in the **intracellular transport of peptide vesicles and organelles**.

b. Neurofilaments (10 nm in diameter)

−consist of spiral protein threads that play a role in **developing and regenerating nerve fibers**.

−degenerate in Alzheimer's disease to form **neurofibrillary tangles**.

−neurofilament protein is exclusive to neurons and their precursors.

c. Microfilaments (5 nm in diameter)

−are composed of **actin**.

−are found in the tips of growing axons.

−facilitate **movement of plasma membrane** and **growth of nerve cell processes**.

4. Inclusion bodies

−include pigment granules:

a. Lipofuscin (lipochrome) granules

−are common pigmented inclusions of cytoplasm that accumulate with aging.

−are considered to be residual bodies derived from lysosomes.

b. Neuromelanin (melanin)

  –is a blackish pigment in the neurons of the substantia nigra and in the locus ceruleus.
  –disappears from the substantia nigra and the locus ceruleus in Parkinson's disease.

5. Dendrites

  –are processes that extend from the cell body.
  –contain cytoplasm similar in composition to that of the cell body; however, no Golgi apparatus is present.
  –conduct in a decremental fashion but may be capable of generating action potentials.
  –**receive synaptic input and transmit it toward the cell body.**

6. Axons

  –arise from either the cell body or the dendrite.
  –originate from the axon hillock, which lacks Nissl substance.
  –give rise to collateral branches.
  –may be myelinated or unmyelinated.
  –**generate, propagate, and transmit action potentials.**
  –end distally in terminal boutons in synapses with neurons, muscle cells, and glands.

7. Nerve fibers (Table 5.1)

  –consist of axons and their glial investments.
  –are classified by function, fiber size, and conduction velocity.

Table 5.1. Classification of Nerve Fibers

Fibers	Diameter (μm)*	Conduction Velocity (m/sec)	Function
Sensory axons			
Ia (A-α)	12–20	70–120	Proprioception, muscle spindles
Ib (A-α)	12–20	70–120	Proprioception, Golgi tendon organs
II (A-β)	5–12	30–70	Touch, pressure, and vibration
III (A-δ)	2–5	12–30	Touch, pressure, fast pain, and temperature
IV (C)	0.5–1	0.5–2	Slow pain and temperature, unmyelinated fibers
Motor axons			
Alpha (A-α)	12–20	15–120	Alpha motor neurons of ventral horn (innervate extrafusal muscle fibers)
Gamma (A-γ)	2–10	10–45	Gamma motor neurons of ventral horn (innervate intrafusal muscle fibers)
Preganglionic autonomic fibers (B)	< 3	3–15	Myelinated preganglionic autonomic fibers
Postganglionic autonomic fibers (C)	1	2	Unmyelinated postganglionic autonomic fibers

*Myelin sheath included if present.

8. Myelin sheath

   −is produced in the peripheral nervous system (PNS) by Schwann cells.
   −is produced in the central nervous system (CNS) by oligodendrocytes.
   −is interruped by the nodes of Ranvier.
   −consists of a spirally wrapped plasma membrane.

9. Synapses

   −are the **sites of functional contact** of a nerve cell with another nerve cell, an effector cell, or a sensory receptor cell.
   −consist of presynaptic membrane, synaptic cleft, and postsynaptic membrane.
   −are classified by the site of contact (e.g., axosomatic, axodendritic, or axoaxonic).
   −are also classified as chemical or electrical:

   #### a. Chemical synapses

   −use neurotransmitters.

   #### b. Electrical (ephapses) synapses

   −consist of gap junctions.
   −allow ions to pass from cell to cell.

III. Neuroglia

−are non-neuronal cells of the CNS and the PNS.
−arise from the neural tube and neural crest.
−are capable of mitotic cell division throughout adult life, especially in response to trauma or disease.
−are best revealed with gold and silver impregnation stains.
−are classified as **macroglia (astrocytes and oligodendrocytes), microglia, and ependyma**. Schwann cells are classified as peripheral neuroglia.

A. Astrocytes

−are the largest glial cells.
−consist of **fibrous astrocytes,** which are found mainly in white matter, and **protoplasmic astrocytes,** which are found mainly in gray matter.
−play a role in the metabolism of certain neurotransmitters (γ-aminobutyric acid [GABA], serotonin, and glutamate).
−buffer the potassium concentration of the extracellular space.
−contain glial filaments and glycogen granules as their most characteristic cytoplasmic components.
−contain or give rise to the following structures:

1. Astrocytic end feet

   −are the processes that form the external glial limiting membrane (interface between the pia mater and the CNS) and the internal glial limiting membrane (interface between the ependyma and the CNS).

   ##### a. Perivascular end feet

   −surround capillaries.

   ##### b. Perineuronal end feet

   −surround neurons.

2. Glial filaments

−contain glial fibrillary acidic protein (**GFAP**), a marker for astrocytes.

3. Glycogen granules

B. Oligodendrocytes

−are small glial cells with few short processes.
−lack glial filaments and glycogen granules.
−are the myelin-forming cells of the CNS; one oligodendrocyte can myelinate numerous (up to 30) axons.
−consist of:

1. Interfascicular oligodendrocytes

−are found in white matter.

2. Satellite cells

−are found in gray matter.

C. Microglia (Hortega cells)

−arise from monocytes, which enter the CNS via abnormal blood vessels.
−are activated by inflammatory and degenerative processes.
−are macrophages, which are migratory and phagocytize debris of nerve tissue.

D. Ependymal cells

−line the central canal of the spinal cord and ventricles of the brain.
−include choroid epithelial cells of the choroid plexus cells and tanycytes of the third ventricle; the choroid plexus cells produce cerebrospinal fluid (CSF).

E. Schwann cells (neurolemmal cells)

−are derivatives of the neural crest.
−are myelin-forming cells of the PNS; a Schwann cell myelinates only one internode (only one peripheral axon).
−invest all unmyelinated axons of the PNS.
−function in regeneration and remyelination of severed axons in the PNS (Figure 5.2).
−are separated from each other by the **node of Ranvier**.

F. Tumors of neuroglial cells (gliomas)

−are derived from the three glial cell types: astrocytes, oligodendrocytes, and ependymocytes.
−result from proliferation of glioblasts, embryonic precursors.
−represent 50% of primary intracranial tumors.

1. Astrocytomas

−are most commonly found in the white matter of the cerebral hemisphere in middle and late life.
−in children, astrocytomas of the cerebellum are the most common intracranial tumor.
−in damaged areas of the brain, astrocytes form glial scars, a condition called **gliosis**.

a. Benign astrocytomas

−are slow growing neoplasms of infiltrative character.

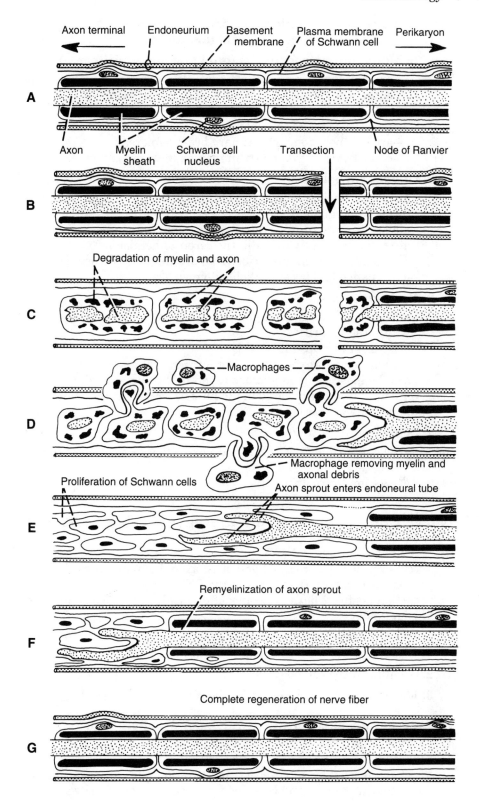

Figure 5.2. Wallerian (anterograde) degeneration and regeneration of a nerve fiber.

–arise from **astroblasts,** embryonic precursors.

–frequently become malignant (**anaplastic astrocytomas**).

b. Malignant astrocytomas (glioblastoma multiforme)

–are rapid growing, fatal astrocytic tumors; less than 20% of patients survive one year.

–arise from **astroblasts**.

–represent 50% of the gliomas.

–are the most common primary brain tumors.

–occur twice as frequently in men as in women.

2. Oligodendrogliomas

–are slow growing, benign tumors that account for approximately 5% of intracranial gliomas.

–may arise from **oligodendroblasts,** embryonic precursors.

–are most frequently found in the cerebral hemisphere.

–are usually well-circumscribed and are frequently calcified.

–may change and become glioblastomas.

3. Ependymomas

–are slow growing, benign circumscribed neoplasms typically found within the ventricles.

–arise from **ependymal cells**.

–account for approximately 5% of intracranial gliomas.

–are the most common gliomas found in the spinal cord.

–are most frequently found in the lumbosacral segments (filum terminale and cauda equina).

4. Schwannomas

–are benign tumors of peripheral nerves (e.g., acoustic neuromas of CN VIII).

–arise from **Schwann cells**.

IV. Nerve Cell Degeneration and Regeneration (see Figure 5.2)

A. Retrograde degeneration

–occurs toward the proximal end of an axon, including the cell body.

–takes place in both the CNS and the PNS.

–reaction begins 2 days or sooner after insult and reaches a maximum in about 20 days.

–involves:

1. Disappearance of Nissl substance (chromatolysis)

2. Swelling of the cell body

3. Flattening and displacement of the nucleus to the periphery

B. Anterograde degeneration (wallerian degeneration) [see Figure 5.2]

–occurs toward the distal end of the axon.

–takes place in both the PNS and the CNS.

–is characterized by successive fragmentation and disappearance of axons and myelin sheaths and by secondary proliferation of Schwann cells.

C. Regeneration of the peripheral nerve fiber (see Figure 5.2)

  −a myelinated peripheral nerve fiber consists of an axon, a myelin sheath and its basement membrane, and a delicate connective sheath, the endoneurium.

  −the severed distal nerve fiber maintains its integrity and provides a tube of basement membrane and endoneurium into which an axon sprout grows.

  −Schwann cells proliferate along a degenerating axon and myelinate a new axon sprout, which grows at the rate of 3 mm/day.

  −if the path of regenerating axons is blocked, a traumatic neuroma forms at the site of obstruction (amputation neuroma); a neuroma consists of a proliferative mass of axons and Schwann cells.

D. Regeneration of axons in the CNS

  −no basement membranes or endoneurial investments surround axons of the CNS.

  −effective regeneration does not occur in the CNS.

E. Transsynaptic (transneuronal) degeneration

  −interruption of certain CNS pathways results in degeneration of denervated neurons.

  −transection of the optic nerve results in degeneration of neurons in the lateral geniculate body.

V. Axonal Transport

  −controls the intracellular distribution of membranes and secretory proteins from the Golgi apparatus to axon terminals (anterograde axonal transport).

  −controls the return of degraded membranes to the cell body for recycling (retrograde axonal transport).

  −fast anterograde (forward-moving) axonal transport is 400 mm/per day.

  −fast retrograde (backward-moving) axonal transport is 200 mm/day.

  −slow axonal transport is concerned with the transport of fibrous cytoskeletal proteins and is conducted at less than 10 mm/day.

  −is used by neurotropic viruses (e.g., herpes simplex and rabies) to reach the CNS via peripheral nerve terminals.

  −is used to **trace neuroanatomic pathways** by the following methods:

A. Horseradish peroxidase (HRP) method (Figure 5.3)

  −HRP is used primarily to study **retrograde transport**.

  1. HRP is injected into a region (nucleus) of the nervous system.

  2. It is taken up by the cell body and transported in an anterograde direction to the axon terminal.

  3. It is taken up by the axon terminal and transported in a retrograde direction to the cell body.

B. Autoradiographic method (see Figure 5.3)

  −is used to trace the axonal pathway in serial autoradiographs.

  1. Radioactive-labeled amino acids are injected into a region (nucleus) of the CNS.

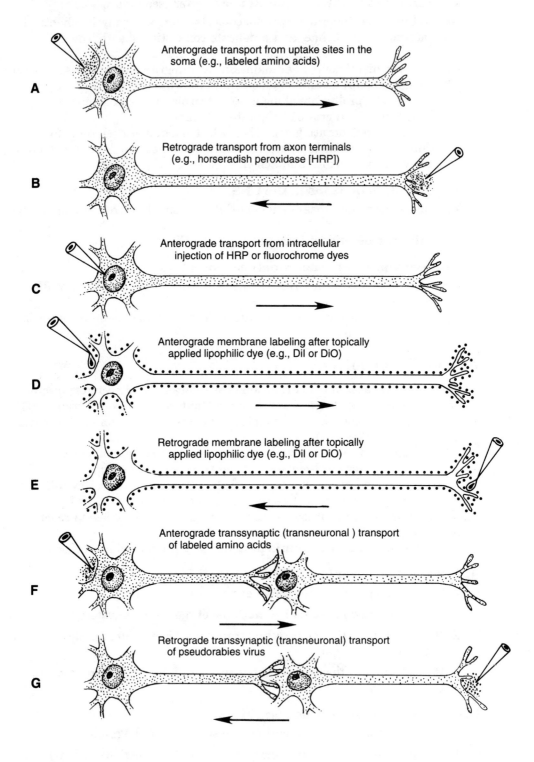

Figure 5.3. Some common tracing methods used to elucidate neuroanatomical pathways by intracellular labeling.

2. The radioactive substance is taken up by the cell body and is transported to the axon terminal. (Only nerve cell bodies take up the label.)

C. Membrane labeling by externally applied carbocyanine dyes (see Figure 5.3)

   −traces neuronal pathways in fixed (dead) tissue.

   1. Commonly used **fluorescent dyes** are DiI, DiO, and DiS.

   2. These **lipophilic dyes** are used to trace neuronal pathways in fixed tissue by diffusion through the plasma membrane of the neuron.

   3. Labeling may be anterograde or retrograde.

VI. Capillaries of the CNS

−have a higher density in gray matter than in white matter and consist of two types:

A. Nonfenestrated capillaries

   −are ubiquitous in white and gray matter.
   −represent the site of the **blood–brain barrier,** which consists of rows of tight junctions between cells of the cerebral capillaries.
   −have endothelial cells with tight junctions surrounded by a continuous basement membrane and an outer investment of astrocytic foot processes.

B. Fenestrated capillaries

   −consist of endothelial cells with fenestrations that permit the free passage of blood-borne substances into the extracellular spaces of the CNS.
   −are located in specialized areas of the brain that lack a blood–brain barrier (e.g., in the circumventricular organs).

Review Test

Directions: Each of the numbered items or incomplete statements in this section is followed by answers or by completions of the statement. Select the **one** lettered answer or completion that is **best** in each case.

1. All of the following statements concerning ependymal cells are correct EXCEPT

(A) they are derived from the neural crest.
(B) they line the central canal.
(C) they are in contact with CSF.
(D) they produce CSF.
(E) they include tanycytes and choroid plexus cells.

2. All of the following statements concerning wallerian degeneration are correct EXCEPT

(A) it occurs in the CNS.
(B) it occurs in the PNS.
(C) it is a retrograde degeneration.
(D) it is characterized by the disappearance of axons and myelin sheaths.
(E) it is characterized by the proliferation of Schwann cells.

3. All of the following statements concerning neurons are correct EXCEPT

(A) they are of neuroectodermal origin.
(B) they have lost the capacity to undergo cell division.
(C) they contain Nissl substance.
(D) they are derived from the neural tube and neural crest.
(E) bipolar neurons are the most common type of neuron.

4. All of the following statements concerning axons are correct EXCEPT they

(A) may arise from the perikaryon.
(B) may arise from a dendrite.
(C) arise from the axon hillock.
(D) contain rough endoplasmic reticulum.
(E) transmit action potentials.

5. All of the following statements concerning myelin are correct EXCEPT

(A) it is produced by the microglia.
(B) it is produced by Schwann cells.
(C) it is produced by oligodendrocytes.
(D) myelinating cells of the PNS myelinate only one internode.
(E) myelinating cells of the CNS myelinate several internodes of different axons.

6. All of the following statements concerning astrocytes are correct EXCEPT

(A) they possess many processes.
(B) they are found in both white and gray matter.
(C) they are considered to be the scavenger cells of the CNS.
(D) they have perivascular end feet.
(E) in damaged brain tissue, astrocytes form glial scars.

7. All of the following statements concerning Schwann cells are correct EXCEPT

(A) they play an important role in peripheral nerve regeneration.
(B) they are derived from the neural tube.
(C) they may give rise to tumors of peripheral nerves.
(D) one Schwann cell myelinates one internode of an axon.
(E) they are neurolemmal cells.

Directions: Each group of items in this section consists of lettered options followed by a set of numbered items. For each item, select the **one** lettered option that is most closely associated with it. Each lettered option may be selected once, more than once, or not at all.

Questions 8–12

Match each of the descriptions below with the corresponding type of nerve cell.

(A) Astrocytes
(B) Oligodendrocytes
(C) Microglial cells
(D) Schwann cells
(E) Tanycytes

8. Are a variety of ependymal cell found in the wall of the third ventricle

9. Arise from monocytes

10. Are neural crest derivatives

11. Contain glial filaments and glycogen granules

12. Are perineuronal satellite cells in the CNS

Questions 13–18

Match each of the descriptions below with the appropriate type of cell.

(A) Pseudounipolar neurons
(B) Bipolar neurons
(C) Multipolar neurons
(D) Betz cells
(E) Purkinje cells

13. Are diagnostic of the cerebellar cortex

14. Are found only in the motor cortex

15. Are found in dorsal root ganglia

16. Are motor neurons of the ventral horn

17. Are found in the olfactory epithelium

18. Are found in the cochlear ganglion

Answers and Explanations

1–A. Ependymal cells are derived from the neural tube, line the central canal and ventricles, and are in contact with CSF. Ependymal cells include choroid plexus cells, which produce CSF. Tanycytes are modified ependymal cells found in the wall of the third ventricle.

2–C. Wallerian degeneration is an anterograde degeneration of nerve fibers, characterized by the disappearance of axons and myelin and by Schwann cell proliferation.

3–E. Neurons are of ectodermal origin, contain Nissl substance, and have lost the capacity to undergo cell division. The neural tube and the neural crest both give rise to neurons. Multipolar neurons are the most common type. Bipolar neurons are found in the olfactory mucous membrane, in the ganglia of the vestibulocochlear nerve, and in the retina.

4–D. Axons may arise from the perikaryon or from a dendrite. They always arise from the axon hillock. Axons do not contain rough endoplasmic reticulum (Nissl substance). Axons generate and transmit action potentials.

5–A. Myelin is produced by Schwann cells in the PNS and by oligodendrocytes in the CNS. Schwann cells myelinate only one internode; oligodendrocytes myelinate several internodes of different axons (up to 30). Microglial cells are the scavenger cells of the CNS; they do not produce myelin.

6–C. Astrocytes have many processes and are found in the gray and white matter. They have perivascular end feet. In the damaged brain, astrocytes form glial scar tissue, known as gliosis or astrogliosis. The microglial cells are the scavenger cells of the CNS.

7–B. Schwann cells (neurolemmal cells) play an important role in peripheral nerve regeneration. They are derived from the neural crest. They may give rise to benign tumors called schwannomas. Schwann cells are the myelin-forming cells of the PNS; they myelinate only one internode of an axon.

8–E. Tanycytes are a variety of ependymal cell found in the wall of the third ventricle. The processes of these cells extend from the lumen of the third ventricle to the capillaries of the hypophyseal portal system and also to the neurosecretory neurons of the arcuate nucleus.

9–C. Microglial cells, the scavenger cells of the CNS, arise from monocytes and enter the CNS via abnormal blood vessels.

10–D. Schwann cells are derived from the neural crest; they myelinate the axons of the PNS.

11–A. Astrocytes are characterized by the presence of glial filaments and glycogen; glial filaments contain glial fibrillary acidic protein (GFAP), a marker for astrocytes.

12–B. Oligodendrocytes are perineuronal satellite cells; they myelinate the axons of the CNS.

13–E. Purkinje cells are diagnostic of the cerebellar cortex. They represent the sole output from the cerebellar cortex and are GABA-ergic inhibitory neurons.

14–D. Betz cells are large pyramidal cells found only in the motor cortex (area 4). They give rise to 3% of the corticospinal tract.

15–A. Pseudounipolar neurons are found in the dorsal root ganglia and in the sensory ganglia of cranial nerves (except CN VIII). They are also found in the mesencephalic nucleus (CN V).

16–C. Ventral horn motor neurons and the motor neurons of the cranial nerves are multipolar neurons.

17–B. The neurosensory cells of the olfactory epithelium are bipolar neurons; their axons, fila olfactoria, constitute the olfactory nerve (CN I).

18–B. The cochlear and vestibular ganglia (CN VIII) contain bipolar neurons.

6

Spinal Cord

I. Introduction—The Spinal Cord

–is derived from the caudal part of the neural tube.
–maintains segmental organization throughout development.
–is surrounded by three membranes, the **meninges**.
–weighs about 30 g, comprising 2% of the adult brain weight.

II. External Morphology

A. Location—the spinal cord (Figure 6.1)

–extends, in adults, from the foramen magnum to the lower border of the first lumbar vertebra; in newborns, it extends to the third lumbar vertebra.
–is continuous with the **medulla oblongata** at the spinomedullary junction, a plane defined by three structures: the foramen magnum, the pyramidal decussation, and the emergence of the first cervical nerve ventral rootlets.
–lies within the **subarachnoid space,** which extends caudally to the level of the second sacral vertebra (see Figure 2.2).

B. Attachments

–suspend and anchor the spinal cord within the dural sac.
–arise from the vascular **pia mater,** which closely invests the spinal cord.

1. Denticulate ligaments

–are two flattened bands of pial tissue that attach to the spinal dura with about 21 teeth.

2. Filum terminale

–is a pial filament extending from the conus medullaris to the end of the dural sac, with which it fuses.

3. Spinal nerve roots

–provide the strongest anchorage and fixation of the spinal cord to the vertebral canal.

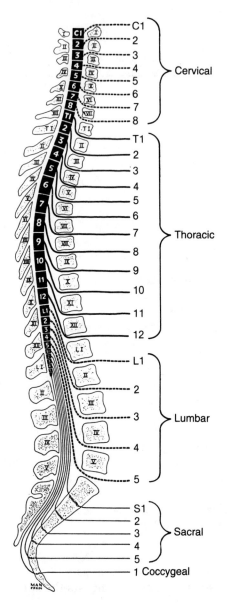

Figure 6.1. Diagram of the position of the spinal cord with reference to the vertebral bodies and spinous processes. The conus medullaris lies in the L1–L2 interspace. The dural cul de sac ends at S2. (Reprinted with permission from Haymaker W and Woodhall B: *Peripheral Nerve Injuries,* 2nd ed. Philadelphia, WB Saunders, 1952, p 32.)

C. Shape—the spinal cord (Figure 6.2)

–is an elongated nearly cylindrical structure, flattened dorsoventrally, and is approximately 1 cm in diameter.

–has **cervical** (C5–T1) and **lumbar** (L1–S2) **enlargements** for the nerve supply of the upper and lower extremities (the brachial and lumbosacral plexuses).

–terminates caudally as the **conus medullaris**.

–averages, in length, 45 cm in males and 42 cm in females.

D. Spinal nerves (see Figures 6.1 and 6.2)

–consist of thirty-one pairs of nerves that emerge from the spinal cord: **8 cervical, 12 thoracic, 5 lumbar, 5 sacral, and 1 coccygeal**.

–contain both motor and sensory fibers.

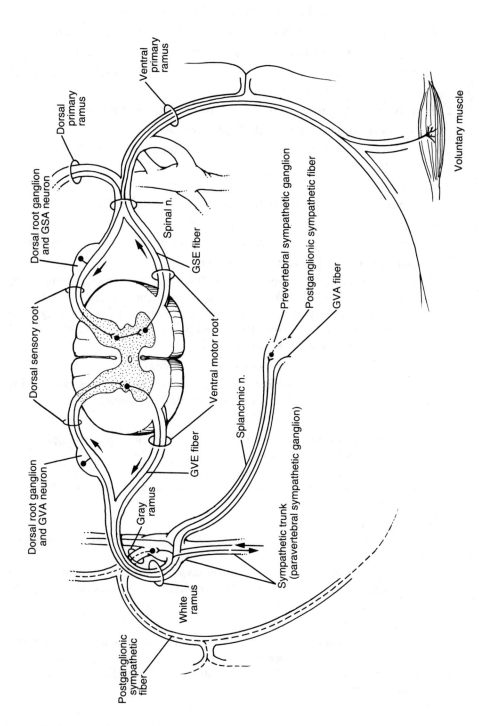

Figure 6.2. The typical thoracic spinal nerve and its branches and reflex connections. White communicating rami are found only at thoracolumbar levels T1–L3. Gray communicating rami are found at all spinal cord levels.

1. Special considerations

a. The first cervical nerve and the coccygeal nerve usually have no dorsal (sensory) roots and no corresponding dermatomes.

b. The first cervical nerve passes between the atlas and the skull.

c. The second cervical nerve passes between the atlas and the axis.

d. With the exception of C1, spinal nerves exit the vertebral canal via intervertebral or sacral foramina.

2. Functional components of spinal nerve fibers (Figure 6.3)

a. General somatic afferent (GSA) fibers

−convey sensory input from skin, muscle, bone, and joints to the central nervous system (CNS).

b. General visceral afferent (GVA) fibers

−convey sensory input from visceral organs to the CNS.

c. General somatic efferent (GSE) fibers

−convey motor output from ventral horn motor neurons to skeletal muscle.

d. General visceral efferent (GVE) fibers

−convey motor output from intermediolateral cell column neurons, via paravertebral or prevertebral ganglia, to glands, smooth muscle, and visceral organs (sympathetic divisions of the autonomic nervous system).

−convey motor output from the sacral parasympathetic nucleus to the pelvic viscera via intramural ganglia.

3. Components and branches of spinal nerves

−the spinal nerve is formed by the union of dorsal and ventral roots within the intervertebral foramen, resulting in a mixed nerve.

a. Dorsal root

−enters the dorsal lateral sulcus as dorsal rootlets, conveying sensory input from the body via the dorsal root ganglion.

−contains, distally, the dorsal root ganglion.

−joins the ventral root distal to the dorsal root ganglion and within the intervertebral foramen to form the spinal nerve.

b. Dorsal root ganglion

−is located within the dorsal root and within the **intervertebral foramen**.

−contains **pseudounipolar neurons** of neural crest origin, which transmit sensory input from the periphery (GSA and GVA) to the spinal cord via the dorsal roots.

c. Ventral root

−emerges as ventral rootlets from the ventral lateral sulcus, conveying motor output from visceral and somatic motor neurons.

−joins the dorsal roots distal to the dorsal root ganglion and within the intervertebral foramen to form the spinal nerve.

d. Cauda equina

−consists of lumbosacral (dorsal and ventral) nerve roots that descend from the spinal cord through the subarachnoid space to exit through their respective intervertebral or sacral foramina.

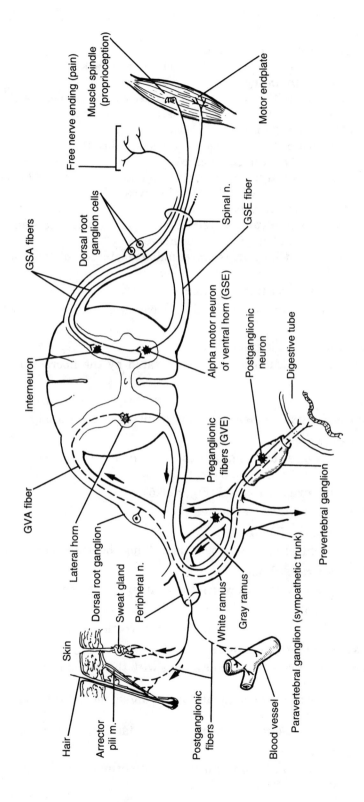

Figure 6.3. Diagram of the four functional components of the thoracic spinal nerve: general visceral afferent (GVA); general somatic afferent (GSA); general somatic efferent (GSE); and general visceral efferent (GVE). Proprioceptive, cutaneous, and visceral reflex arcs are shown. The muscle stretch (myotatic) reflex includes the muscle spindle, GSA dorsal root ganglion cell, GSE ventral horn motor neuron, and skeletal muscle.

e. Spinal nerve rami

–include:

(1) Dorsal primary ramus

–innervates the skin and muscles of the back.

(2) Ventral primary ramus

–innervates the ventral lateral muscles and skin of the trunk, extremities, and visceral organs.

(3) Meningeal ramus

–innervates the meninges and vertebral column.

(4) Gray communicating rami

–contain **unmyelinated** postganglionic sympathetic fibers.

–are associated with *all* spinal nerves.

(5) White communicating rami

–contain **myelinated** preganglionic sympathetic fibers and myelinated GVA fibers (splanchnic nerves).

–are found only in thoracolumbar segments of the spinal cord (T1–L3).

E. Spinal nerve innervation (Figure 6.4)

–one spinal nerve innervates the derivatives from one **somite,** which includes:

1. Dermatome (see Figure 6.4)

–consists of a **cutaneous area** innervated by the fibers of one spinal nerve.

2. Myotome

–consists of **muscles** innervated by the fibers of one spinal nerve.

3. Sclerotome

–consists of **bones and ligaments** innervated by the fibers of one spinal nerve.

F. Surface structures and sulci (Figure 6.5)

–underlie the pia mater and include:

1. Ventral median fissure

–is a deep ventral midline groove underlying the ventral spinal artery.

2. Ventral lateral sulcus

–is a shallow groove from which the ventral rootlets emerge.

3. Dorsal lateral sulcus

–is a shallow groove into which the dorsal rootlets enter.

4. Dorsal intermediate sulcus

–is a shallow groove that is continuous with the dorsal intermediate septum.

–is found between the dorsal lateral and dorsal medial sulci but only rostral to T6.

–separates the fasciculus gracilis from the fasciculus cuneatus.

5. Dorsal median sulcus

–is a shallow dorsal midline groove that is continuous with the dorsal median septum.

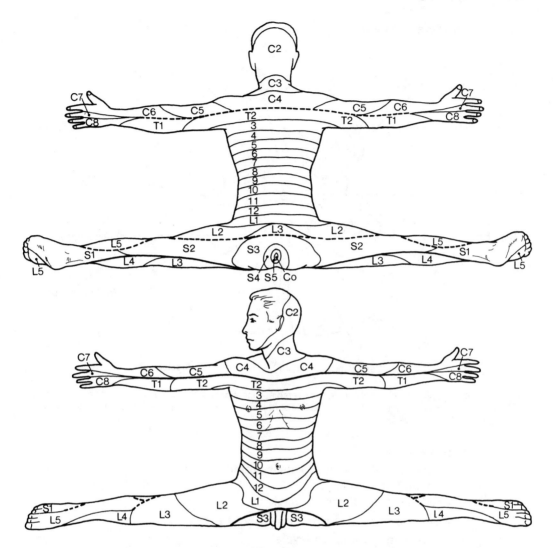

Figure 6.4. Cutaneous distribution of spinal nerves, the dermatomes. (Reprinted with permission from Haymaker W and Woodhall B: *Peripheral Nerve Injuries,* 2nd ed. Philadelphia, WB Saunders, 1952, p 32.)

III. Internal Morphology (see Figure 6.5)

–in transverse sections, the spinal cord consists of central gray matter and peripheral white matter.

A. Gray matter

–is located centrally within the spinal cord.

–is butterfly- or **H-shaped** in a configuration that varies according to spinal cord level.

–contains a central canal.

–is divided into cytoarchitectural areas called **Rexed laminae,** expressed with Roman numerals (see Figure 6.5).

–is divided into three horns or cell columns on each side:

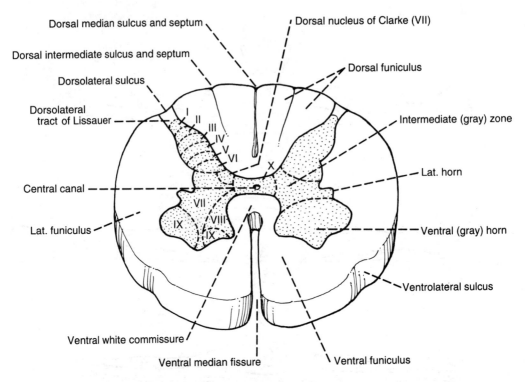

Figure 6.5. Topography of the spinal cord in transverse section: horns (columns), sulci, funiculi, and Rexed laminae. The lateral horn is only found at thoracolumbar cord levels (T1–L3). The posterior intermediate sulcus and septum are only found above T6.

1. Dorsal horn (column)

—receives and processes sensory input.
—is found at all levels.
—includes the following nuclei:

a. Dorsomarginal nucleus (Rexed lamina I)

—is found at all cord levels.
—is associated with light touch, pain, and temperature sensation and is one site of origin of the ventral and lateral spinothalamic tracts.

b. Substantia gelatinosa (Rexed lamina II)

—is found at all cord levels.
—is homologous to the spinal trigeminal nucleus.
—is associated with light touch, pain, and temperature sensation and integrates input for the ventral and lateral spinothalamic tracts.

c. Nucleus proprius (Rexed laminae III and IV)

—is found at all cord levels.
—is associated with light touch, pain, and temperature sensation and gives rise (from Rexed lamina IV) to the ventral and lateral spinothalamic tracts.

d. Nucleus dorsalis of Clarke (Rexed lamina VII)

—is found at the base of the dorsal horn.
—extends from (C8) T1 to L3.

−is homologous to the **accessory cuneate nucleus** of the medulla.

−subserves unconscious proprioception from muscle spindles and Golgi tendon organs and is the origin of the dorsal spinocerebellar tract.

2. Lateral horn (column) [Rexed lamina VII]

−receives viscerosensory input.

−is found between the dorsal and ventral horns.

−extends from (C8) T1 to L3.

−contains the **intermediolateral nucleus** (column), a visceromotor nucleus that extends from T1 to L3.

−contains preganglionic sympathetic neurons (GVE).

−contains, at T1–T2, the ciliospinal **center of Budge** (sympathetic innervation of the eye).

3. Ventral horn (column) [Rexed laminae VII, VIII, and IX]

−contains predominately motor nuclei.

−is found at all levels.

−includes the following nuclei:

a. Spinal border cells (Cooper-Sherrington)

−extend from L2 to S3.

−subserve unconscious proprioception from Golgi tendon organs and muscle spindles.

−are the origin of the ventral spinocerebellar tract.

b. Sacral parasympathetic nucleus (Rexed lamina VII)

−extends from S2 to S4.

−gives rise to preganglionic parasympathetic fibers that innervate the pelvic viscera via the pelvic nerve.

c. Somatic motor nuclei (Rexed lamina IX)

−are found at all levels.

−are subdivided into medial and lateral groups that innervate axial and appendicular muscles, respectively.

d. Spinal accessory nucleus (Rexed lamina IX)

−extends from C1 to C6.

−gives rise to the spinal root of the **spinal accessory nerve (CN XI)**.

−innervates the sternocleidomastoid and trapezius muscles.

e. Phrenic nucleus (Rexed lamina IX)

−extends from C3 to C6.

−innervates the diaphragm.

B. White matter (see Figure 6.5)

−consists of bundles of myelinated fibers that surround the central gray matter.

−consists of ascending and descending fiber pathways called tracts.

−is divided bilaterally by sulci into three major divisions and contains the ventral white commissure.

1. Dorsal funiculus (dorsal column)

−is located between the dorsal median sulcus and the dorsal lateral sulcus.

−is subdivided above T6 into two fasciculi:

a. Fasciculus gracilis

–is located between the dorsal median sulcus and the dorsal intermediate sulcus and septum.
–is found at all cord levels.

b. Fasciculus cuneatus

–is located between the dorsal intermediate sulcus and septum and the dorsal lateral sulcus.
–is found only at the upper thoracic and cervical cord levels (C1–T6).

2. Lateral funiculus

–is located between the dorsal lateral and ventral lateral sulci.

3. Ventral funiculus

–is located between the ventral median fissure and the ventral lateral sulcus.

4. Ventral white commissure

–is located between the central canal and the ventral medial fissure.
–contains decussating spinothalamic tracts.

C. Determination of spinal cord levels

–is based on regional variation in the shape of gray matter and on the presence of dorsal intermediate sulci and septa.

1. Cervical cord

–dorsal intermediate sulci and septa are present.
–ventral horns are massive from C3 to C8.

2. Thoracic cord

–dorsal intermediate sulci and septa are present from T1 to T6.
–the nucleus dorsalis of Clarke is present at all thoracic levels but is most prominent at T11 and T12.
–lateral horns are present at all thoracic levels.
–dorsal and ventral horns are typically slender and H-shaped.

3. Lumbar cord

–the nucleus dorsalis of Clarke is very prominent at L1 and L2.
–both ventral and dorsal horns are massive from L2 to L5; the substantia gelatinosa is greatly enlarged.
–the lumbar section is difficult to distinguish from upper sacral segments.
–the lateral horn is prominent only at L1.

4. Sacral cord

–the ventral and dorsal horns are massive; the substantia gelatinosa is greatly enlarged.
–the sacral cord is greatly reduced in diameter from S3 to S5.

5. Coccygeal segment

–the dorsal horns are more voluminous than the ventral horns.
–the diameter of the segment is greatly reduced.

IV. The Myotatic Reflex (see Figure 6.3)

–is a monosynaptic and ipsilateral muscle stretch reflex.

–is incorrectly called a deep tendon reflex.

–has an afferent and an efferent limb, like all reflexes.

–interruption of either limb results in areflexia.

A. Afferent limb

–includes a muscle spindle (receptor) and a dorsal root ganglion neuron and its Ia fiber.

B. Efferent limb

–includes a ventral horn motor neuron that innervates striated muscle (effector).

Review Test

Directions: Each of the numbered items or incomplete statements in this section is followed by answers or by completions of the statement. Select the **one** lettered answer or completion that is **best** in each case.

1. All of the following statements concerning the substantia gelatinosa are correct EXCEPT

(A) it is found at all spinal cord levels.
(B) it is a sensory nucleus.
(C) it plays a role in mediating pain and temperature.
(D) it is homologous to the spinal trigeminal nucleus.
(E) it is greatly reduced in size at sacral levels.

2. Which statement concerning the dorsal root ganglion is false?

(A) It contains pseudounipolar neurons.
(B) It is located within the intervertebral foramen.
(C) It contains neurons of neural crest origin.
(D) It usually is missing at C1.
(E) It lies within the subarachnoid space.

3. Which statement concerning the lateral horn is false?

(A) It receives viscerosensory input.
(B) It is found at the level of the phrenic nucleus.
(C) It is coextensive with the nucleus dorsalis of Clarke.
(D) It contains a visceromotor nucleus.
(E) It corresponds to Rexed lamina VII.

4. All of the following statements concerning the spinal cord are correct EXCEPT it

(A) represents 2% of brain weight.
(B) terminates in the adult at VL1–VL2.
(C) lies within the subarachnoid space.
(D) terminates in the newborn at VS2.
(E) contains 31 pairs of spinal nerves.

5. All of the following statements concerning spinal nerves are correct EXCEPT

(A) dorsal roots contain sensory input.
(B) ventral roots contain motor output.
(C) all spinal nerves have gray communicating rami.
(D) all spinal nerves have white communicating rami.
(E) the first cervical nerves frequently have no dorsal roots.

6. All of the following statements concerning the cauda equina are correct EXCEPT it

(A) contains motor fibers.
(B) contains sensory fibers.
(C) is found in the subarachnoid space.
(D) is derived from the pia.
(E) is found below the first lumbar vertebra.

7. All of the following statements concerning nuclei of the spinal cord are correct EXCEPT

(A) the nucleus dorsalis of Clark extends from C8 to L3.
(B) the phrenic nucleus extends from C3 to C6.
(C) the spinal parasympathetic nucleus extends from S1 to S5.
(D) the spinal accessory nucleus extends from C1 to C6.
(E) the intermediolateral nucleus (cell column) extends from T1 to L3.

8. All of the following statements concerning the myotatic reflex are correct EXCEPT

(A) it is a monosynaptic and ipsilateral reflex.
(B) it is a muscle stretch reflex.
(C) it includes a muscle spindle.
(D) it includes a ventral horn motor neuron.
(E) the cell body of afferent nerve fiber is found in the dorsal horn.

Directions: Each group of items in this section consists of lettered options followed by a set of numbered items. For each item, select the **one** lettered option that is most closely associated with it. Each lettered option may be selected once, more than once, or not at all.

Questions 9–13

Match each of the statements below to the structure most closely associated with it.

(A) Dorsal intermediate septum
(B) Ventral lateral sulcus
(C) Dorsal median sulcus
(D) Dorsal lateral sulcus
(E) Ventral median fissure

9. Contains the sulcal branch of an artery

10. Receives dorsal roots

11. Is not found at lumbar levels

12. Is located between the fasciculus gracilis and the fasciculus cuneatus

13. Is the zone of emergence for ventral roots

Questions 14–16

Match each characteristic below with the spinal cord area it best describes.

(A) Cervical cord
(B) Upper thoracic cord
(C) Lumbar cord
(D) Lower thoracic cord
(E) Coccygeal cord
(F) Sacral cord

14. Contains preganglionic parasympathetic neurons

15. Contains massive ventral horns and dorsal intermediate sulcus

16. Has a ciliospinal center of Budge

Answers and Explanations

1–E. The substantia gelatinosa is greatly enlarged at sacral levels. It is a sensory nucleus found at all cord levels, mediates pain and temperature, and is homologous to the spinal trigeminal nucleus.

2–E. The dorsal root ganglion contains large (proprioception) and small (pain and temperature) pseudounipolar neurons of neural crest origin and lies within the intervertebral foramen. It usually is absent in the first cervical nerve and in the coccygeal nerve.

3–B. The lateral horn extends from (C8) T1 to L3. The phrenic nucleus extends from C3 to C6. The nucleus dorsalis of Clarke is coextensive with the lateral horn and its intermediolateral nucleus or cell column. Rexed lamina VII (lamina intermedia) includes the sympathetic intermediolateral nucleus, the parasympathetic sacral nucleus (S2–S4), and the nucleus dorsalis of Clarke.

4–D. In the newborn, the spinal cord ends at the level of the third lumbar vertebra (VS3). In the adult, the spinal cord ends at the level of the interspace between the first and second lumbar vertebrae (VL1–VL2). In the adult, the dural cul-de-sac ends at the level of the second sacral vertebra (VS2).

5–D. White communicating rami are found only at thoracolumbar levels of the spinal cord (T1–L3); they contain myelinated preganglionic sympathetic fibers and myelinated GVA fibers (from splanchnic nerves). Gray communicating rami contain unmyelinated postganglionic sympathetic fibers and contribute to all spinal nerves. The first cervical nerve and the coccygeal nerve usually have no dorsal (sensory) roots.

6–D. The cauda equina consists of lumbosacral nerve roots that descend below the level of the conus medullaris, within the subarachnoid space, to exit through their respective intervertebral or sacral foramina. Dorsal roots contain sensory fibers; ventral roots contain motor fibers. The cauda equina syndrome affects the lumbosacral nerve roots, producing both sensory and motor symptoms.

7–C. The spinal parasympathetic nucleus extends over three sacral segments, S2 to S4.

8–E. The myotatic reflex is a monosynaptic and ipsilateral muscle stretch reflex (incorrectly called a deep tendon reflex). The afferent limb consists of a muscle spindle (receptor) and a Ia fiber (axon) of a dorsal root ganglion neuron; the efferent limb consists of the axon of a ventral horn alpha motor neuron and the innervated striated muscle fibers (effector). The quadriceps (patellar) and triceps surae (ankle) muscle stretch reflexes are examples of myotatic reflexes.

9–E. The ventral median fissure contains the sulcal branch of ventral (anterior) spinal artery.

10–D. The dorsal lateral sulcus receives the dorsal roots.

11–A. The dorsal intermediate septum extends from C1 to T6. It is diagnostic for cervical and upper thoracic cord segments.

12–A. The dorsal intermediate septum separates the fasciculus gracilis from the fasciculus cuneatus. It is diagnostic of the cervical and upper thoracic cord.

13–B. The ventral lateral sulcus is the zone of emergence for the ventral roots.

14–F. The sacral cord contains the sacral parasympathetic nucleus (S2–S4); this gives rise to preganglionic fibers that synapse in the intramural ganglia of the pelvic viscera.

15–A. The cervical cord contains massive ventral horns, which give rise to the brachial plexus (C5–C8). The dorsal intermediate sulcus and septum are also diagnostic of cervical cord levels.

16–B. The ciliospinal center of Budge is found in the lateral horn at T1. This sympathetic nucleus innervates the radial muscle of the iris (dilatator pupillae) and the nonstriated superior and inferior tarsal (Müller) muscles.

7

Tracts of the Spinal Cord

I. Introduction—Tracts of the Spinal Cord

—consist of fiber bundles that have a common origin and a common termination.

—are somatotopically organized.

—are divided into **ascending and descending pathways**.

II. Ascending Spinal Tracts

—represent functional pathways that convey sensory information from soma or viscera to higher levels of the neuraxis.

—usually consist of a chain of three neurons: first-, second-, and third-order neurons. The first-order neuron is always in the dorsal root ganglion.

—usually decussate before reaching their final destination.

—give rise to collateral branches that serve in local spinal reflex arcs.

—include six major tracts:

A. Dorsal column–medial lemniscus pathway (Figure 7.1)

—mediates tactile discrimination, vibration, form recognition, and joint and muscle sensation.

—mediates conscious proprioception.

—receives input from Pacini's and Meissner's corpuscles, joint receptors, muscle spindles, and Golgi tendon organs.

1. First-order neurons

—are located in dorsal root ganglia at all levels.

—give rise to the **fasciculus gracilis** from the lower extremity.

—give rise to the **fasciculus cuneatus** from the upper extremity.

—give rise to axons that ascend in the dorsal columns and terminate in the gracile and cuneate nuclei of the medulla.

2. Second-order neurons

—are located in the gracile and cuneate nuclei of the caudal medulla.

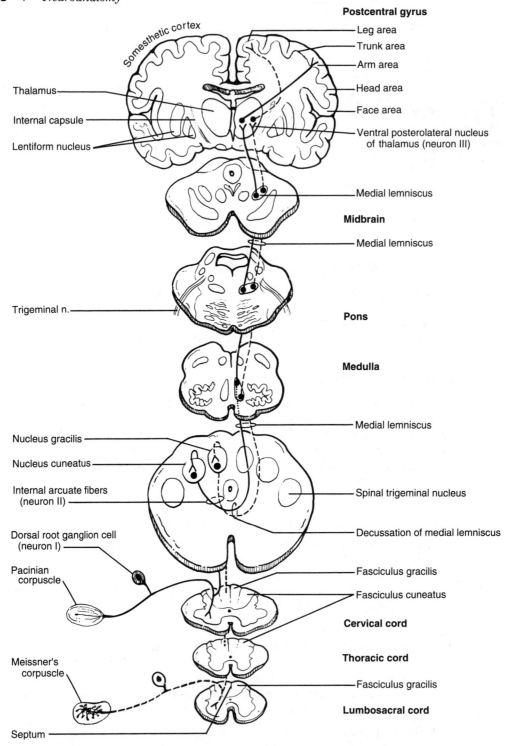

Figure 7.1. Schematic diagram of the dorsal column–medial lemniscus pathway. Impulses conducted by this pathway mediate discriminatory tactile sense (touch, vibration, and pressure) and kinesthetic sense (position and movement). The dorsal column system mediates conscious proprioception. (Adapted with permission from Carpenter MB and Sutin J: *Human Neuroanatomy*. Baltimore, Williams & Wilkins, 1983, p 266.)

−give rise to axons, **internal arcuate fibers** that decussate and form a compact fiber bundle, the **medial lemniscus**. The medial lemniscus ascends through the contralateral brainstem to terminate in the ventral posterolateral (**VPL**) nucleus of the thalamus.

3. Third-order neurons

−are located in the VPL nucleus of the thalamus.

−project via the posterior limb of the internal capsule to the postcentral gyrus, the **somatesthetic cortex** (areas 3, 1, and 2).

B. Ventral spinothalamic tract*

−is concerned with **light touch,** the sensation produced by stroking glabrous skin with a wisp of cotton.

−receives input from free nerve endings and from Merkel's tactile disks.

1. First-order neurons

−are found in dorsal root ganglia at all levels.

−project axons into the medial root entry zone to second-order neurons in the dorsal horn.

2. Second-order neurons

−are located in the **dorsal horn**.

−give rise to axons that decussate in the ventral white commissure and ascend in the contralateral ventral funiculus.

−terminate in the VPL nucleus of the thalamus.

3. Third-order neurons

−are found in the **VPL nucleus** of the thalamus.

−project via the posterior limb of the internal capsule and corona radiata to the postcentral gyrus (areas 3, 1, and 2).

C. Lateral spinothalamic tract (Figure 7.2)

−mediates pain and temperature sensation.

−receives input from free nerve endings and thermal receptors.

−receives input from A-δ and C fibers (i.e., fast- and slow-conducting pain fibers, respectively).

−is somatotopically organized with sacral fibers dorsolaterally and cervical fibers ventromedially.

1. First-order neurons

−are found in dorsal root ganglia at all levels.

−project axons via the **dorsolateral tract of Lissauer** to second-order neurons in the dorsal horn.

−synapse with second-order neurons in the dorsal horn.

2. Second-order neurons

−are found in the dorsal horn.

−give rise to axons that decussate in the **ventral white commissure** and ascend in the ventral half of the lateral funiculus.

−project collaterals to the reticular formation.

---

*Some authors refer to the spinothalamic tracts as the anterolateral system.

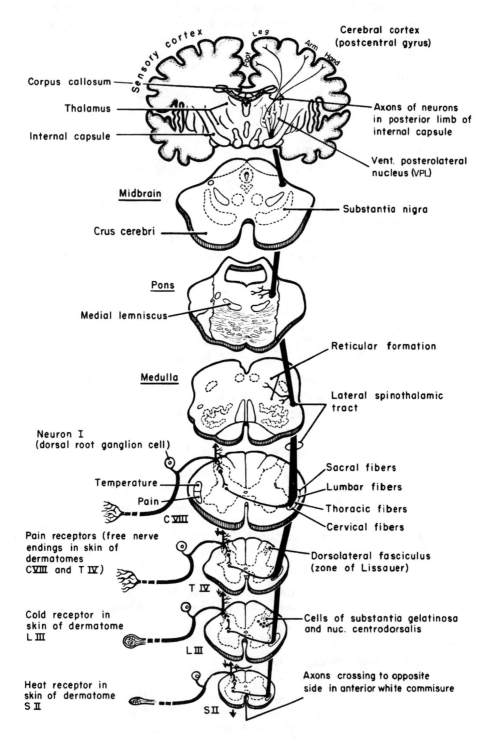

Figure 7.2. Schematic diagram of the lateral spinothalamic tract. Impulses conducted by this tract mediate pain and thermal sense. Numerous collaterals are distributed to the brainstem reticular formation. (Reprinted with permission from Carpenter MB and Sutin J: *Human Neuroanatomy.* Baltimore, Williams & Wilkins, 1983, p 274.)

−terminate contralaterally in the VPL nucleus and bilaterally in the intralaminar nuclei of the thalamus.

3. Third-order neurons

−are found in the VPL nucleus and in the intralaminar nuclei.

a. VPL neurons

−project via the posterior limb of the internal capsule to the somatesthetic cortex of the postcentral gyrus (areas 3, 1, and 2).

b. Intralaminar neurons

−project to the caudatoputamen and to the frontal and parietal cortex.

D. Dorsal spinocerebellar tract (Figure 7.3)

−transmits unconscious proprioceptive information to the cerebellum.
−receives input from muscle spindles, Golgi tendon organs, and pressure receptors.
−is involved in fine coordination of posture and the movement of individual muscles of the lower extremity.
−is an uncrossed tract.

1. First-order neurons

−are found in dorsal root ganglia from C8 to S3.
−provide the afferent limb for muscle stretch reflexes (e.g., the patellar reflex).
−project via the medial root entry zone to synapse in the **nucleus dorsalis of Clarke**.

2. Second-order neurons

−are found in the nucleus dorsalis of Clarke (C8 to L3).
−give rise to axons that ascend in the lateral funiculus and reach the cerebellum via the inferior cerebellar peduncle.
−contain axons that terminate ipsilaterally as mossy fibers in the cortex of the rostral and caudal cerebellar vermis.

E. Ventral spinocerebellar tract (see Figure 7.3)

−transmits unconscious proprioceptive information to the cerebellum.
−is concerned with coordinated movement and posture of the entire lower extremity.
−receives input from muscle spindles, Golgi tendon organs, and pressure receptors.
−is a crossed tract.

1. First-order neurons

−are found in the dorsal root ganglia from L1 to S2.
−provide the afferent limb for muscle stretch reflexes (e.g., the patellar reflex).
−synapse on **spinal border cells**.

2. Second-order neurons

−are spinal border cells found in the ventral horns (L1–S2).
−give rise to axons that decussate in the ventral white commissure and ascend lateral to the lateral spinothalamic tract in the lateral funiculus.

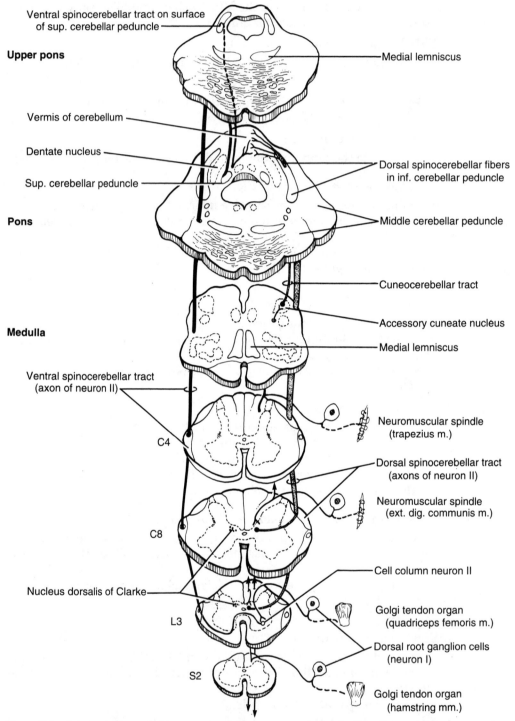

Figure 7.3. Schematic diagram of the ventral and dorsal spinocerebellar tracts and the cuneocerebellar tract. Impulses conducted by these tracts arise from the muscle spindles and the Golgi tendon organs and are conveyed to the spinocerebellum. These tracts mediate unconscious proprioception. Their first-order neurons mediate the myotatic reflexes. (Adapted with permission from Carpenter MB and Sutin J: *Human Neuroanatomy*. Baltimore, Williams & Wilkins, 1983, p 277.)

−give rise to axons that enter the cerebellum via the **superior cerebellar peduncle** and terminate contralaterally as mossy fibers in the cortex of the rostral cerebellar vermis.

F. **Cuneocerebellar tract** (see Figure 7.3)

−is the upper extremity equivalent of the dorsal spinocerebellar tract.

1. **First-order neurons**

−are found in the dorsal root ganglia from C2 to T7.
−project their axons via the fasciculus cuneatus to the caudal medulla, where they synapse in the **accessory cuneate nucleus,** a homolog of the nucleus dorsalis of Clarke.

2. **Second-order neurons**

−are located in the accessory cuneate nucleus of the medulla.
−give rise to axons that project to the cerebellum via the **inferior cerebellar peduncle**. These axons terminate ipsilaterally in the arm region of the anterior lobe of the cerebellum.

III. Descending Spinal Tracts (Figures 7.4 and 7.5)

−are concerned with somatic and visceral motor activities.
−have their cells of origin in the cerebral cortex or in the brainstem.

A. **Lateral corticospinal (pyramidal) tract** (see Figure 7.4)

−is not fully myelinated until the end of the second year.

1. **Function—the lateral corticospinal tract**

−is concerned with **voluntary skilled motor activity,** primarily of the limbs.
−modulates the transmission of sensory input via the ascending sensory pathways.
−receives input from the **paracentral lobule,** a medial continuation of the motor and sensory cortices, and subserves the muscles of the contralateral leg and foot.

2. **Origin and termination—the lateral corticospinal tract**

−arises from lamina V of the cerebral cortex from three cortical areas, in equal proportions: the **premotor cortex** (area 6); the **precentral motor cortex** (area 4); and the **postcentral sensory cortex** (areas 3, 1, and 2).
−terminates via interneurons on ventral horn motor neurons and sensory neurons of the dorsal horn.

3. **Course—the lateral corticospinal tract**

−passes through the posterior limb of the internal capsule.
−passes through the middle three-fifths of the **crus cerebri** (basis pedunculi) of the midbrain.
−passes through the base of the pons.
−constitutes the pyramid of the medulla.
−undergoes a 90% decussation in the caudal medulla.
−lies in the dorsal quadrant of the lateral funiculus of the spinal cord.

4. **Transection**

−results in **spastic hemiparesis** with Babinski's sign.

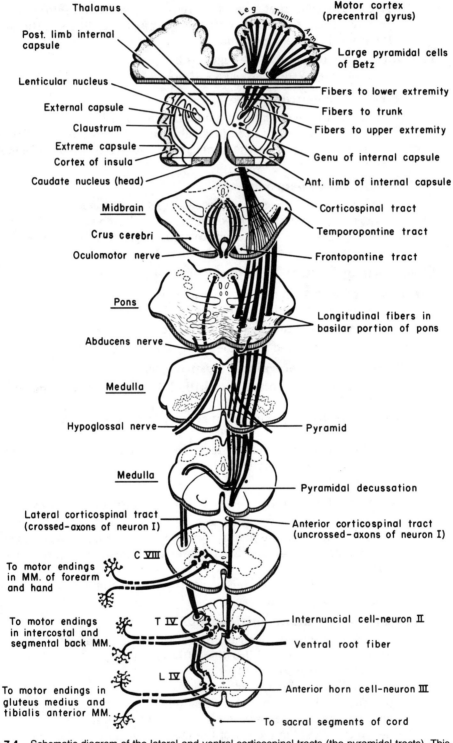

Figure 7.4. Schematic diagram of the lateral and ventral corticospinal tracts (the pyramidal tracts). This major descending motor pathway mediates willed volitional motor activity. The cells of origin are located in the premotor, the motor, and the sensory cortices. (Reprinted with permission from Carpenter MB and Sutin J: *Human Neuroanatomy.* Baltimore, Williams & Wilkins, 1983, p 285.)

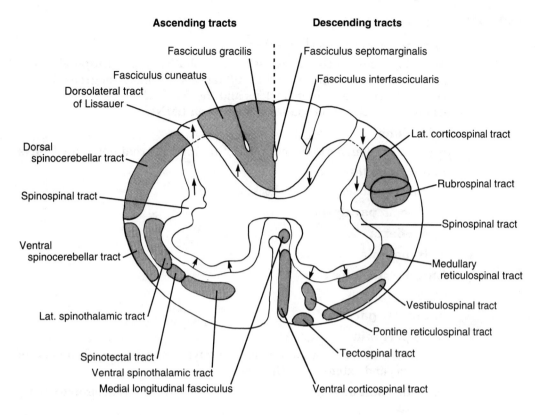

Ascending tracts

Descending tracts

Fasciculus gracilis

Fasciculus septomarginalis

Fasciculus cuneatus

Fasciculus interfascicularis

Dorsolateral tract of Lissauer

Dorsal spinocerebellar tract

Lat. corticospinal tract

Spinospinal tract

Rubrospinal tract

Ventral spinocerebellar tract

Spinospinal tract

Lat. spinothalamic tract

Medullary reticulospinal tract

Spinotectal tract

Vestibulospinal tract

Ventral spinothalamic tract

Pontine reticulospinal tract

Medial longitudinal fasciculus

Tectospinal tract

Ventral corticospinal tract

Figure 7.5. Schematic diagram of the major ascending and descending pathways of the spinal cord. The spinospinal system surrounds the spinal gray. Ascending tracts are shown on the left; descending tracts are shown on the right. (Adapted with permission from Carpenter MB: *Core Text of Neuroanatomy,* 3rd ed. Baltimore, Williams & Wilkins, 1985, p 97.)

B. Ventral corticospinal tract (see Figure 7.4)

—is a small uncrossed tract that decussates at spinal cord levels in the ventral white commissure.

—is concerned with the control of axial muscles.

C. Rubrospinal tract (see Figure 7.5)

—arises in the contralateral red nucleus of the midbrain.

—plays a role in the control of flexor tone.

—is located ventral to the lateral corticospinal tract.

D. Vestibulospinal tract (see Figure 7.5)

—arises in the ipsilateral lateral vestibular nucleus.

—plays a role in the control of extensor tone.

—is located in the ventral funiculus.

E. Descending autonomic tracts

—project to sympathetic (T1–L3) and parasympathetic (S2–S4) centers in the spinal cord.

—innervate the ciliospinal center (T1–T2).

—interruption of this tract (found in the dorsal quadrant of the lateral funiculus) results in **Horner's syndrome**.

VI. Clinical Correlations

A. Upper motor neurons (UMNs)

–are cortical neurons that give rise to corticobulbar or corticospinal tracts.

–are found in brainstem nuclei that influence lower motor neurons (LMNs) [e.g., the lateral vestibular nucleus and the red nucleus].

–terminate directly on or via interneurons on LMNs.

B. UMN lesions

–are caused by damage to the neurons (or their axons) that innervate UMNs.

1. Acute stage lesions

–result in transient spinal shock, including:

a. Flaccid paralysis

b. Areflexia

c. Hypotonia

2. Chronic stage lesions

–result in:

a. Spastic paresis

b. Hypertonia

–occurs with increased tone in antigravity muscles (i.e., flexors of the arms and extensors of the legs).

c. Reduction or loss of superficial abdominal and cremasteric reflexes

d. Extensor toe response (Babinski's sign)

e. Clonus

–is a repetitive, sustained stretch reflex (e.g., ankle clonus).

C. LMNs

–are neurons that directly innervate skeletal muscles.

–are found in the ventral horns of the spinal cord.

–are found in the motor nuclei of cranial nerves III–VII and IX–XII.

D. LMN lesions

–result from damage to motor neurons or their peripheral axons.

–result in:

1. Flaccid paralysis with muscle atrophy

2. Areflexia

3. Muscle atrophy

4. Fasciculations and fibrillations

Review Test

Directions: Each of the numbered items or incomplete statements in this section is followed by answers or by completions of the statement. Select the **one** lettered answer or completion that is **best** in each case.

1. All of the following statements concerning the dorsal spinocerebellar tract are correct EXCEPT

(A) it is an uncrossed tract.
(B) it enters the cerebellum via the superior cerebellar peduncle.
(C) it subserves unconscious proprioception.
(D) it terminates in the cerebellar vermis.
(E) it receives input from muscle spindles and Golgi tendon organs.

2. All of the following statements concerning the corticospinal tracts are correct EXCEPT

(A) they arise from lamina V of the cerebral cortex.
(B) they arise from UMNs.
(C) they descend through the anterior limb of the internal capsule.
(D) they undergo a 90% decussation in the caudal medulla.
(E) they descend through the base of the pons.

3. The ability to recognize an unseen familiar object placed in the hand depends on the integrity of which pathway?

(A) Spinospinal tract
(B) Dorsal columns
(C) Dorsal spinocerebellar tract
(D) Spino-olivary tract
(E) Spinothalamic tract

4. Which statement concerning the rubrospinal tract is false?

(A) It lies ventral to the lateral corticospinal tract in the spinal cord.
(B) It arises from the red nucleus of the midbrain.
(C) It is an UMN tract.
(D) It is a crossed tract.
(E) It plays a role in the control of extensor tone.

5. Destruction of the ventral horn results in all of the following deficits EXCEPT

(A) loss of muscle stretch reflexes.
(B) loss of muscle bulk.
(C) flaccid paralysis.
(D) Babinski's sign.
(E) loss of superficial abdominal reflexes.

6. All of the following tracts decussate in the ventral white commissure EXCEPT the

(A) lateral spinothalamic tract.
(B) ventral spinocerebellar tract.
(C) ventral corticospinal tract.
(D) dorsal spinocerebellar tract.
(E) ventral spinothalamic tract.

7. The corticospinal tracts receive contributions from all of the following areas EXCEPT the

(A) prefrontal cortex.
(B) premotor cortex.
(C) motor cortex.
(D) somatesthetic cortex.
(E) paracentral lobule.

8. All of the following statements concerning the lateral spinothalamic tract are correct EXCEPT

(A) it projects collaterals to the reticular formation.
(B) it projects to intralaminar nuclei of the thalamus.
(C) it projects to the ventral posteromedial (VPM) nucleus of the thalamus.
(D) it mediates pain and temperature.
(E) its cells of origin are in the dorsal horn.

9. All of the following statements concerning the dorsal column–medial lemniscus pathway are correct EXCEPT

(A) it has second-order neurons in the medulla.
(B) it receives input from Pacini's and Meissner's corpuscles.
(C) it decussates in the spinal cord.
(D) it mediates kinesthetic sensation.
(E) it mediates vibration sensation.

Directions: Each group of items in this section consists of lettered options followed by a set of numbered items. For each item, select the **one** lettered option that is most closely associated with it. Each lettered option may be selected once, more than once, or not at all.

Questions 10–14

Match each characteristic below with the nuclear structure it best describes.

(A) Nucleus gracilis
(B) Spinal accessory nucleus
(C) Intermediolateral nucleus
(D) Accessory cuneate nucleus
(E) Thalamic intralaminar nuclei

10. Contains LMNs

11. Subserves unconscious proprioception

12. Gives rise to internal arcuate fibers

13. Contains visceromotor neurons

14. Receives nociceptive input

Questions 15–22

Match each description of a spinal cord tract with the appropriate lettered structure shown in the illustration.

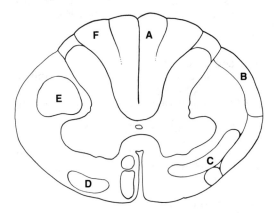

15. Projects to the cerebellum via the inferior cerebellar peduncle

16. Mediates pain and temperature sensation

17. Cells of origin are found in the precentral gyrus

18. Mediates two-point tactile discrimination from the hand

19. Myelination not fully achieved until the end of the second year

20. Transection results in spasticity

21. Plays a role in regulating extensor tone

22. Transmits vibration sensation from the ankle

Answers and Explanations

1–B. The uncrossed dorsal spinocerebellar tract enters the cerebellum via the inferior cerebellar peduncle and terminates in the cerebellar vermis. It receives input from muscle spindles and Golgi tendon organs and subserves unconscious proprioception.

2–C. The corticospinal tracts arise from UMNs found in lamina V of the cerebral cortex. They descend through the posterior limb of the internal capsule, the middle third of the crus cerebri (basis pedunculi) of the midbrain, and the base of the pons and constitute the medullary pyramids. Ninety percent of the corticospinal fibers decussate in the caudal medulla as the pyramidal decussation.

3–B. The ability to recognize the form and texture of an unseen familiar object is called stereognosis. This is an important function of the dorsal column–medial lemniscus system.

4–E. The rubrospinal tract, an UMN tract, originates in the red nucleus of the midbrain, crosses in the ventral tegmental decussation of the midbrain, traverses the tegmentum of the pons and medulla, and terminates in the ventral horn of the spinal cord. In the spinal cord, the tract lies in the lateral funiculus ventral to the lateral corticospinal tract. It plays a role in regulating flexor tone.

5–D. Destruction of ventral horn motor neurons results in a LMN lesion and is characterized by flaccid paralysis, muscle atrophy (loss of muscle bulk), and areflexia (loss of muscle stretch and superficial abdominal reflexes). Babinski's sign is not seen in LMN disease.

6–D. The dorsal spinocerebellar tract is an uncrossed tract.

7–A. The corticospinal (pyramidal) tracts receive contributions from the premotor (area 6), motor (area 4), and the sensory or somatesthetic (areas 3, 1, and 2) cortices. They receive approximately one-third of their axons from each of these cortical areas. The paracentral lobule represents a continuation of the motor and somatesthetic cortices onto the medial aspect of the hemisphere. The prefrontal cortex lies rostral to the premotor cortex.

8–C. The lateral spinothalamic tract mediates pain and temperature sensation and projects to the reticular formation of the brainstem and to the VPL and intralaminar nuclei of the thalamus. First-order neurons are in the dorsal root ganglion, second-order neurons (cells of origin) are in the dorsal horn, and third-order neurons lie in the VPL nucleus of the thalamus.

9–C. The uncrossed dorsal columns consist of the fasciculus gracilis and the fasciculus cuneatus and mediate tactile discrimination, form recognition, vibration, movement, and joint and muscle sensation (proprioception). They receive input from tactile receptors (Pacini's and Meissner's corpuscles), muscle spindles, joint receptors, and Golgi tendon organs. The dorsal column–medial lemniscus pathway decussates in the caudal medulla (decussation of the medial lemniscus). First-order neurons are in the dorsal root ganglion; second-order neurons are in the gracile and cuneate nuclei of the medulla; and third-order neurons are in the VPL nucleus of the thalamus.

10–B. The spinal accessory nucleus is found within the ventral horn and extends from C1 to C6. It contains LMNs that give rise to the spinal root of the spinal accessory nerve (CN IX). The spinal division of this nerve innervates the sternocleidomastoid muscle and the upper parts of the trapezius muscle.

11–D. The accessory cuneate nucleus is a homolog of the nucleus dorsalis of Clarke. Located in the caudal medulla, it gives rise to the uncrossed cuneocerebellar tract and mediates unconscious proprioception to the cerebellum.

12–A. The nucleus gracilis, located in the caudal "closed medulla," receives proprioceptive and tactile input from the fasciculus gracilis and gives rise to the decussating internal arcuate fibers, which ascend to the thalamus as the medial lemniscus.

13–C. The intermediolateral nucleus is found in the lateral horn and extends from C8 to L3. It contains visceromotor neurons that give rise to preganglionic sympathetic fibers (general visceral efferent fibers).

14–E. The intralaminar nuclei of the thalamus receive nociceptive (pain) input from the spinothalamic and the spinoreticulothalamic tracts.

15–B. The dorsal spinocerebellar tract projects unconscious proprioceptive information (muscle spindles and Golgi tendon organs) to the cerebellum via the inferior cerebellar peduncle.

16–C. The lateral spinothalamic tract lies between the ventral spinocerebellar tract and the ventral horn. It mediates pain and temperature sensation.

17–E. The lateral corticospinal tract has its cells of origin in the premotor, motor, and sensory cortices. The precentral gyrus and the anterior paracentral lobule are motor cortex and contain the motor homunculus; it gives rise to one-third of the fibers of the corticospinal (pyramidal) tract.

18–F. The fasciculus cuneatus mediates two-point tactile discrimination from the hand.

19–E. The corticospinal (pyramidal) tracts are not fully myelinated until the end of the second year. For this reason, Babinski's sign may be elicited in young children.

20–E. Transection of the lateral corticospinal tract results in spastic paresis (exaggerated muscle stretch reflexes and clonus).

21–D. The vestibulospinal (lateral) tract, found ventral to the ventral horn, plays a role in regulating extensor tone.

22–A. The fasciculus gracilis transmits vibratory sensation (pallesthesia) from the lower extremities.

8

Lesions of the Spinal Cord

I. Overview—Pathways and Lesions of the Spinal Cord

–are shown in Figure 8.1. Clinically important pathways are shown on the left side; clinical deficits are shown on the right side.

–spinal cord lesions affecting these pathways may be classified according to the area of origin or the area affected.

A. Lower motor neuron (LMN) lesions

B. Upper motor neuron (UMN) lesions

C. Sensory pathway lesions

D. Peripheral nervous system lesions

E. Combined upper and lower motor neuron lesions

F. Combined motor and sensory lesions

G. Herniations of the intervertebral disk

II. Lower Motor Neuron Lesions (Figure 8.2A)

–result from damage to motor neurons of the ventral horns or motor neurons of the cranial nerve nuclei.

–result from interruption of the final common pathway connecting the neuron via its axon with the muscle fibers it innervates (the motor unit).

A. Neurologic deficits resulting from LMN lesions

1. Flaccid paralysis

2. Muscle atrophy (amyotrophy)

3. Hypotonia

4. Areflexia

–consists of loss of muscle stretch reflexes (knee and ankle jerks) and loss of superficial reflexes (abdominal and cremasteric reflexes).

5. Fasciculations (visible muscle twitches)

6. Fibrillations (seen only on an electromyogram [EMG])

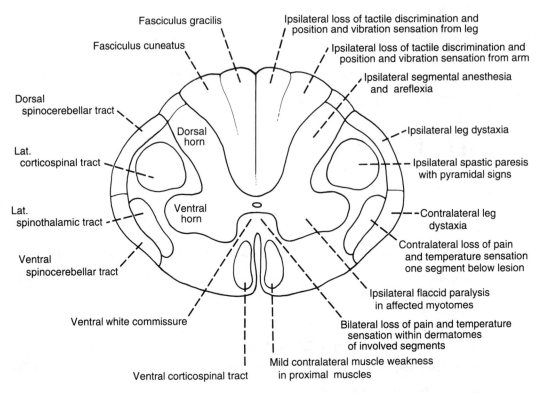

Figure 8.1. Transverse section of the cervical spinal cord showing, on the left side, the clinically important ascending and descending pathways. Clinical deficits resulting from the interruption of these pathways are shown on the right side. Destructive lesions of the dorsal horns result in anesthesia and areflexia; destructive lesions of the ventral horns result in lower motor neuron lesions and areflexia. Destruction of the ventral white commissure interrupts the central transmission of pain and temperature impulses bilaterally via the lateral spinothalamic tracts.

B. Diseases of LMNs (see Figure 8.2*A*)

1. Poliomyelitis

– is an acute inflammatory viral infection affecting the LMNs and is caused by an enterovirus.

– results in a flaccid paralysis.

2. Progressive infantile muscular atrophy

– is known as **Werdnig-Hoffmann disease**.

– is a heredofamilial degenerative disease of infants that affects LMNs.

III. Upper Motor Neuron Lesions

– result from damage to cortical neurons that give rise to corticospinal and corticobulbar tracts.

– are lesions of the corticospinal and corticobulbar tracts called **pyramidal tract lesions**.

– may occur at all levels of the neuraxis from the cerebral cortex to the spinal cord.

– when rostral to the pyramidal decussation of the caudal medulla, they result in deficits below the lesion and on the contralateral side.

– when caudal to the pyramidal decussation, they result in deficits below the lesion and on the ipsilateral side.

A. Lateral corticospinal tract lesion (see Figure 8.2*B*)

−results in the following ipsilateral motor deficits found below the lesion:

1. Spastic hemiparesis with muscle weakness

2. Hyperreflexia (exaggerated muscle stretch reflexes)

3. Clasp-knife spasticity

−when a joint is moved briskly, resistance is felt initially and then fades (like the opening of a pocketknife blade).

4. Loss of superficial (abdominal and cremasteric) reflexes

5. Clonus

−consists of rhythmic contractions of muscles in response to sudden, passive movements (wrist, patellar, or ankle clonus).

6. Babinski's sign

−consists of plantar reflex response that is extensor (dorsiflexion of big toe).

B. Ventral corticospinal tract lesion

−results in **mild contralateral motor deficit**. Ventral corticospinal tract fibers decussate at spinal levels in the ventral white commissure.

C. Hereditary spastic paraplegia or diplegia (see Figure 8.2*B*)

−is caused by bilateral degeneration of the corticospinal tracts.

−results in gradual development of **spastic weakness of the legs** with increased difficulty in walking.

IV. Sensory Pathway Lesions

A. Dorsal columns syndrome (see Figure 8.2*C*)

−includes the fasciculi gracilis (T6–S5) and cuneatus (C2–T6) and the dorsal roots.

−is seen in subacute combined degeneration (vitamin B_{12} neuropathy).

−is seen in neurosyphilis as **tabes dorsalis** and in nonsyphilitic sensory neuropathies.

−results in the following **ipsilateral sensory deficits** found below the lesion:

1. Loss of tactile discrimination

2. Loss of position (joint) and vibratory sensation

3. Stereoanesthesia (astereognosis)

4. Sensory (dorsal column) dystaxia

5. Paresthesias and pain (dorsal root irritation)

6. Hyporeflexia or areflexia (dorsal root deafferentation)

7. Urinary incontinence, constipation, and impotence (dorsal root deafferentation)

8. Romberg's sign (sensory dystaxia) [standing patient is more unsteady with eyes closed]

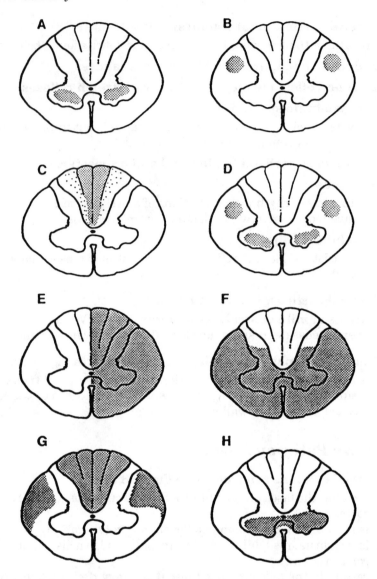

Figure 8.2. Lesions of the spinal cord: (*A*) poliomyelitis and progressive infantile muscular atrophy (Werdnig-Hoffman disease); (*B*) hereditary spastic paraplegia or diplegia; (*C*) dorsal column disease (*tabes dorsalis*); (*D*) amyotrophic lateral sclerosis (ALS); (*E*) hemisection of the spinal cord (Brown-Séquard syndrome); (*F*) complete ventral spinal artery occlusion of the spinal cord; (*G*) subacute combined degeneration (vitamin B$_{12}$ neuropathy); and (*H*) syringomyelia.

B. Lateral spinothalamic tract lesion

  –results in contralateral loss of pain and temperature sensation one segment below the level of the lesion.

C. Ventral spinothalamic tract lesion

  –results in contralateral loss of light (crude) touch sensation three or four segments below the level of the lesion.

  –does not appreciably reduce touch sensation if the dorsal columns are intact.

D. Dorsal spinocerebellar tract lesion

 —results in ipsilateral leg dystaxia; patient has difficulty performing the heel-to-shin test.

E. Ventral spinocerebellar tract lesion

 —results in contralateral leg dystaxia; patient has difficulty performing the heel-to-shin test.

V. Peripheral Nervous System (PNS) Lesions

 —may be sensory, motor, or combined.
 —affect spinal roots, dorsal root ganglia, and peripheral nerves.

A. Herpes zoster (shingles)

 —is a common **viral infection** of the nervous system.
 —consists of an acute inflammatory reaction in the dorsal root or cranial nerve ganglia.
 —is usually limited to the territory of one dermatome; the most common sites are **T5–T10**.
 —causes irritation of dorsal root ganglion cells, resulting in pain, itching, and burning sensations in the involved dermatomes.
 —produces the characteristic vesicular eruption in the affected dermatome.

B. Acute idiopathic polyneuritis (Guillain-Barré syndrome)

 —is also called **postinfectious polyneuritis**.
 —usually follows an infectious illness.
 —results from a cell-mediated–immunologic reaction directed at peripheral nerves.
 —affects primarily motor fibers and causes segmental demyelination and wallerian degeneration.
 —produces **LMN symptoms** (muscle weakness, flaccid paralysis, and areflexia).
 —results in symmetric paralysis that begins in the lower extremities and ascends to involve the trunk and upper extremities; the facial nerve frequently is involved bilaterally.

VI. Combined Upper and Lower Motor Neuron Lesions

A. Characteristics

 —are muscle weakness and wasting without sensory deficits.

B. Prototypic disease—amyotrophic lateral sclerosis (see Figure 8.2*D*)

 —is also called **Lou Gehrig's disease,** motor neuron disease, or motor system disease; it often is referred to as **ALS**.
 —usually occurs in persons 50 to 70 years of age.
 —affects twice as many men as women.
 —involves both LMNs and UMNs; either component may dominate the clinical picture.
 —progressive (spinal) muscular atrophy or progressive bulbar palsy refers to a LMN component.
 —pseudobulbar palsy or primary lateral sclerosis refers to an UMN component.

VII. Combined Motor and Sensory Lesions

A. Spinal cord hemisection (Brown-Séquard syndrome) [see Figures 8.1 and 8.2E)

1. Dorsal column transection

–results in ipsilateral loss of tactile discrimination, form perception, and position and vibration sensation below the lesion.

2. Lateral spinothalamic tract transection

–results in contralateral loss of pain and temperature sensation, starting one segment below the lesion.

3. Ventral spinothalamic tract transection

–results in contralateral loss of crude touch sensation starting three or four segments below the lesion.

4. Dorsal spinocerebellar tract transection

–results in ipsilateral leg dystaxia.

5. Ventral spinocerebellar tract transection

–results in contralateral leg dystaxia.

6. Hypothalamospinal tract transection rostral to T2

–results in **Horner's syndrome**.

7. Lateral corticospinal tract transection

–results in ipsilateral spastic paresis below the UMN lesion with Babinski's sign.

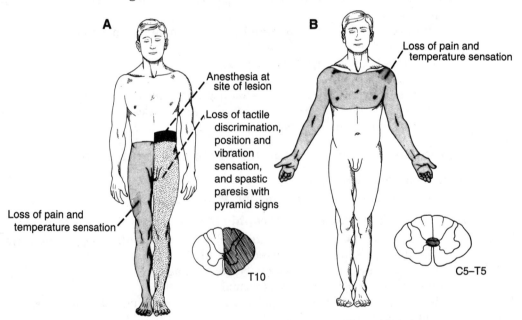

Figure 8.3. (*A*) Brown-Séquard syndrome, resulting from spinal cord hemisection at T10. Patient also would have hyperreflexia of the muscle stretch reflexes and Babinski's sign (extensor toe sign) on the side of the lesion. Note also the dissociated sensory loss (ipsilateral loss of tactile discrimination and vibration sensation) and contralateral loss of pain and temperature sensation. (*B*) Syringomyelia. Central cavitation of the spinal cord interrupts the decussating spinothalamic tracts and results in a bilateral loss of pain and temperature sensation. Note the cape-like sensory loss.

8. Ventral corticospinal tract transection

−results in minor contralateral muscle weakness below the lesion.

9. Ventral horn destruction

−results in ipsilateral flaccid paralysis of somitic muscles (LMN lesion).

10. Dorsal horn destruction

−results in ipsilateral dermatomic anesthesia and areflexia.

B. Complete transection of the spinal cord

−results in the following conditions:

1. Exitus lethalis between C1 and C3

2. Quadriplegia between C4 and C5

3. Paraplegia below T1

4. Spastic paralysis of all voluntary movements below the lesion

5. Complete anesthesia below the lesion

6. Urinary and fecal incontinence, although reflex emptying may occur

7. Anhidrosis and loss of vasomotor tone

8. Paralysis of volitional and automatic breathing if the transection is above C5 (the phrenic nucleus is found at C3–C5)

C. Ventral (anterior) spinal artery occlusion (see Figure 8.2*F*)

−causes infarction of the ventral two-thirds of the spinal cord.

−usually spares the dorsal columns and dorsal horns.

−results in paralysis of voluntary and automatic respiration in cervical segments; it also results in bilateral Horner's syndrome.

−results in loss of voluntary bladder and bowel control, with preservation of reflex emptying.

−results in anhidrosis and loss of vasomotor tone.

1. Ventral horn destruction

−results in complete flaccid paralysis and areflexia at the level of the lesion.

2. Corticospinal tract transection

−results in a spastic paresis below the lesion.

3. Spinothalamic tract transection

−results in loss of pain and temperature sensations starting one segment below the lesion.

4. Dorsal spinocerebellar tract and ventral spinocerebellar tract transection

−results in cerebellar incoordination, which is masked by LMN and UMN paralysis.

D. Conus medullaris and epiconus syndromes

−include neurologic deficits and signs that are most always bilateral.

1. Conus medullaris syndrome

−involves segments S3–Co.

–is usually caused by small intramedullary tumor metastases or hemorrhagic infarcts.

–results in destruction of the sacral parasympathetic nucleus, which
causes paralytic bladder, fecal incontinence, and impotence.

–causes perianogenital sensory loss in dermatomes S3–Co (saddle anesthesia).

–shows an absence of motor deficits in the lower limbs.

2. Epiconus syndrome

–includes segments L4–S2.

–results in reflex functioning of the bladder and rectum but loss of voluntary control.

–is characterized by considerable **motor disability** (external rotation
and extension of the thigh are most affected).

–affects the ventral horns and long tracts.

–is associated with absent Achilles tendon reflex.

E. Cauda equina syndrome

–classically involves spinal roots L3–Co.

–produces neurologic deficits similar to those seen in conus or epiconus lesions.

–results in signs that frequently predominate on one side.

–may result from intervertebral disk herniation.

–severe spontaneous radicular pain is common.

F. Filum terminale (tethered cord) syndrome

–results from a thickened and shortened filum terminale that adheres to the
sacrum and causes traction on the conus medullaris.

–results in sphincter dysfunction, gait disorders, and deformities of the feet.

G. Subacute combined degeneration (vitamin B_{12} neuropathy) [see Figure 8.2G]

–is a spinal cord disease associated with pernicious anemia.

–consists of demyelination of dorsal columns, resulting in loss of vibration
and position sensation.

–consists of demyelination of spinocerebellar tracts, resulting in arm and leg
dystaxia.

–consists of demyelination of corticospinal tracts resulting in spastic paresis
(UMN signs).

H. Syringomyelia (see Figures 8.2H and 8.3B)

–is a central cavitation of the cervical spinal cord of unknown etiology.

–results in destruction of the ventral white commissure and interruption of
decussating spinothalamic fibers, causing bilateral loss of pain and temperature sensation.

–can result in extension of the syrinx into the ventral horn, causing a LMN
lesion with muscle wasting and hyporeflexia. Atrophy of lumbricals and in-
terosseous muscles of the hand is a common finding.

–can result in extension of the syrinx into the lateral funiculus, affecting the
lateral corticospinal tract and resulting in spastic paresis (an UMN lesion).

–can result in caudal extension of the syrinx into the lateral horn at T1 or lateral extension into the lateral funiculus (interruption of descending autonomic pathways), resulting in Horner's syndrome.

VIII. Intervertebral Disk Herniation

–consists of prolapse or herniation of the **nucleus pulposus** through the defective **anulus fibrosus** into the vertebral canal. The nucleus pulposus impinges on spinal roots, resulting in root pain (radiculopathy) or muscle weakness.

–may compress the spinal cord with a large central protrusion (above VL1).

–is recognized as the major cause of severe and chronic low back and leg pain.

–appears in 90% of cases at the L4–L5 or L5–S1 interspaces; usually a single nerve root is compressed but several may be involved at the L5–S1 interspace (cauda equina).

–appears in 10% of cases in the cervical region, usually at the C5–C6 or C6–C7 interspaces.

–is characterized by **spinal root symptoms,** which include paresthesias, pain, sensory loss, hyporeflexia, and muscle weakness.

Review Test

Directions: Each of the numbered items or incomplete statements in this section is followed by answers or by completions of the statement. Select the **one** lettered answer or completion that is **best** in each case.

1. All of the following statements concerning amyotrophic lateral sclerosis (ALS) are correct EXCEPT

(A) it is associated with UMN lesions.
(B) it is associated with LMN lesions.
(C) it results in sensory deficits.
(D) its onset usually occurs between 50 to 70 years of age.
(E) it results in muscle weakness.

2. All of the following statements concerning syringomyelia are correct EXCEPT

(A) it is a central cavitation of the spinal cord.
(B) it usually is found at lumbosacral levels.
(C) it usually includes a LMN lesion.
(D) it usually results in a bilateral loss of pain and temperature sensation.
(E) it may result in Horner's syndrome.

3. All of the following statements concerning subacute combined degeneration are correct EXCEPT

(A) it causes demyelination of the dorsal columns.
(B) it causes demyelination of spinocerebellar tracts.
(C) it is associated with pernicious anemia.
(D) it is characterized by pyramidal tract signs.
(E) it is characterized by LMN symptoms.

4. Hemisection of the spinal cord at T1 on the left side results in all of the following signs or symptoms EXCEPT

(A) plantar response flexor on the left side.
(B) loss of vibration sensation in the left leg.
(C) leg dystaxia on the right side.
(D) exaggerated knee jerk reflex on the left side.
(E) normal pain and temperature sensation on the left side.

5. UMN lesions can be found in all of the following clinical syndromes EXCEPT

(A) amyotrophic lateral sclerosis (ALS).
(B) subacute combined degeneration.
(C) syringomyelia.
(D) cauda equina syndrome.
(E) ventral spinal artery occlusion.

6. LMN lesions result in all of the following deficits or signs EXCEPT

(A) loss of muscle stretch reflexes.
(B) loss of superficial reflexes.
(C) fasciculations.
(D) muscle wasting.
(E) plantar reflex extensor.

7. All of the following statements concerning poliomyelitis are correct EXCEPT

(A) it is a viral infection.
(B) it is a LMN disease.
(C) it affects dorsal root ganglion cells.
(D) it affects motor cranial nerve nuclei and ventral horn motor neurons.
(E) it results in hypertonia.

8. Which of the following statements concerning UMN lesions is false?

(A) They are found above the pyramidal decussation.
(B) They result in the presence of Babinski's sign.
(C) They result in the absence of the knee jerk reflex.
(D) They are commonly caused by cerebrovascular accidents.
(E) They frequently involve the internal capsule.

9. All of the following neurologic deficits are associated with transection of the lateral corticospinal tract EXCEPT

(A) it results in ipsilateral spastic paresis below the lesion.
(B) it results in ipsilateral loss of vibration sensation below the lesion.
(C) it results in an ipsilateral extensor plantar reflex.
(D) it results in an ipsilateral hyperreflexia below the lesion.
(E) it results in a loss of superficial abdominal and cremasteric reflexes.

10. All of the following statements concerning Horner's syndrome are correct EXCEPT

(A) it is seen in spinal cord lesions above T1.
(B) it is ipsilateral to the lesion.
(C) it results from interruption of descending autonomic pathways.
(D) it results in mydriasis and mild ptosis.
(E) it results in facial hemianhydrosis.

11. Ventral spinal artery occlusion results in all of the following deficits EXCEPT

(A) areflexia at the level of the lesion.
(B) loss of vibration and position sensation below the lesion.
(C) bilateral loss of pain and temperature sensation below the lesion.
(D) bilateral spastic paralysis below the lesion.
(E) urinary incontinence.

12. All of the following statements concerning cauda equina syndrome are correct EXCEPT

(A) its signs are frequently unilateral.
(B) it may result from a herniated disk.
(C) it classically involves spinal roots L3–Co.
(D) it may result in profound motor deficits.
(E) it may result in Babinski's sign.

13. Which of the following statements concerning conus medullaris syndrome is false?

(A) Plantar reflexes are usually extensor.
(B) It involves spinal segments S3–Co.
(C) It may result in perianogenital sensory loss.
(D) It may result in a paralytic bladder.
(E) It may result in impotence.

14. All of the following statements concerning intervertebral disk herniation are correct EXCEPT

(A) it results from prolapse of the nucleus pulposus through a defective anulus fibrosus into the vertebral canal.
(B) it may involve the cauda equina.
(C) it usually involves a single nerve root.
(D) it most frequently appears in the L4–L5 interspace.
(E) it usually results in urinary incontinence.

Questions 15–17

Neuropathologic examination of the spinal cord reveals two lesions labeled A and B on the illustration below. Lesion A is restricted to five segments. Answer the following questions relating to this case study by selecting the **one** best choice.

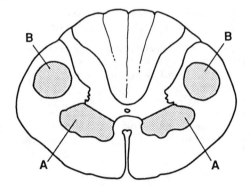

15. The result of lesion A is best described as

(A) bilateral arm dystaxia with dysdiadocho-kinesia.
(B) spastic paresis of the legs.
(C) flaccid paralysis of the upper extremities.
(D) loss of pain and temperature sensation below the lesion.
(E) urinary and fecal incontinence.

16. The result of lesion B is best described as

(A) dyssynergia of movements affecting both arms and legs.
(B) flaccid paralysis of the upper extremities.
(C) impaired two-point tactile discrimination in both arms.
(D) spastic paresis affecting primarily the muscles distal to the knee joint.
(E) none of the above.

17. Lesions A and B result from

(A) an intramedullary tumor.
(B) an extramedullary tumor.
(C) thrombosis of a spinal artery.
(D) multiple sclerosis.
(E) amyotrophic lateral sclerosis (ALS).

Directions: Each group of items in this section consists of lettered options followed by a set of numbered items. For each item, select the **one** lettered option that is most closely associated with it. Each lettered option may be selected once, more than once, or not at all.

Questions 18–23

A patient's spinal cord has been transected on the left side at T10. The extent of the motor and sensory deficits is indicated and labeled on the following illustration. Match each neurologic symptom described below with its territory of involvement.

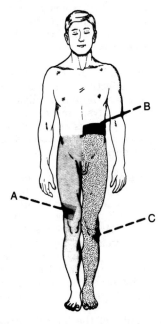

18. Loss of pain and temperature sensation

19. Loss of all sensory modalities

20. Loss of position sensation

21. Exaggerated muscle stretch reflexes

22. Loss of vibration sensation

23. Demonstrable muscle weakness

Questions 24–31

Match each statement below with the lesion that corresponds best to it.

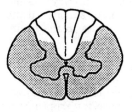
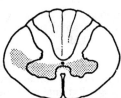

(A) Lesion limited to five segments

(B) Lesion limited to four segments

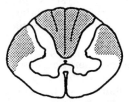
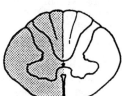

(C) Lesion extends the length of the spinal cord

(D) Lesion limited to one segment

24. Neurologic manifestation of vitamin B_{12} deficiency

25. Lesion due to vascular occlusion

26. Loss of vibration sensation on the right side; loss of pain and temperature sensation on the left side

27. Bilateral loss of pain and temperature sensation in the legs

28. Bilateral loss of pain and temperature sensation in the hands; muscle atrophy in both hands; spastic paresis on the right side only

29. Urinary incontinence and quadriplegia

30. No muscle atrophy or fasciculations

31. Demyelinating disease

Answers and Explanations

1–C. ALS is a motor system disease and does not involve sensory systems. Onset is usually after the age of 50 years. ALS affects the corticospinal and corticobulbar tracts (UMN lesion) and the ventral horn cells of the spinal cord and their cranial nerve equivalents in the brainstem (LMN lesion).

2–B. Syringomyelia is a central cavitation of the cervical spinal cord and is of unknown etiology. Expansion of the syrinx typically affects the ventral white commissure, interrupting the decussating fibers of the spinothalamic tracts and resulting in a bilateral loss of pain and temperature sensation at the level of involvement. Lateral extension involves one or both of the ventral horns and results in a LMN lesion with muscle wasting and flaccid paralysis. Caudal extension to (C8) T1–T2 may involve the lateral horn (ciliospinal center of Budge) and produce Horner's syndrome.

3–E. Subacute combined degeneration, associated with pernicious anemia, results in demyelination of the dorsal columns (the fasciculus gracilis more often than the fasciculus cuneatus), the spinocerebellar tracts, and the lateral corticospinal tracts. LMNs are not involved.

4–A. Hemisection of the spinal cord is known as Brown-Séquard syndrome. Transection of the left lateral corticospinal tract would result in an extensor plantar response on the left side (Babinski's sign). Leg dystaxia on the right side results from interruption of the crossed ventral spinocerebellar tract.

5–D. UMN lesions by definition are lesions in which the corticospinal or corticobulbar tracts have been damaged. ALS, subacute combined degeneration, syringomyelia (with extension into the lateral funiculus), and ventral spinal artery occlusion all cause UMN lesions with spastic paresis. The cauda equina lies external to the spinal cord; lesions of this structure do not cause UMN lesions.

6–E. LMN lesions result from destruction of ventral horn (or cranial nerve) motor neurons or transection of their axons. LMN lesions interrupt the final common pathway to skeletal muscles; they result in flaccid paralysis and atrophy (muscle wasting) and a loss of all reflex action (areflexia). Fasciculations (visible muscle twitching) and fibrillations (seen on an electromyogram) are signs of LMN disease. Babinski's sign, an extensor plantar reflex, is not seen in LMN lesions.

7–C. Poliomyelitis is an acute inflammatory viral infection affecting LMNs in the spinal cord and brainstem (bulbar paralysis) and results in flaccid paralysis, muscle atrophy, and areflexia. There is a loss of muscle tone (atonia). The poliovirus does not attack the sensory neurons of the dorsal root ganglia.

8–C. UMN lesions result from destruction of cortical neurons (or their axons) that give rise to the corticospinal and corticobulbar tracts. UMNs are found in the cerebral cortex and in the brainstem. UMN lesions result in spastic paralysis (hyperreflexia, hypertonia, claspknife phenomenon, clonus, muscle weakness, and Babinski's sign). UMN lesions are commonly caused by cerebrovascular accidents and frequently damage the internal capsule.

9–B. Transection of the lateral corticospinal tract results in an UMN lesion. The deficits are ipsilateral and caudal to the lesion. Plantar stimulation results in extension of the great toe and abduction of the other toes—this is Babinski's sign. Loss of vibration sensation results from interruption of the dorsal column–medial lemniscus system.

10–D. Interruption of descending autonomic pathways found in the lateral funiculi of the spinal cord result in Horner's syndrome. Horner's syndrome is ipsilateral to the lesion and consists of miosis, ptosis, facial hemianhydrosis, and apparent enophthalmos.

11–B. The ventral (anterior) spinal artery irrigates the ventral two-thirds of the spinal cord including the ventral horns, the corticospinal tracts, and the spinothalamic tracts. LMN deficits (flaccid paralysis and areflexia) are seen only at the level of infarction. Bilateral destruction of the lateral spinothalamic tracts results in bilateral loss of pain and temperature sensation caudal to the lesion. Vibration and position sensation are not affected because the dorsal columns are intact. Bilateral lesions of the anterior quadrants of the lateral funiculi interrupt corticosacral fibers that control bladder function (urinary incontinence).

12–E. Pure cauda equina syndrome involves the descending dorsal and ventral roots, classically spinal roots L3–S5. A herniated nucleus pulposus compressing the spinal roots may cause sensory and/or motor deficits, urinary and fecal incontinence, and impotence. Disk prolapse usually occurs unilaterally, producing symptoms on the ipsilateral side. Profound motor deficits may be seen. Babinski's sign is seen in UMN lesions, not in LMN lesions.

13–A. Conus medullaris syndrome involves spinal segments S3–Co and results in perianogenital sensory loss, a paralytic bladder, and impotence. The plantar reflex is flexor (no Babinski's sign). Also, epiconus syndrome is found at segments L4–S2; this syndrome is characterized by considerable motor disability and an absent Achilles tendon reflex, in addition to urinary incontinence.

14–E. Intervertebral disk herniation results from the prolapse of the nucleus pulposus through a defective anulus fibrosus into the vertebral canal. In 90% of cases, it appears at the L4–L5 or the L5–S1 interspace. In 10% of cases, it appears at the cervical region, usually at the C5–C6 or C6–C7 interspace. Intervertebral disk herniation may involve the cauda equina; usually it involves a single nerve root. Urinary incontinence is not seen with unilateral root lesions.

15–C. Lesion A involves degeneration of the ventral horns bilaterally at midcervical levels, resulting in flaccid paralysis in the upper extremities.

16–D. Lesion B involves degeneration of the lateral corticospinal tracts bilaterally, resulting in spastic paresis of the lower extremities and primarily affecting the muscles distal to the knee. Spastic paresis of the upper extremities is masked by flaccid paralysis resulting from lesion A.

17–E. Lesions A and B are the result of ALS, a pure motor disease.

18–A. Hemisection of the spinal cord results in a contralateral loss of pain and temperature sensation, starting one segment below the lesion.

19–B. Hemisection of the spinal cord results in a loss of all sensory modalities at the level of transection.

20–C. Hemisection of the spinal cord results in a loss of dorsal column modalities (including position sensation) below the lesion on the ipsilateral side.

21–C. Hemisection of the spinal cord results in corticospinal tract deficits below the transection on the ipsilateral side, including exaggerated muscle stretch reflexes (hyperreflexia).

22–C. Hemisection of the spinal cord results in dorsal column deficits (including vibration sense) below the lesion on the ipsilateral side.

23–C. Transection of the lateral corticospinal tract results in spastic paresis and muscle weakness below the lesion on the ipsilateral side.

24–C. A neurologic manifestation of vitamin B_{12} deficiency is subacute combined degeneration. There is no involvement of LMNs.

25–A. Lesion A shows the territory of infarction resulting from occlusion of the ventral (anterior) spinal artery.

26–D. A spinal cord hemisection (Brown-Séquard syndrome) on the right side results in a loss of vibration sensation on the right side and a loss of pain and temperature sensation on the left side (dissociated sensory loss).

27–A. Total occlusion of the ventral spinal artery, involving five cervical segments, results in infarction of the ventral two-thirds of the spinal cord and interrupts both lateral spinothalamic tracts. The patient would have a loss of pain and temperature sensation caudal to the lesion.

28–B. Lesion A shows a cervical syringomyelic lesion involving the ventral white commissure, both ventral horns, and the right corticospinal tract. The patient would have a bilateral loss of pain and temperature sensation in the hands, muscle wasting in both hands, and a spastic paresis on the right side.

29–A. In lesion A, both lateral and ventral funiculi have been infarcted by arterial occlusion. Bilateral destruction of the lateral corticospinal tracts at upper cervical levels results in quadriplegia (spastic paresis in upper and lower extremities). Bilateral destruction of the ventrolateral quadrants results in urinary and fecal incontinence.

30–C. In lesion C, subacute combined degeneration, there is no involvement of LMNs, hence no flaccid paralysis, muscle atrophy, or fasciculations.

31–C. In lesion C, subacute combined degeneration, there is symmetric degeneration of the white matter, both in the dorsal columns (fasciculi gracilis) and in the lateral funiculi (corticospinal tracts). In this degenerative disease, both the myelin sheaths and the axis cylinders are involved. Subacute combined degeneration is classified under nutritional diseases (in this case a vitamin B_{12} neuropathy). In true demyelinative diseases (e.g., multiple sclerosis), the myelin sheaths are involved but the axis cylinders and nerve cells are relatively spared.

9

Brainstem

I. Introduction—The Brainstem (Figure 9.1)

–includes the **medulla, pons,** and **mesencephalon** (midbrain).
–extends from the pyramidal decussation to the posterior commissure.
–gives rise to cranial nerves III–XII.
–receives its blood supply from the vertebrobasilar system.

II. Medulla Oblongata (Myelencephalon)

A. Overview—the medulla

–contains autonomic centers that regulate respiration, circulation, and gastrointestinal motility.
–extends from the pyramidal decussation to the inferior pontine sulcus.
–gives rise to CN IX–CN XII. The nuclei of CN V and CN VIII extend caudally into the medulla.
–is connected to the cerebellum by the inferior cerebellar peduncle.

B. Internal structures of the medulla (Figures 9.2–9.5)

1. Ascending sensory pathways and relay nuclei

a. Fasciculus gracilis and fasciculus cuneatus

–convey dorsal column modalities.
–terminate in the nucleus gracilis and nucleus cuneatus.

b. Nucleus gracilis and nucleus cuneatus

–contain second-order neurons of the dorsal column–medial lemniscus pathway.
–give rise to internal arcuate fibers.
–project via the medial lemniscus to the ventral posterolateral nucleus of the thalamus.

c. Internal arcuate fibers

–arise from the nucleus gracilis and nucleus cuneatus and form the contralateral medial lemniscus.

117

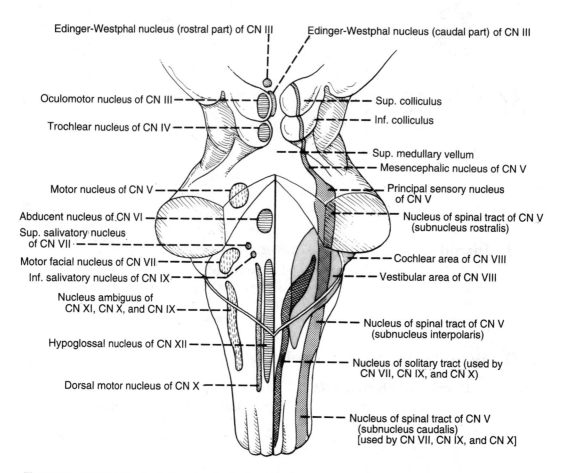

Figure 9.1. Outline of the brainstem showing the location of motor and sensory cranial nerve nuclei. Motor nuclei are shown on the left side of the figure and sensory nuclei are shown on the right side.

d. Decussation of the medial lemniscus (see Figure 9.3)

–is formed by decussating internal arcuate fibers.

e. Medial lemniscus

–conveys dorsal column modalities to the ventral posterolateral nucleus.

f. Spinal lemniscus (see Figures 9.3–9.9)

–contains the lateral and ventral spinothalamic tracts and the spinotectal tract.

2. Descending motor pathways

a. Pyramidal decussation (see Figure 9.2)

–is located at the spinomedullary junction.
–consists of crossing corticospinal fibers.

b. Pyramids (see Figures 9.3–9.5)

–constitute the base of the medulla.
–contain uncrossed corticospinal fibers.

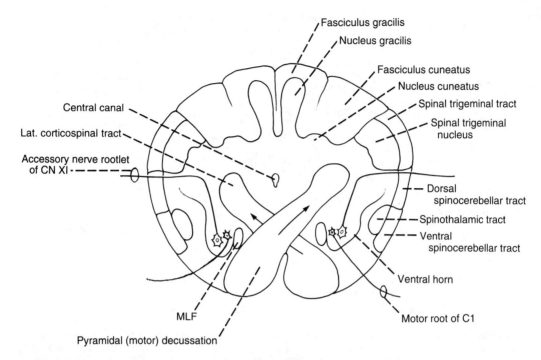

Fasciculus gracilis
Nucleus gracilis
Fasciculus cuneatus
Nucleus cuneatus
Spinal trigeminal tract
Spinal trigeminal nucleus
Central canal
Lat. corticospinal tract
Accessory nerve rootlet of CN XI
Dorsal spinocerebellar tract
Spinothalamic tract
Ventral spinocerebellar tract
Ventral horn
MLF
Motor root of C1
Pyramidal (motor) decussation

Figure 9.2. Transverse section of the caudal medulla at the level of the pyramidal (motor) decussation. The nucleus of the accessory nerve (CN XI) is located in the ventral horn and gives rise to the spinal root of CN XI. Ventral horn neurons from the spinal nucleus give rise to the ventral roots of C1.

3. Cerebellar pathways and relay nuclei

a. Accessory (lateral) cuneate nucleus
  −contains second-order neurons of the cuneocerebellar tract.
  −projects to the cerebellum via the inferior cerebellar peduncle.

b. Inferior olivary nucleus
  −underlies the olive.
  −is a cerebellar relay nucleus that projects olivocerebellar fibers via the inferior cerebellar peduncle to the contralateral cerebellar cortex and cerebellar nuclei.
  −receives input from the red nucleus.

c. Central tegmental tract
  −extends from the midbrain to the inferior olivary nucleus.
  −contains rubro-olivary and reticulothalamic fibers.

d. Lateral reticular nucleus
  −is a cerebellar relay nucleus that projects via the inferior cerebellar peduncle to the cerebellum.

e. Arcuate nucleus
  −is located on the ventral surface of the pyramids.
  −gives rise to arcuatocerebellar fibers that become the striae medullares of the rhomboid fossa.

f. Dorsal spinocerebellar tract
  −mediates unconscious proprioception from the lower extremities to the cerebellum via the inferior cerebellar peduncle.

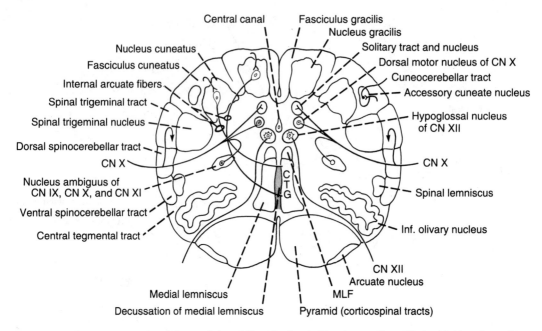

Figure 9.3. Transverse section of the caudal medulla at the level of the decussation of the medial lemniscus. The internal arcuate fibers decussate and form the medial lemniscus. *CTG* = **C**uneate (arm), **T**runk, and **G**racile (leg) components of the medial lemniscus. General somatic afferent (GSA) fibers of the vagal nerve (CN X) enter the spinal trigeminal tract of CN V (*arrow*).

g. Ventral spinocerebellar tract

—mediates unconscious proprioception from the lower extremities to the cerebellum via the superior cerebellar peduncle.

h. Inferior cerebellar peduncle

—connects the medulla to the cerebellum.

4. Cranial nerve nuclei and associated tracts

a. Medial longitudinal fasciculus (MLF)

—contains vestibular fibers of CN VIII that coordinate eye movements via CN III, CN IV, and CN VI.
—mediates nystagmus and lateral conjugate gaze.

b. Solitary tract

—receives general visceral afferent (GVA) input from CN IX and CN X.
—receives special visceral afferent (SVA) [taste] input from CN VII, CN IX, and CN X.

c. Solitary nucleus

—projects GVA and SVA input ipsilaterally via the central tegmental tract to the parabrachial nucleus of the pons and then to the posteromedial nucleus of the thalamus.

d. Dorsal motor nucleus of CN X (see Figures 9.1, 9.3, and 9.4)

—gives rise to vagal preganglionic parasympathetic general visceral efferent (GVE) fibers that synapse in the terminal (intramural) ganglia of the thoracic and abdominal viscera.

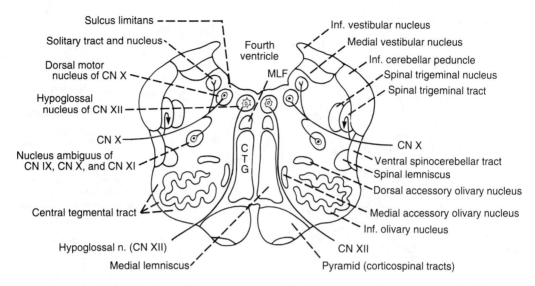

Figure 9.4. Transverse section of the medulla at the midolivary level. The vagal (CN X), hypoglossal (CN XII), and vestibular (CN VIII) nerves are prominent in this section. The nucleus ambiguus gives rise to special visceral efferent (SVE) fibers to CN IX, CN X, and CN XI. The dorsal spinocerebellar tract is in the inferior cerebellar peduncle.

e. Inferior salivary nucleus of CN IX

–gives rise to preganglionic parasympathetic (GVE) fibers that synapse in the otic ganglion.

f. Hypoglossal nucleus of CN XII (see Figures 9.1, 9.3, and 9.4)

–gives rise to general somatic efferent (GSE) fibers that innervate the intrinsic and extrinsic muscles of the tongue.

g. Nucleus ambiguus of CN IX, CN X, and CN XI (see Figures 9.1 and 9.3–9.5)

–represents a special visceral efferent (SVE) cell column whose axons innervate branchial arch muscles of the larynx and pharynx. These fibers contribute to parts of CN IX, CN X, and CN XI; they exit the medulla via the postolivary sulcus.

–gives rise to vagal preganglionic parasympathetic GVE fibers that synapse in the terminal ganglia of the heart (sinoatrial and atrioventricular nodes) [see Figure 18.2].

h. Ventral horn of CN XI (see Figure 9.2)

–is located at the level of the pyramidal decussation.

–contains motor neurons of the spinal accessory nerve.

i. Spinal trigeminal tract (Figure 9.6; see Figures 9.1–9.5)

–replaces the dorsolateral tract of Lissauer.

–contains first-order neuron general somatic afferent (GSA) fibers that mediate pain, temperature, and light touch sensations from the face via CN V, CN VII, CN IX, and CN X.

–projects to the spinal trigeminal nucleus.

j. Spinal trigeminal nucleus (see Figures 9.1–9.6)

–replaces the substantia gelatinosa of the spinal cord.

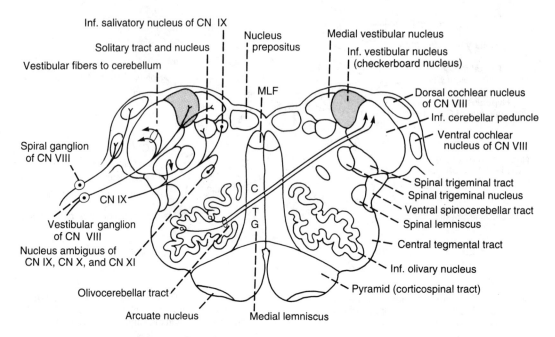

Figure 9.5. Rostral medulla at the level of the dorsal and ventral cochlear nuclei (of CN VIII). The glossopharyngeal nerve (CN IX) is also found at this level. The hypoglossal nucleus (of CN XII) has been replaced by the nucleus prepositus. General somatic afferent (GSA) fibers of the glossopharyngeal nerve (CN IX) enter the spinal trigeminal tract of CN V (*arrow*).

  –gives rise to decussating axons that form the ventral trigeminothalamic tract. This tract terminates in the ventral posteromedial nucleus of the thalamus.

5. Area postrema

  –lies rostral to the obex in the floor of the fourth ventricle.

  –is a circumventricular organ with no blood–brain barrier (see Chapter 2).

III. Pons

A. Overview—the pons

  –contains auditory relay nuclei and vestibular nuclei; the latter regulate postural mechanisms and vestibulo-ocular reflexes.

  –contains, in its caudal portion, the facial motor nucleus of CN VII, which innervates the muscles of facial expression.

  –contains, in the midpons, the trigeminal motor nucleus of CN V; its axons innervate the muscles of mastication.

  –contains a center for lateral gaze.

  –extends from the inferior pontine sulcus to the superior pontine sulcus.

  –consists of the **base,** which contains corticobulbar, corticospinal, and corticopontine tracts and pontine nuclei; and the **tegmentum,** which contains cranial nerve nuclei, reticular nuclei, and the major ascending sensory pathways.

  –is connected to the cerebellum by the middle cerebellar peduncle.

  –gives rise to CN V–CN VIII.

B. Internal structures of the pons (Figure 9.7; see Figure 9.6)

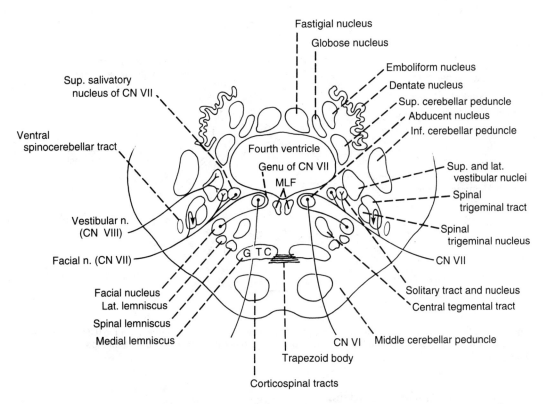

Figure 9.6. Caudal pons at the level of the abducent (CN VI) and facial (CN VII) nuclei. Note that the intra-axial abducent fibers pass through the medial lemniscus and the descending corticospinal fibers. Note the looping course of the intra-axial facial nerve fibers that exit the brainstem in the cerebellopontine sulcus. The four cerebellar nuclei overlie the fourth ventricle. Note also the looping course of the facial nerve fibers.

1. Ascending sensory pathways and relay nuclei

a. Dorsal and ventral cochlear nuclei (see Figure 9.5)

–receive auditory input from the cochlea through special somatic afferent (SSA) fibers via the cochlear branch of CN VIII.

–are auditory relay nuclei that give rise to the contralatral lateral lemniscus.

b. Trapezoid body

–is formed by decussating fibers of the ventral cochlear nuclei.

–contains the acoustic striae, medial lemnisci, exiting abducent fibers, and aberrant corticobulbar fibers.

c. Superior olivary nucleus

–is an auditory relay nucleus located at the level of the trapezoid body.

–receives input from the cochlear nuclei.

–contributes to the lateral lemniscus.

d. Lateral lemniscus

–is a pontine auditory pathway extending from the trapezoid body to the nucleus of the inferior colliculus.

–conducts a preponderance of contralateral cochlear input.

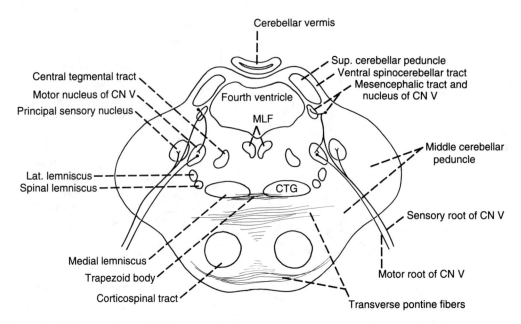

Figure 9.7. Midpons at the level of the motor and principal sensory nuclei of the trigeminal nerve (CN V). The mesencephalic tract and nucleus provide the afferent limb of the myotatic jaw jerk reflex; the motor trigeminal nucleus is the efferent limb.

e. Medial lemniscus

–mediates contralateral dorsal column modalities to the ventral posterolateral nucleus of the thalamus.

f. Spinal lemniscus

–contains lateral and ventral spinothalamic tracts and the spinotectal tract.

2. Descending motor pathways (base of the pons)

a. Corticobulbar tract

–synapses in the motor nuclei of the cranial nerves except in the ocular motor nuclei of CN III, CN IV, and CN VI.

b. Corticospinal tract (pyramidal tract)

–synapses in the ventral horn of the spinal cord.

c. Corticopontine tract

–synapses in the pontine nuclei.

3. Cerebellar pathways and relay nuclei

a. Central tegmental tract

–extends from the midbrain to the inferior olivary nucleus.
–contains rubro-olivary and reticulothalamic fibers.

b. Juxtarestiform body

–forms part of the inferior cerebellar peduncle.
–contains vestibulocerebellar, cerebellovestibular, and cerebelloreticular fibers.

c. Middle cerebellar peduncle

–contains pontocerebellar fibers.

–connects the pons to the cerebellum.

d. Superior cerebellar peduncle

–connects the cerebellum to the pons and midbrain.

–contains the dentatorubrothalamic fibers and the ventral spinocerebellar tract.

e. Pontine nuclei

–are cerebellar relay nuclei found in the base of the pons.

–give rise to pontocerebellar fibers that constitute the middle cerebellar peduncle.

4. Cranial nerve nuclei and associated tracts

a. Dorsal and ventral cochlear nuclei of CN VIII

–are found at the medullopontine junction.

b. Medial, lateral, and superior vestibular nuclei of CN VIII (see Figure 9.6)

–receive proprioceptive (SSA) input from the semicircular ducts, utricle, saccule, and the cerebellum.

–project to the cerebellum and the MLF.

–the lateral vestibular nucleus gives rise to the lateral vestibulospinal tract.

c. Medial longitudinal fasciculus

–contains vestibular fibers of CN VIII that coordinate eye movements.

–mediates nystagmus and lateral conjugate gaze.

d. Abducent nucleus of CN VI (see Figure 9.6)

–underlies, in the caudal medial pontine tegmentum, the facial colliculus of the rhomboid fossa.

–projects exiting fibers through the trapezoid body and through the corticospinal tract of the base of the pons.

–gives rise to GSE fibers that innervate the lateral rectus muscle.

–gives rise to fibers that project, via the MLF, to the contralateral medial rectus subnucleus of the oculomotor nucleus of CN III.

–is the **pontine center for lateral conjugate gaze,** which receives commands from the contralateral frontal eye field (area 8). It innervates, via the MLF, the contralateral medial rectus muscle and, via abducent fibers, the ipsilateral lateral rectus muscle to execute conjugate lateral gaze.

e. Facial nucleus of CN VII (see Figure 9.6)

–gives rise to SVE fibers that innervate the muscles of facial expression.

–contains axons that project dorsomedially, encircle the abducent nucleus as a genu, and pass ventrolaterally between the facial nucleus and spinal trigeminal nucleus to exit the brainstem at the cerebellopontine angle.

f. Superior salivatory nucleus of CN VII

–includes the lacrimal nucleus.

–gives rise to GVE preganglionic parasympathetic fibers that synapse in the pterygopalatine and submandibular ganglia.

g. Spinal trigeminal tract and nucleus of CN V

h. Motor nucleus of CN V

–lies in the lateral midpontine tegmentum at the level of entrance of the trigeminal nerve.

–lies medial to the principal sensory nucleus of the trigeminal nerve.

–receives bilateral corticobulbar input.

–gives rise to SVE fibers that innervate muscles of mastication.

i. Principal sensory nucleus of CN V

–lies lateral to the motor nucleus of CN V.

–receives discriminative tactile and pressure sensation input from the face.

–gives rise to trigeminothalamic fibers that join the contralateral ventral trigeminothalamic tract.

–gives rise to the uncrossed dorsal trigeminothalamic tract, which terminates in the ventral posteromedial nucleus of the thalamus.

j. Mesencephalic nucleus and tract of CN V (Figures 9.8 and 9.9; see Figure 9.7)

–extend from the upper pons to the upper midbrain.

–contain pseudounipolar neurons.

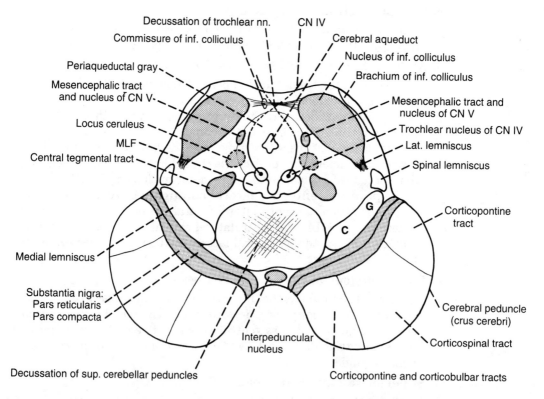

Figure 9.8. Midbrain at the level of the inferior colliculus, the decussation of the superior cerebellar peduncles, and the trochlear nucleus (of CN IV). Note that trochlear fibers decussate and exit the brainstem on the dorsal surface.

−receive input from muscle spindles and pressure receptors (muscles of mastication and extraocular muscles).

5. Locus ceruleus

−is a melanin-containing nucleus located in the pons and midbrain.
−is an important nucleus of the monoamine system that projects noradrenergic axons to all parts of the central nervous system.
−is thought to play a role in non-REM sleep and in the control of cortical activation (tone).

IV. Mesencephalon (Midbrain) [see Figures 9.8 and 9.9]

A. Overview—the midbrain

−mediates auditory and visual reflexes.
−contains the oculomotor nerve (CN III) and the trochlear nerve (CN IV), which innervate the extraocular muscles of the eye.
−contains a center for vertical conjugate gaze in its rostral extent.
−contains the **substantia nigra,** the largest nucleus of the midbrain; degeneration of this extrapyramidal motor nucleus results in Parkinson's disease.
−contains the **paramedian reticular formation;** lesions of this formation result in coma.
−extends from the superior medullary velum to the posterior commissure.
−gives rise to two cranial nerves: **CN III** (oculomotor) and **CN IV** (trochlear).
−consists dorsoventrally of three parts: the **tectum,** the **tegmentum,** and the **base (basis pedunculi).**

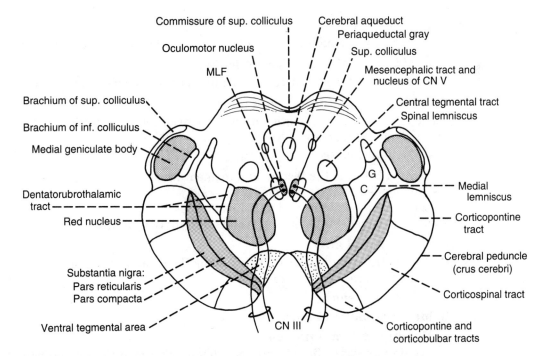

Figure 9.9. Midbrain at the level of the superior colliculus, the oculomotor nucleus (of CN III), and the red nucleus. Note that oculomotor fibers pass laterally through the red nucleus and basis pedunculi and exit in the interpeduncular fossa.

B. Structures of the midbrain

1. Tectum

–is located dorsal to the cerebral aqueduct.

–forms the roof of the midbrain, including the superior and inferior colliculi.

2. Tegmentum

–is located between the tectum and the base (basis pedunculi).

–contains cranial nerve nuclei and sensory pathways.

3. Basis pedunculi (crus cerebri)

–forms the base of the midbrain and contains corticospinal, corticobulbar, and corticopontine tracts.

4. Pedunculus cerebri (cerebral peduncle)

–includes the tegmentum and basis pedunculi.

5. Pretectum (pretectal area)

–is located between the superior colliculus and the habenular trigone.

C. Inferior collicular level of the midbrain (see Figure 9.8)

1. Inferior colliculus

–contains the nucleus of the inferior colliculus.

2. Nucleus of the inferior colliculus

–is an auditory relay nucleus that receives binaural input from the lateral lemniscus.

–projects to the medial geniculate body via the brachium of the inferior colliculus.

3. Lateral lemniscus

–projects binaural auditory information to the inferior collicular nucleus.

4. Commissure of the inferior colliculus

–interconnects the inferior collicular nucleus and its opposite partner.

5. Brachium of the inferior colliculus

–conducts auditory information from the inferior collicular nucleus to the medial geniculate body.

6. Cerebral aqueduct

–is located between the tectum and tegmentum.

–is surrounded by the periaqueductal gray.

–interconnects the third and fourth ventricles.

–blockage (aqueductal stenosis) results in **hydrocephalus**.

7. Periaqueductal gray

–is the central gray matter that surrounds the cerebral aqueduct.

–contains several nuclear groups:

a. Locus ceruleus

b. Mesencephalic nucleus and tract

c. Dorsal tegmental nucleus

–contains enkephalinergic neurons that play a role in endogenous pain control.

d. Dorsal nucleus of raphe
    —contains serotonergic neurons.

8. Trochlear nucleus of CN IV (see Figure 9.8)
    —gives rise to GSE fibers, which encircle the periaqueductal gray, decussate in the superior medullary velum, and exit the midbrain from its dorsal aspect to innervate the superior oblique muscle.

9. Medial longitudinal fasciculus
    —contains vestibular fibers that coordinate eye movements.
    —interconnects the ocular motor nuclei of CN III, CN IV, and CN VI.

10. Decussation of the superior cerebellar peduncles (see Figure 9.8)
    —is the most conspicuous structure of this level.

11. Interpeduncular nucleus
    —receives input from the habenular nuclei via the habenulointerpeduncular tract (fasciculus retroflexus of Meynert).

12. Substantia nigra (see Figures 9.8 and 9.9)
    —is divided into the dorsal **pars compacta,** which contains large pigmented (melanin) cells, and the ventral **pars reticularis**.
    —receives GABA-ergic input from the caudatoputamen (striatonigral fibers).
    —projects dopaminergic fibers to the caudatoputamen (nigrostriatal fibers).
    —projects nondopaminergic fibers to the ventral anterior nucleus and the ventral lateral nucleus of the thalamus (nigrothalamic fibers).

13. Medial lemniscus
    —mediates dorsal column modalities to the ventral posterolateral nucleus.

14. Spinal lemniscus
    —contains the lateral and ventral spinothalamic tracts and the spinotectal tract.

15. Central tegmental tract
    —contains rubro-olivary and reticulothalamic fibers.

16. Basis pedunculi (crus cerebri) [see Figures 9.8 and 9.9]

D. Superior collicular level of the midbrain (see Figure 9.9)

1. Superior colliculus
    —receives visual input from the retina and from frontal (area 8) and occipital (area 19) eye fields.
    —receives auditory input from the inferior colliculus to mediate audiovisual reflexes.
    —is concerned with detection of movement in visual fields, thus facilitating visual orientation, searching, and tracking.

2. Commissure of the superior colliculus
    —interconnects the two superior colliculi.

3. Brachium of the superior colliculus
    —conducts retinal and corticotectal fibers to the superior colliculus and to the pretectum, thus mediating optic and pupillary reflexes.

4. Cerebral aqueduct and periaqueduct gray

5. Oculomotor nucleus of CN III (see Figure 9.9)

–gives rise to GSE fibers that innervate four extraocular muscles (medial, inferior, superior recti, and inferior oblique) and the superior levator palpebrae.

–projects crossed fibers to the superior rectus.

–projects crossed and uncrossed fibers to the levator palpebrae.

6. Edinger-Westphal nucleus of CN III

–gives rise to GVE preganglionic parasympathetic fibers that terminate in the ciliary ganglion.

–postganglionic fibers from the ciliary ganglion innervate the ciliary body (accommodation) and the sphincter muscle of the iris (pupillary light reflex).

7. Medial longitudinal fasciculus

–contains vestibular fibers that coordinate eye movements.

–interconnects the ocular motor cranial nerves (CN III, CN IV, and CN VI).

8. Central tegmental tract

–contains rubro-olivary and reticulothalamic fibers.

9. Red nucleus (see Figure 9.9)

–is located in the tegmentum at the level of the oculomotor nucleus (the level of the superior colliculus).

–receives bilateral input from the cerebral cortex.

–receives contralateral input from the cerebellar nuclei.

–gives rise to the crossed rubrospinal tract.

–gives rise to the uncrossed rubro-olivary tract.

–exerts facilitatory influence on flexor muscles.

10. Medial lemniscus

–mediates dorsal column modalities to the ventral posterolateral nucleus of the thalamus.

11. Spinal lemniscus

–contains the lateral and ventral spinothalamic tracts.

12. Substantia nigra

13. Basis pedunculi (crus cerebri)

E. Posterior commissural level (pretectal region)

–is a transition area between the mesencephalon and the diencephalon.

1. Posterior commissure

–marks the caudal extent of the third ventricle.

–marks the rostral extent of the cerebral aqueduct.

–interconnects pretectal nuclei, thus mediating consensual pupillary light reflexes.

2. Pretectal nucleus

–receives retinal input via the brachium of the superior colliculus.

–projects to the ipsilateral and contralateral Edinger-Westphal nucleus, thus mediating the pupillary light reflexes.

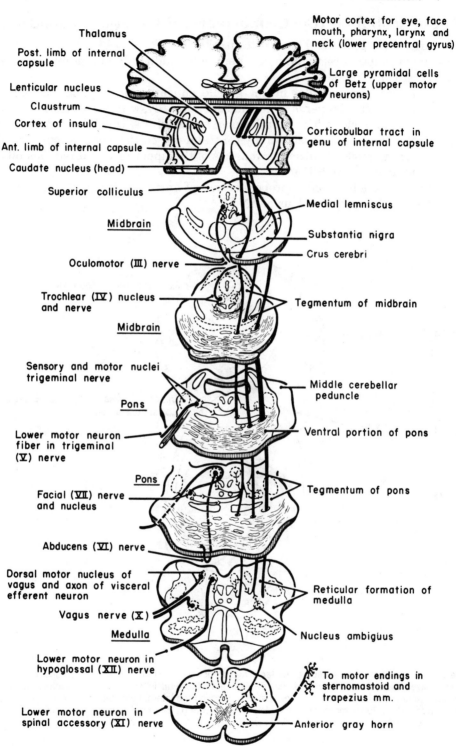

Thalamus

Post. limb of internal capsule

Lenticular nucleus

Claustrum

Cortex of insula

Ant. limb of internal capsule

Caudate nucleus (head)

Superior colliculus

Midbrain

Oculomotor (III) nerve

Trochlear (IV) nucleus and nerve

Midbrain

Sensory and motor nuclei trigeminal nerve

Pons

Lower motor neuron fiber in trigeminal (V) nerve

Pons

Facial (VII) nerve and nucleus

Abducens (VI) nerve

Dorsal motor nucleus of vagus and axon of visceral efferent neuron

Vagus nerve (X)

Medulla

Lower motor neuron in hypoglossal (XII) nerve

Lower motor neuron in spinal accessory (XI) nerve

Motor cortex for eye, face mouth, pharynx, larynx and neck (lower precentral gyrus)

Large pyramidal cells of Betz (upper motor neurons)

Corticobulbar tract in genu of internal capsule

Medial lemniscus

Substantia nigra

Crus cerebri

Tegmentum of midbrain

Middle cerebellar peduncle

Ventral portion of pons

Tegmentum of pons

Reticular formation of medulla

Nucleus ambiguus

To motor endings in sternomastoid and trapezius mm.

Anterior gray horn

Figure 9.10. Corticobulbar pathways of the brainstem. Corticobulbar fibers arise from the face area of the motor cortex and innervate motor (GSE and SVE) cranial nerve nuclei of CN V, CN VII, CN IX, CN X, CN XI, and CN XII. Direct corticobulbar fibers to the ocular motor nerves, CN III, CN IV, and CN VI have not been demonstrated. Interruption of corticobulbar fibers results in an upper motor neuron (UMN) lesion. (Reprinted with permission from Carpenter MC: *Core Text of Neuroanatomy,* 3rd ed. Baltimore, Williams & Wilkins, 1985, p 129.)

V. Corticobulbar (Corticonuclear) Fibers (Figures 9.10 and 9.11)

–arise from precentral and postcentral gyri.
–may synapse directly on motor neurons or indirectly via interneurons (corticoreticular fibers).
–innervate sensory relay nuclei (gracile, cuneate, solitary, and trigeminal).
–innervate cranial nerve motor nuclei bilaterally, with the exception of part of the facial nucleus. The **facial nerve subnucleus,** which innervates muscles of the lower face, receives only contralateral corticobulbar input. The facial nerve subnucleus subserves muscles of the upper face and receives bilateral input (see Figure 9.11).
–project, it is believed, a preponderance of uncrossed indirect corticobulbar fibers to the spinal nucleus of CN IX.

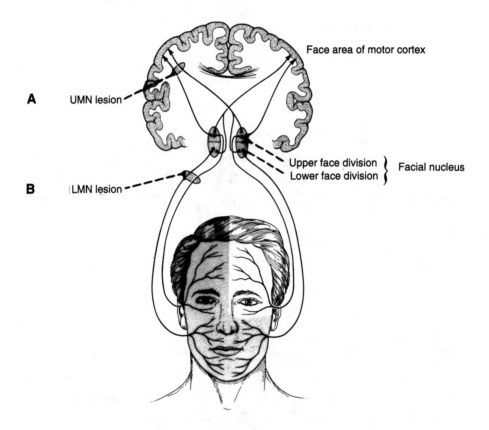

Figure 9.11. Corticobulbar innervation of the facial nerve nucleus of CN VII. The upper face division of the facial nucleus receives bilateral input. The lower face division of the facial nucleus receives only contralateral input. An upper motor neuron (UMN) lesion at *A* (e.g., a stroke involving the internal capsule), therefore, spares the contralateral upper face. A lower motor neuron (LMN) lesion at *B* (e.g., Bell's palsy) results in ipsilateral paralysis of facial muscles in both the upper and the lower face.

Review Test

Directions: Each of the numbered items or incomplete statements in this section is followed by answers or by completions of the statement. Select the **one** lettered answer or completion that is **best** in each case.

1. The base of the pons contains all of the following nuclei and fibers EXCEPT the

(A) cerebellar relay nuclei.
(B) arcuate nuclei.
(C) corticospinal fibers.
(D) corticobulbar fibers.
(E) exiting fibers of the abducent nucleus.

2. All of the following statements concerning the trapezoid body are correct EXCEPT

(A) it is found in the ventral pontine tegmentum.
(B) it contains the MLF.
(C) it contains the medial lemniscus.
(D) it contains aberrant corticobulbar fibers.
(E) it contains auditory fibers.

3. All of the following statements concerning the spinal trigeminal nucleus are correct EXCEPT

(A) it is a homolog of the substantia gelatinosa.
(B) it gives rise to the dorsal trigeminothalamic tract.
(C) it receives input from free nerve endings.
(D) it projects to the contralateral ventral posteromedial nucleus of the thalamus.
(E) it is found in the lateral pontine tegmentum.

4. Which one of the following nuclei does not project to the cerebellum?

(A) Lateral reticular nucleus
(B) Arcuate nucleus
(C) Inferior olivary nucleus
(D) Accessory (lateral) cuneate nucleus
(E) Nucleus ambiguus

5. The cerebral aqueduct is found in which part of the brain?

(A) Telencephalon
(B) Diencephalon
(C) Mesencephalon
(D) Metencephalon
(E) Myelencephalon

6. Decussation of the superior cerebellar peduncles occurs in which area of the brain?

(A) Rostral midbrain
(B) Caudal midbrain
(C) Rostral pons
(D) Caudal pons
(E) Cerebellum

7. All of the following statements concerning the medulla oblongata are correct EXCEPT

(A) it extends from the pyramidal decussation to the inferior pontine sulcus.
(B) it contains the facial nucleus.
(C) it contains the medial and inferior vestibular nuclei.
(D) it contains the inferior olivary nucleus.
(E) it contains the nucleus ambiguus.

8. All of the following statements concerning the hypoglossal nucleus are correct EXCEPT

(A) it gives rise to SVE fibers.
(B) it has axons that exit the medulla between the olive and the pyramid.
(C) it lies dorsal to the MLF.
(D) it innervates the intrinsic musculature of the tongue.
(E) its intra-axial root fibers lie adjacent to the medial lemniscus.

9. All of the following statements concerning the abducent nucleus are correct EXCEPT

(A) it is found in the pontine tegmentum.
(B) it underlies the facial colliculus.
(C) it exits the brainstem at the superior pontine sulcus.
(D) it gives rise to fibers that traverse the cavernous sinus.
(E) it gives rise to fibers that traverse the corticospinal tracts.

10. All of the following statements concerning the motor nucleus of the trigeminal nerve are correct EXCEPT

(A) it plays a role in the corneal reflex.
(B) it lies medial to the principal sensory nucleus of CN V.
(C) it is located in the rostral pontine tegmentum.
(D) it receives bilateral input from corticobulbar fibers.
(E) it gives rise to SVE fibers.

11. All of the following statements concerning the trochlear nerve are correct EXCEPT

(A) it has its nucleus in the midbrain tegmentum.
(B) it exits the brainstem caudal to the inferior colliculus.
(C) it decussates in the superior medullary velum.
(D) it innervates a muscle that depresses the globe.
(E) it innervates a muscle that extorts the globe.

12. All of the following statements concerning the locus ceruleus are correct EXCEPT

(A) its neurons contain melanin.
(B) its neurons contain dopamine.
(C) it is located in the pons and midbrain.
(D) it projects to the spinal cord.
(E) it projects to the cerebral cortex.

13. All of the following statements concerning the oculomotor nuclear complex are correct EXCEPT

(A) stimulation of its parasympathetic component results in mydriasis.
(B) damage to its GSE fibers results in severe ptosis.
(C) it is found in the midbrain at the level of the superior colliculus.
(D) its preganglionic parasympathetic fibers synapse in the ciliary ganglion.
(E) its exiting GSE fibers pass through the crus cerebri.

Directions: Each group of items in this section consists of lettered options followed by a set of numbered items. For each item, select the **one** lettered option that is most closely associated with it. Each lettered option may be selected once, more than once, or not at all.

Questions 14–23

Match each description with the nuclear structure it best describes.

(A) Cochlear nuclei
(B) Nucleus gracilis
(C) Inferior olivary nucleus
(D) Superior salivatory nucleus
(E) Substantia nigra
(F) Mesencephalic nucleus

14. Neurons that contain melanin

15. Contains pseudounipolar ganglion cells

16. Gives rise to the lateral lemniscus

17. Projects to the contralateral cerebellum

18. Is the afferent limb of the jaw jerk reflex

19. Projects to the pterygopalatine ganglion

20. Gives rise to the medial lemniscus

21. Projects dopaminergic fibers to the caudatoputamen (striatum)

22. Projects to the ventral posterolateral nucleus

23. Receives input from the red nucleus

Answers and Explanations

1–B. The base of the pons contains corticospinal, corticobulbar, and corticopontine fibers and pontine nuclei (cerebellar relay nuclei). Exiting intra-axial abducent fibers of CN VI pass through the corticospinal fibers in the base of the pons. Arcuate nuclei are displaced pontine nuclei found in the pyramids.

2–B. The trapezoid body contains auditory fibers from the cochlear and superior olivary nuclei, the medial lemniscus, and corticobulbar fibers. Exiting intra-axial abducent fibers pass through the trapezoid body. The MLF lies dorsal to this structure.

3–B. The spinal trigeminal nucleus of CN V extends from C3 to the caudal pole of the principal sensory nucleus of the trigeminal nerve. It is considered a homolog of the substantia gelatinosa. It lies in the lateral medulla and lateral pontine tegmentum and gives rise to the crossed ventral trigeminothalamic tract. The dorsal trigeminothalamic tract arises from the principal sensory nucleus of CN V.

4–E. The nucleus ambiguus is a SVE cell column that gives rise to the motor components of CN IX, CN X, and CN XI. The nucleus ambiguus also contains GVE (parasympathetic) neurons with axons that innervate the heart via the vagal nerve.

5–C. The cerebral aqueduct is found in the mesencephalon; it connects the third ventricle to the fourth ventricle.

6–B. Decussation of the superior cerebellar peduncles occurs in the caudal midbrain tegmentum at the level of the inferior colliculus.

7–B. On its ventral aspect, the medulla extends from the pyramidal decussation to the inferior pontine sulcus (pontobulbar sulcus); on its dorsal aspect, it extends from the pyramidal decussation to the striae medullares of the rhomboid fossa. The medial and inferior vestibular nuclei are found in the medulla and extend into the caudal pontine tegmentum. The inferior olivary nucleus, a cerebellar relay nucleus, is the most prominent nucleus of the medulla. The nucleus ambiguus is found in the medulla; it gives rise to SVE fibers of CN IX, CN X, and CN XI. The facial nucleus is found in the caudal pontine tegmentum.

8–A. The hypoglossal nucleus of CN XII gives rise to GSE fibers. The hypoglossal nucleus lies dorsal to the medial longitudinal fasciculus, gives rise to fibers that exit the medulla in the preolivary sulcus, and innervates the intrinsic and extrinsic muscles of the tongue (except the palatoglossus muscle, which is innervated by CN X). Intra-axial root fibers lie between the medial lemniscus and the inferior olivary nucleus.

9–C. The abducent nucleus of CN VI underlies the facial colliculus in the caudal pontine tegmentum. It gives rise to GSE fibers that innervate the lateral rectus muscle. It exits the brainstem at the inferior pontine sulcus (pontobulbar sulcus). Exiting abducent fibers pass through the corticospinal tracts, which traverse the base of the pons.

10–A. The motor nucleus of the trigeminal nerve (CN V) is a component of the SVE cell column, lies medial to the principal sensory nucleus of CN V, is found in the rostral pontine tegmentum, and receives bilateral corticobulbar input. The afferent limb of the corneal reflex is the ophthalmic nerve (CN V-1); the efferent limb is the facial nerve (CN VII), which innervates the orbicularis oculi muscle.

11–E. The trochlear nerve (CN IV) has its nucleus in the midbrain tegmentum at the level of the inferior colliculus. It decussates in the superior medullary velum and exits the brainstem lateral to the frenulum of the superior medullary velum. It is the only cranial nerve to exit the brainstem from the dorsal surface. It innervates the superior oblique muscle, which depresses, intorts, and abducts the eyeball.

12–B. The locus ceruleus is a pigmented (melanin-containing) nucleus found in the rostral pontine tegmentum that extends into the midbrain. Its cells contain catecholamines (noradrenaline). It projects to all parts of the central nervous system, including the cerebral cortex and the spinal cord. Dopamine is found in the substantia nigra of the midbrain.

13–A. Stimulation of the parasympathetic component results in miosis (sphincter pupillae muscle). Preganglionic parasympathetic fibers synapse in the ciliary ganglion. The oculomotor nuclear complex is found in the midbrain at the level of the red nucleus and the superior colliculus. Exiting oculomotor fibers pass through the crus cerebri. Transection of these fibers results in severe ptosis, a dilated pupil, paralysis of the medial, superior, and inferior recti muscles and paralysis of the inferior oblique and the levator palpebrae muscles. The paralytic eye "looks down and out."

14–E. Dopaminergic neurons in the pars compacta of the substantia nigra contain melanin.

15–F. The mesencephalic nucleus of CN V contains pseudounipolar ganglion cells.

16–A. The cochlear nuclei give rise to the lateral lemniscus.

17–C. The inferior olivary nucleus projects via the inferior cerebellar peduncle to the contralateral cerebellum.

18–F. The mesencephalic nucleus provides the afferent limb of the jaw jerk reflex.

19–D. The superior salivatory nucleus of CN VII projects to the pterygopalatine (sphenopalatine) ganglion.

20–B. The nucleus gracilis and the nucleus cuneatus give rise, via internal arcuate fibers, to the medial lemniscus.

21–E. The substantia nigra projects dopaminergic fibers to the caudatoputamen (striatum).

22–B. The nucleus gracilis projects to the ventral posterolateral nucleus of the thalamus.

23–C. The inferior olivary nucleus receives input from the red nucleus via the ipsilateral central tegmental tract; the rubro-olivary tract is a component of the central tegmental tract.

10

Trigeminal System

I. Trigeminal Nerve (CN V) [Figure 10.1; see Figures 1.1, 9.1, and 9.7]

—is the largest cranial nerve.
—exits the brainstem from the pons.
—is the nerve of the first branchial arch (mandibular).
—contains sensory (general somatic afferent [GSA]) and motor (special visceral efferent [SVE]) fibers.
—provides sensory innervation to the face and oral cavity.
—innervates the dura of the anterior and middle cranial fossae.
—innervates the muscles of mastication.
—consists of a large ganglion that gives rise to three major divisions: **ophthalmic, maxillary, and mandibular**.

A. Trigeminal (or semilunar or gasserian) ganglion

—is located in the trigeminal fossa of the petrous bone in the middle cranial fossa.
—is enclosed by a duplication of the dura (Meckel's cave).
—contains pseudounipolar ganglion cells, which are first-order neurons for the trigeminothalamic tracts.
—consists of the following divisions:

1. Ophthalmic nerve (CN V-1)

—lies in the lateral wall of the **cavernous sinus**.
—enters the orbit via the **superior orbital fissure**.
—innervates the forehead, dorsum of the nose, upper eyelid, orbit (cornea and conjunctiva), mucous membranes of the nasal vestibule and frontal sinus, and the cranial dura.
—mediates the afferent limb of the **corneal reflex**.

2. Maxillary nerve (CN V-2)

—lies in the lateral wall of the **cavernous sinus**.
—exits the skull via the **foramen rotundum**.

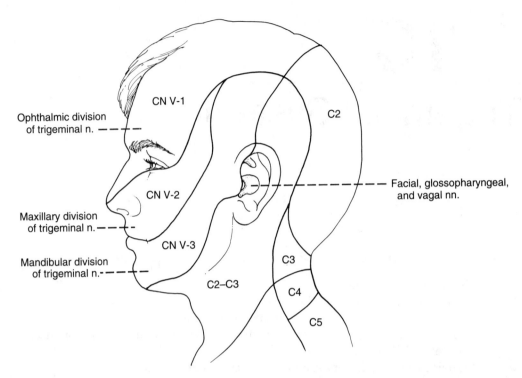

Figure 10.1. The cutaneous innervation of the head and upper neck. There is very little overlap between the three dermatomes of the trigeminal nerve (CN V). Note that the angle of the jaw is innervated by the cervical plexus (C2–C3). CN V-1 is the ophthalmic nerve; CN V-2 is the maxillary nerve; and CN V-3 is the mandibular nerve.

–innervates the upper lip and cheek, lower eyelid, anterior portion of the temple, paranasal sinuses, oral mucosa of the upper mouth, nose, pharynx, gums, teeth and palate of the upper jaw, and the cranial dura.

3. Mandibular nerve (CN V-3)

–exits the skull via the **foramen ovale**.

–consists of a motor component that innervates the **muscles of mastication** (temporalis, masseter, lateral and medial pterygoids); the mylohyoid and anterior belly of the **digastric muscles;** and the **tensores tympani** and **veli palatini**.

–consists of a sensory component that innervates the lower lip and chin, posterior portion of the temple, external auditory meatus and tympanic membrane, external ear, teeth of the lower jaw, oral mucosa of the cheeks and the floor of the mouth, anterior two-thirds of the tongue, temporomandibular joint, and the cranial dura.

B. Cranial nerves VII, IX, and X

–contribute GSA fibers from the external ear to the trigeminal system.

–use the spinal trigeminal tract and nucleus.

C. Spinal trigeminal tract

–extends from C3 to the level of the trigeminal nerve in the midpons.

–is a homolog of the dorsolateral tract of Lissauer.

–receives pain, temperature, and light touch input from CN V, CN VII, CN IX, and CN X.

−transection (**tractotomy**) results in ipsilateral facial anesthesia.

−projects to the spinal trigeminal nucleus as follows:

1. **Pain fibers** terminate in the caudal one-third of the spinal trigeminal nucleus.

2. **Corneal reflex fibers** terminate in the rostral two-thirds of the spinal trigeminal nucleus.

II. Ascending Trigeminothalamic Tracts

−convey GSA information from the face, oral cavity, and dura mater to the thalamus.

−consist of chains of three neurons.

−have their first-order neurons, pseudounipolar ganglion cells, in the trigeminal ganglion and in the sensory ganglia of CN VII, CN IX, and CN X.

A. Ventral trigeminothalamic tract (Figure 10.2)

−serves as a pain, temperature, and light touch pathway from the face and oral cavity.

−contains GSA fibers from CN VII, CN IX, and CN X (ear and external auditory meatus).

−receives input from free nerve endings and Merkel's tactile disks.

−receives discriminative tactile and pressure input from the contralateral principal sensory nucleus of CN V, which terminates in the ventral posteromedial (**VPM**) nucleus of the thalamus.

−ascends to the contralateral sensory cortex via three neurons:

1. First-order neurons

−are located in the trigeminal ganglion.

−mediate pain and temperature sensation and give rise to axons that descend in the spinal trigeminal tract.

−mediate light touch sensation and give rise to bifurcating axons that ascend and descend in the spinal trigeminal tract.

−synapse with second-order neurons in the spinal trigeminal nucleus.

2. Second-order neurons

−are located in the spinal trigeminal nucleus.

−give rise to decussating axons that terminate in the contralateral VPM nucleus of the thalamus.

−project axons to the reticular formation and to motor cranial nerve nuclei to mediate reflexes (e.g., tearing and corneal reflexes).

−mediate painful stimuli and are found in the caudal one-third of the spinal trigeminal nucleus.

3. Third-order neurons

−are located in the VPM nucleus.

−project via the posterior limb of the internal capsule to the face area of the postcentral gyrus (areas 3, 1, and 2).

B. Dorsal trigeminothalamic tract (see Figure 10.2)

−subserves discriminative tactile and pressure sensation from the face and oral cavity via the GSA fibers of CN V.

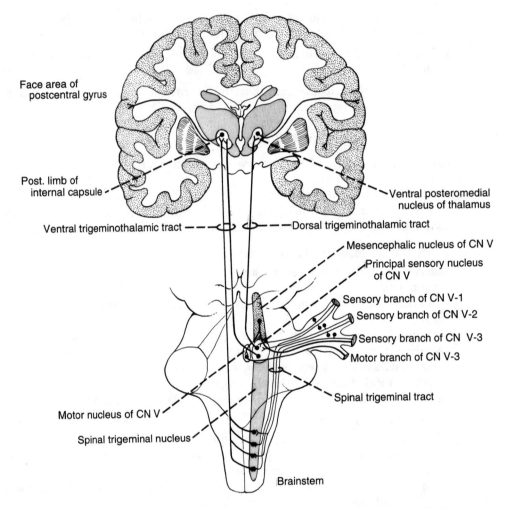

Figure 10.2. Diagram of the ventral (pain and temperature) and dorsal (discriminative touch) trigeminothalamic pathways.

—contains some discriminative **GSA fibers** from CN VII, CN IX, and CN X (ear).
—receives input from Meissner's and Pacini's corpuscles.
—is an uncrossed tract.
—is the rostral equivalent of the dorsal column–medial lemniscus system.
—ascends to the sensory cortex via three neurons:

1. First-order neurons

—are located in the trigeminal ganglion.
—synapse in the principal sensory nucleus of CN V.

2. Second-order neurons

—are located in the principal sensory nucleus of CN V.
—project to the ipsilateral VPM nucleus of the thalamus.

3. Third-order neurons

—are located in the VPM nucleus.

−project via the posterior limb of the internal capsule to the face area of the postcentral gyrus (areas 3, 1, and 2).

III. Trigeminal Sensory Nuclei (see Figures 9.1, 9.7–9.9, and 10.2)

A. Principal (or chief) sensory nucleus

−is located in the rostral pontine tegmentum at the level of the trigeminal motor nucleus of CN V.

−receives discriminative tactile input from the face.

−projects via the uncrossed dorsal trigeminothalamic tract to the VPM nucleus of the thalamus.

−projects via the crossed ventral trigeminothalamic tract to the VPM nucleus of the thalamus.

−is a homolog of the dorsal column nuclei of the medulla.

B. Spinal trigeminal nucleus

−is located in the spinal cord (C1–C3), medulla, and pons.

−receives pain and temperature input from the face and oral cavity.

−projects via the crossed ventral trigeminothalamic tract to the VPM nucleus of the thalamus.

C. Mesencephalic nucleus (see Figures 9.1, 9.7–9.9, and 10.2)

−subserves **GSA proprioception** from the head.

−consists of large pseudounipolar neurons similar to those found in the trigeminal and dorsal root ganglia.

−receives input from muscle spindles and pressure and joint receptors.

−receives input from the muscles of mastication and extraocular muscles, the teeth and hard palate, and the temporomandibular joint.

−projects to the trigeminal motor nucleus to mediate the muscle stretch (jaw jerk) reflex and regulate the force of bite.

D. Trigeminal motor nucleus (SVE) [see Figures 9.1, 9.7–9.9, and 10.2]

−is located in the rostral pontine tegmentum at the level of the principal sensory nucleus of CN V.

−innervates the muscles of mastication.

−receives bilateral corticobulbar input.

−receives input from the mesencephalic tract.

IV. Trigeminocerebellar Fibers

−project from the mesencephalic nucleus of CN V via the superior cerebellar peduncle to the dentate nucleus.

−project from the principal sensory and spinal trigeminal nuclei via the inferior cerebellar peduncle to the cerebellar vermis.

V. Trigeminal Reflexes

A. Jaw jerk (masseter) reflex

−is a monosynaptic myotatic reflex.

1. The **afferent limb** is the mandibular nerve (**CN V-3**).

2. The **efferent limb** is the mandibular nerve (**CN V-3**).

B. Corneal reflex

–is a consensual and disynaptic reflex.

–has its first-order neuron (afferent limb) in the trigeminal ganglion.

–has its second-order neuron in the rostral two-thirds of the spinal trigeminal nucleus.

–has its third-order neuron (efferent limb) in the facial nucleus.

1. The **afferent limb** is the ophthalmic nerve (**CN V-1**).

2. The **efferent limb** is the facial nerve (**CN VII**).

C. Lacrimal (tearing) reflex

1. The **afferent limb** is the ophthalmic nerve (**CN V-1**); it receives impulses from the cornea and conjunctiva.

2. The **efferent limb** is the facial nerve (**CN VII**): It transmits impulses via the superior salivatory nucleus, greater petrosal nerve, pterygopalatine ganglion, and the zygomatic (CN V-2) and lacrimal (CN V-1) nerves to the lacrimal gland (see Figure 13.3).

VI. Clinical Correlations

A. Trigeminal neuralgia

–is also called **tic douloureux**.

–is characterized by recurrent paroxysms of **sharp, stabbing pain** in one or more branches of the trigeminal nerve on one side of the face.

–usually occurs after 50 years of age and is more common in women than in men.

–can result from a redundant loop of the anterior inferior cerebellar artery that impinges on the trigeminal root; surgical treatment is the therapy of choice.

B. Central lesions of the spinal trigeminal tract and nucleus

–may result in a **loss of sensation,** occurring in an onion-peel distribution.

–the face is represented in the spinal trigeminal nucleus as a number of semicircular territories that extend from the perioral region to the ear.

–fibers innervating the mouth area terminate near the obex; fibers innervating the back of the head terminate in the upper cervical levels.

C. Acoustic neuroma (Schwannoma)

–is an extramedullary tumor of the vestibulocochlear nerve (CN VIII) that is found in the cerebellopontine angle or in the internal acoustic meatus.

–results in initial symptoms that include unilateral **tinnitus** and unilateral **hearing loss** as a result of a CN VIII lesion.

–results in symptoms that include **facial weakness and loss of corneal reflex** (efferent limb) due to facial nerve (CN VII) involvement.

–affects the trigeminal nerve (CN V) as the tumor expands, resulting in ipsilateral **loss of pain and temperature sensation and loss of the corneal reflex** (spinal trigeminal tract).

D. Cavernous sinus syndrome (Figure 10.3)

–may be caused by an aneurysm of the cavernous sinus.

–may involve any or all of the following cranial nerves:

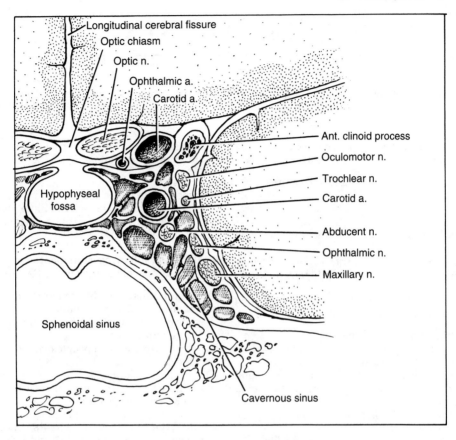

Figure 10.3. Diagram of the contents of the cavernous sinus. The ophthalmic (CN V-1) and maxillary (CN V-2) divisions of the trigeminal nerve (CN V) lie in the wall of the cavernous sinus. Other structures include CN III, CN IV, and CN VI, sympathetic fibers (not shown), and the internal carotid artery (cut twice).

1. **Ocular motor nerves of CN III, CN IV, and CN VI**
   –destruction of CN III results in complete **internal ophthalmoplegia** (parasympatheticoparesis).
2. **Trigeminal nerve branches of CN V-1 and CN V-2**
3. **Postganglionic sympathetic fibers to the orbit**
   –interruption results in **Horner's syndrome**.

Review Test

Directions: Each of the numbered items or incomplete statements in this section is followed by answers or by completions of the statement. Select the **one** lettered answer or completion that is **best** in each case.

1. All of the following statements concerning the spinal trigeminal tract are correct EXCEPT

(A) it contains axons from the trigeminal ganglion.
(B) it mediates pain and temperature sensation.
(C) it is equivalent to the dorsolateral tract of Lissauer.
(D) it is the afferent limb of the jaw jerk reflex.
(E) it extends from C3 to a midpontine level.

2. All of the following statements concerning the corneal reflex are correct EXCEPT

(A) it is a bisynaptic reflex.
(B) it is abolished ipsilaterally by transection of the facial nerve.
(C) it is abolished by a transection of the spinal trigeminal tract made within its caudal medullary extent.
(D) it is mediated via axons found in the spinal trigeminal tract.
(E) it is mediated via axons arising from the spinal trigeminal nucleus.

3. All of the following statements concerning the ventral tigeminothalamic tract are correct EXCEPT

(A) it transmits pain and temperature information.
(B) it consists of axons from the spinal trigeminal nucleus.
(C) it receives axons from the principal sensory nucleus of CN V.
(D) it projects to the contralateral VPM nucleus of the thalamus.
(E) first-order neurons are located in the mesencephalic nucleus.

4. The trigeminal motor nucleus innervates all of the following muscles EXCEPT the

(A) tensor tympani muscle.
(B) posterior belly of the digastric muscle.
(C) mylohyoid muscle.
(D) temporalis muscle.
(E) lateral and medial pterygoid muscles.

5. An aneurysm of the cavernous sinus could result in all of the following EXCEPT

(A) ptosis.
(B) anesthesia of the tongue.
(C) paralysis of the superior oblique muscle.
(D) complete internal ophthalmoplegia.
(E) diplopia.

6. All of the following statements concerning trigeminal neuralgia are correct EXCEPT

(A) it is characterized by recurrent paroxysms of sharp, lancinating pain.
(B) it occurs in any of the three divisions of the trigeminal nerve.
(C) it usually occurs in people over 50 years of age.
(D) it is more common in men than in women.
(E) it may result from pressure on the nerve from a nearby artery.

7. All of the following statements concerning the trigeminal ganglion are correct EXCEPT

(A) it lies in Meckel's cave.
(B) it lies in the middle cranial fossa.
(C) it contains bipolar ganglion cells.
(D) it contains first-order neurons of the dorsal trigeminothalamic tract.
(E) its destruction results in abolition of the corneal reflex and the jaw jerk reflex.

8. All of the following statements concerning the maxillary nerve are correct EXCEPT

(A) it runs in the lateral wall of the cavernous sinus.
(B) it exits the cranial vault via the foramen rotundum.
(C) it contains only GSA fibers.
(D) it innervates the skin of the dorsum of the nose.
(E) it innervates the palate.

9. All of the following statements concerning the mesencephalic nucleus are correct EXCEPT

(A) it projects to the cerebellum.
(B) it is located in the pons.
(C) it mediates the afferent limb of the jaw jerk reflex.
(D) it contains bipolar neurons.
(E) it receives input from muscle spindles.

10. All of the following statements concerning the dorsal trigeminothalamic tract are correct EXCEPT

(A) it is an uncrossed tract.
(B) it mediates two-point tactile discrimination.
(C) it mediates the corneal reflex.
(D) it projects to the VPM nucleus of the thalamus.
(E) its first-order neurons are found in the trigeminal ganglion.

11. All of the following statements concerning the principal sensory nucleus of CN V are correct EXCEPT

(A) it projects to the ipsilateral VPM nucleus of the thalamus.
(B) it projects to the contralateral VPM nucleus of the thalamus.
(C) it receives input from Meissner's and Pacini's corpuscles.
(D) it is located in the medulla and pons.
(E) it is a homolog to the dorsal column nuclei.

12. All of the following statements concerning the trigeminal nerve are correct EXCEPT

(A) it is the nerve of the first branchial arch (mandibular).
(B) it contains only GSA and SVE fibers.
(C) it innervates the stapedius muscle.
(D) it innervates the dura of the anterior and middle cranial fossae.
(E) it mediates the afferent limb of the corneal reflex.

Answers and Explanations

1–D. The afferent limb of the jaw jerk reflex, a myotactic (muscle stretch) reflex, is mediated by the pseudounipolar neurons of the mesencephalic nucleus; the efferent limb is mediated by the motor neurons of the trigeminal motor nucleus.

2–C. The afferent corneal reflex pathway is as follows: First-order neurons of the ophthalmic nerve (CN V-1) are found in the trigeminal ganglion. Their axons enter the pons and descend in the spinal trigeminal tract. They enter the spinal trigeminal nucleus in its rostral portion and synapse on second-order neurons, which project to the ipsilateral and contralateral facial nuclei. Axons from third-order neurons in the facial nuclei innervate the orbicularis oculi muscles bilaterally (directly and consensually). Trigeminal tractotomy at caudal levels produces facial anesthesia without interruption of the corneal reflex.

3–E. The mesencephalic nucleus does not contribute to the ventral trigeminothalamic tract. The ventral trigeminothalamic tract consists of axons from the spinal trigeminal nucleus that transmit pain and temperature information to the contralateral VPM nucleus. In addition, it receives and transmits tactile discriminatory input from the principal sensory nucleus of CN V to the VPM nucleus.

4–B. The posterior belly of the digastric muscle is innervated by the facial nerve (CN VII); the anterior belly of the digastric muscle is innervated by the trigeminal nerve (CN V).

5–B. An aneurysm of the cavernous sinus would not involve the mandibular nerve (CN V-3), which does not pass through the wall of the sinus. The mandibular nerve provides the sensory innervation of the anterior two-thirds of the tongue. Involvement of the oculomotor nerve (CN III), if complete, would result in internal ophthalmoplegia because of interruption of preganglionic parasympathetic fibers (a fixed, dilated, unresponsive pupil).

6–D. Trigeminal neuralgia is more common in women than in men, and it occurs most often on the right side of the face. A redundant loop of the anterior inferior cerebellar artery may impinge on the trigeminal nerve, causing electric "chatter," which is felt as pain. This type of trigeminal neuralgia has been successfully treated by placing a small sponge between the artery and the nerve. Classic idiopathic trigeminal neuralgia is treated with carbamazapine (Tegretol), an anticonvulsant drug.

7–C. The trigeminal (gasserian) ganglion lies within a dural duplication, Meckel's cave, located in the trigeminal fossa of the petrous portion of the temporal bone in the middle cranial fossa. It contains pseudounipolar ganglion cells similar to those found in the dorsal root ganglia. These first-order neurons give rise to the ventral and dorsal trigeminothalamic tracts. Destruction of the trigeminal ganglion interrupts the afferent limbs of the corneal (CN V-1) and jaw jerk (CN V-3) reflexes. The motor root of CN V lies between the ganglion and the petrous bone.

8–D. The maxillary nerve (CN V-2) contains only GSA fibers, runs in the lateral wall of the cavernous sinus, and exits the cranial vault via the foramen rotundum and canalis rotundus. It innervates the palate via the palatine nerves. The dorsum of the nose is innervated by the ophthalmic nerve (CN V-1).

9–D. The mesencephalic nucleus of CN V contains pseudounipolar neurons that mediate the afferent limb of the jaw jerk reflex. It is located in the rostral pons and in the mesencephalon and gives rise to collaterals that project to the cerebellum via the superior cerebellar peduncle. It receives input from muscle spindles and pressure and joint receptors.

10–C. The dorsal trigeminothalamic tract mediates discriminative tactile and pressure sensation (including two-point discrimination), is an uncrossed tract, and projects to the VPM nucleus. First-order neurons are in the trigeminal ganglion, second-order neurons lie in the principal sensory nucleus of the rostral pons, and third-order neurons are located in the VPM nucleus of the thalamus. This tract corresponds in function to the dorsal column–medial lemniscus system. The dorsal trigeminothalamic tract does not mediate the corneal reflex.

11–D. The principal sensory nucleus of CN V is located in the rostral pons at the level of the motor trigeminal nucleus; it receives input from Meissner's and Pacini's corpuscles. It projects to the ipsilateral VPM nucleus of the thalamus via the dorsal trigeminothalamic tract and to the contralateral VPM nucleus of the thalamus via the ventral trigeminothalamic tract. The principal sensory nucleus is homologous to the dorsal column nuclei (gracile and cuneate nuclei).

12–C. The trigeminal nerve (CN V) is the nerve of the first branchial arch (mandibular) and contains only GSA and SVE fibers. It innervates the supratentorial dura of the anterior and middle cranial fossae. The dura of the posterior cranial fossa is innervated by the vagal nerve (CN X) and the second and third spinal nerves (C2 and C3), which hitchhike with the hypoglossal nerve (CN XII). The tensor tympani muscle is innervated by the trigeminal nerve; the stapedius muscle is innervated by the facial nerve (CN VII). The ophthalmic nerve (CN V-1) mediates the afferent limb of the corneal reflex; the facial nerve (CN VII) mediates the efferent limb of the corneal reflex (orbicularis oculi muscle).

11

Auditory System

I. Introduction—The Auditory System

—is an exteroceptive special somatic afferent (SSA) system.
—detects sound frequencies from 20 Hz to 20,000 Hz.
—functions over an intensity range of 120 decibels (dB) and can discriminate changes in intensity between 1 dB and 2 dB.
—is characterized by tonotopic (pitch) localization at all levels of the neuraxis.

II. Outer, Middle, and Inner Ear

A. Outer ear

—consists of an **auricle** and an external auditory **meatus**.
—is separated from the middle ear by the tympanic membrane.
—conducts sound waves to the tympanic membrane.
—blockage (with wax) causes conduction deafness.

B. Middle ear (tympanic cavity)

—is located within the temporal bone.
—serves as an amplifier and impedance matching device.
—communicates with the nasopharynx via the auditory tube.
—receives its blood supply from the stylomastoid branch of the occipital or posterior auricular artery.
—receives sensory innervation mediated by the glossopharyngeal nerve (CN IX).
—contains the **chorda tympani** of CN VII, which mediates taste sensation and parasympathetic input into the submandibular and sublingual glands.
—pathology results in conduction deafness.
—contains the following auditory structures:

1. Tympanic membrane

—receives airborne sound vibrations and transmits energy to the middle ear ossicles.

2. Middle ear ossicles

—consist of the **malleus, incus, and stapes**.

—vibration of the tympanic membrane forces the footplate of the stapes into the oval window, creating a traveling wave in the perilymph-filled scala vestibuli.

3. Tensor tympani and stapedius muscles

—are innervated by the trigeminal and facial nerves, respectively.
—dampen vibrations of the ossicular chain, thus protecting the cochlea from loud low-frequency sounds (<1,000 Hz).

C. Inner ear (membranous labyrinth) [Figure 11.1]

—is derived from the otic placode of the rhombencephalon.
—is located within the **bony labyrinth** of the temporal bone.

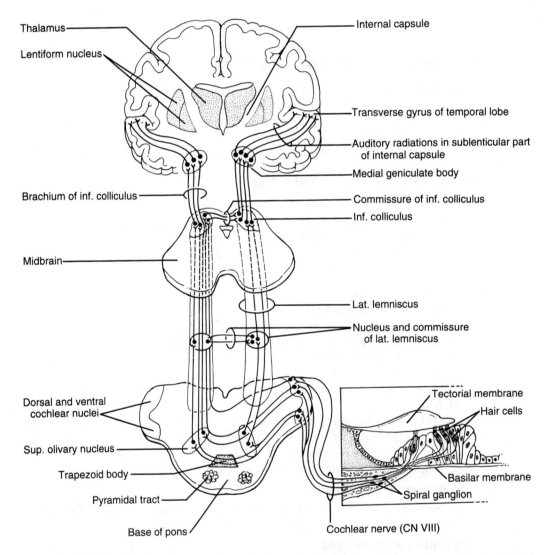

Figure 11.1. Peripheral and central connections of the auditory system. This system arises from the hair cells of the organ of Corti and terminates in the transverse temporal gyri of Heschl of the superior temporal gyrus. It is characterized by bilaterality of projections and tonotopic localization of pitch at all levels (e.g., high pitch, 20,000 Hz, is localized at the base of the cochlea and in the posteromedial part of the transverse temporal gyri).

—receives its blood supply from the labyrinthine artery, usually a branch of the anterior inferior cerebellar artery.

—contains the **cochlea,** which houses the following structures:

1. Scala vestibuli

—contains **perilymph**.

—transmits traveling waves toward the **helicotrema, scala tympani,** and **round window;** traveling waves extend to the portion of the basilar membrane that has the same resonant frequency, through the basilar membrane, and via the scala tympani to the round window.

2. Cochlear duct (scala media)

—contains the organ of Corti.

—contains **endolymph**.

—lies between the scala vestibuli and scala tympani.

3. Organ of Corti

—contains hair cells and the tectorial membrane.

—rests on and is supported by the basilar membrane.

—is a frequency analyzer.

4. Hair cells

—are auditory receptor cells that have **stereocilia** (microvilli) and no kinocilium. The stereocilia are embedded in the overlying tectorial membrane.

—are mechanoreceptors that transduce mechanical (sound) energy into generator potentials.

—are stimulated by vibrations of the basilar membrane.

—are innervated by bipolar neurons of the spiral ganglion.

—receive efferent input via the olivocochlear bundle.

5. Basilar membrane

—separates the cochlear duct from the scala tympani.

—has a pitch localization along its length: 20 Hz at the apex and 20,000 Hz at the base of the cochlea.

—vibration results in deformation of the hair cell microvilli against the tectorial membrane; this action serves as the adequate stimulus.

6. Spiral ganglion (of CN III)

—is located in the **bony modiolus** of the cochlea.

—consists of bipolar neurons of the cochlear division of the vestibulocochlear nerve (CN VIII).

III. Auditory Pathway (see Figure 11.1)

—is characterized by reciprocal connections throughout its caudorostral extent and by multiple decussations at all levels.

—consists of the following structures:

A. Hair cells of the organ of Corti

—are innervated by peripheral processes of bipolar cells of the spiral ganglion.

—consist of two types:

1. Inner hair cells

–synapse with numerous afferent fibers, each of which makes contact with only one hair cell; the majority of fibers in the cochlear nerve come from the inner hair cells.

2. Outer hair cells

–synapse with afferent fibers that contact numerous other outer hair cells.
–outnumber the inner hair cells three to one.

B. Bipolar cells of the spiral (cochlear) ganglion

–project peripherally to hair cells of the organ of Corti.
–project centrally as the **cochlear nerve** to the dorsal and ventral cochlear nuclei of the medullopontine junction.

C. Cochlear nerve (CN VIII) [see Figures 1.1, 9.5, and 11.1]

–extends from the spiral ganglion to the cerebellopontine angle, where it enters the brainstem.

D. Dorsal cochlear nucleus

–underlies the acoustic tubercle of the floor of the fourth ventricle.
–receives input from the cochlear nerve (CN VIII).
–projects contralaterally to the lateral lemniscus.

E. Ventral cochlear nucleus

–receives input from the cochlear nerve (CN VIII).
–projects bilaterally to the superior olivary nuclei.
–projects contralaterally to the lateral lemniscus.
–gives rise to the trapezoid body (ventral acoustic striae).

F. Superior olivary nucleus

–is located in the pons at the level of the facial nucleus.
–receives input from ventral cochlear nuclei.
–projects bilaterally to the lateral lemniscus.
–plays a role in sound localization and binaural processing.
–gives rise to the efferent olivocochlear bundle, a cochlear feedback pathway.

G. Trapezoid body

–is located in the caudal pontine tegmentum at the level of the abducent nucleus.
–is transversed by intra-axial abducent fibers of CN VI.
–contains decussating fibers from the ventral cochlear nucleus.

H. Lateral lemniscus

–receives input from the contralateral cochlear nuclei.
–receives input from the superior olivary nuclei.
–is connected to the contralateral lateral lemniscus via commissural fibers.
–projects to the nucleus of the inferior colliculus.

I. Nucleus of the inferior colliculus

–receives input from the lateral lemniscus.
–projects via the **brachium of the inferior colliculus** to the medial geniculate body.
–projects to the superior colliculus to mediate audiovisual reflexes.

J. Medial geniculate body (see Figures 1.6 and 11.1)

−receives input from the nucleus of the inferior colliculus.

−projects via the **auditory radiation** to the primary auditory cortex, the transverse gyri of Heschl (areas 41 and 42).

K. Auditory radiation (see Figures 11.1 and 16.3)

−extends from the medial geniculate body via the posterior limb of the internal capsule to the transverse gyri of Heschl.

L. Transverse temporal gyri of Heschl (see Figure 11.1)

−contain the primary auditory cortex (areas 41 and 42).

−are located in the depths of the lateral sulcus.

−receive auditory input via the auditory radiation.

−project to the auditory association cortex (area 22).

IV. Efferent Cochlear (Olivocochlear) Bundle

−is a crossed and uncrossed tract that arises from the superior olivary nucleus and projects to the hair cells of the organ of Corti.

−suppresses auditory nerve activity when stimulated.

−plays a role, through inhibition, in "auditory sharpening."

V. Hearing Defects

−may be classified as:

A. Conduction deafness

−is caused by interruption of the passage of sound waves through the external or middle ear.

−includes the following causes:

1. Obstruction by wax (cerumen) or a foreign body in the external auditory meatus

2. Otosclerosis

−is produced by neogenesis of the labyrinthine spongy bone around the oval window, resulting in fixation of the stapes.

−is the most frequent cause of progressive conduction deafness.

3. Otitis media

−is an **inflammation of the middle ear**.

−is the most common cause of meningitis (excluding meningococcus) and the most common cause of brain abscesses.

B. Nerve deafness (sensorineural or perceptive deafness)

−is due to **disease** of the cochlea, cochlear nerve, or central auditory connections (acoustic neuroma).

−may result from the **action of drugs and toxins** (e.g., quinine, aspirin, and streptomycin).

−may result from **prolonged exposure to loud noise** (industrial noise or rock music [high frequency loss]).

−may result from **rubella infection in utero**.

−includes the following:

1. Presbycusis

–is **hearing loss occurring with aging**. It results from degenerative disease of the organ of Corti in the first few millimeters of the basal coil of the cochlea (high frequency loss of 4000 Hz to 8000 Hz).

–is the most common cause of hearing loss.

2. Acoustic neuroma

–consists of a **schwannoma** (neurilemoma) of the vestibulocochlear nerve (CN VIII).

–is located in the internal auditory meatus or in the cerebellopontine angle of the posterior cranial fossa.

–symptoms include **unilateral deafness** and **tinnitus** (ear ringing)

VI. Tuning Fork Tests

–are used to distinguish between conduction deafness and nerve deafness (sensorineural deafness).

–compare air conduction with bone conduction.

A. Weber test

–is performed by placing a vibrating tuning fork on the vertex of the skull.

–normal subject hears equally on both sides.

–patient with unilateral conduction deafness hears the vibration louder in the diseased ear.

–patient with unilateral partial nerve deafness hears the vibration louder in the normal ear.

B. Rinne test

–compares air and bone conduction.

–is performed by placing a vibrating tuning fork on the mastoid process until it is no longer heard; then it is held in front of the ear.

–normal subject hears vibration in the air after bone conduction is gone.

–patient with unilateral conduction deafness fails to hear vibrations in the air after bone conduction is gone.

–patient with unilateral partial nerve deafness hears vibration in the air after bone conduction is gone.

C. Schwabach test

–compares bone conduction of a patient with that of a person with normal hearing.

–shows bone conduction to be better than normal in cases of conduction deafness.

–shows bone conduction to be less than normal in cases of nerve deafness.

Review Test

Directions: Each of the numbered items or incomplete statements in this section is followed by answers or by completions of the statement. Select the **one** lettered answer or completion that is **best** in each case.

1. All of the following statements concerning conduction deafness are correct EXCEPT

(A) the sound of a vibrating tuning fork placed on the vertex is heard best in the deaf ear.
(B) it may be the result of an acoustic neuroma.
(C) it may be the result of otosclerosis.
(D) it may be the result of otitis media.
(E) it may be the result of wax in the external auditory meatus.

2. All of the following statements concerning nerve deafness are correct EXCEPT

(A) in patients with partial nerve deafness, air conduction is better than bone conduction.
(B) it may result from a middle ear infection.
(C) it may result from a tumor in the internal auditory meatus.
(D) it may result from toxins and drugs.
(E) it may result from degenerative disease of the organ of Corti.

3. The auditory pathway includes all of the following structures EXCEPT the

(A) trapezoid body.
(B) nucleus of the inferior colliculus.
(C) inferior olivary nucleus.
(D) lateral lemniscus.
(E) medial geniculate body.

4. All of the following statements concerning the auditory system are correct EXCEPT

(A) the membranous labyrinth is irrigated by a branch of the anterior inferior cerebellar artery.
(B) it is characterized by multiple decussations at all levels.
(C) it is characterized by pitch localization at all levels.
(D) it detects sound frequencies from 20 Hz to 50 kHz.
(E) it can discriminate intensity changes between 1 dB and 2 dB.

5. All of the following statements concerning the tympanic cavity are correct EXCEPT

(A) it contains the chorda tympani.
(B) it contains parasympathetic input to the submandibular and sublingual glands.
(C) it contains two striated muscles.
(D) it communicates with the nasopharynx.
(E) it receives sensory innervation by the vagal nerve.

6. All of the following statements concerning the organ of Corti are correct EXCEPT

(A) it receives input from the brainstem.
(B) it is innervated by bipolar neurons of the spiral ganglion.
(C) it contains mechanoreceptors.
(D) it contains inner and outer hair cells.
(E) it is a structure of the middle ear.

7. All of the following statements concerning the basilar membrane are correct EXCEPT

(A) it separates the cochlear duct from the scala tympani.
(B) it has a pitch localization along its length.
(C) it is in contact with endolymph.
(D) it gives rise to the tectorial membrane.
(E) its destruction at the apex of the cochlea results in a hearing loss in the low frequency range.

8. All of the following statements concerning the hair cells of the organ of Corti are correct EXCEPT

(A) they are mechanoreceptors.
(B) they project centrally to the cochlear nuclei.
(C) they are stimulated by vibrations of the basilar membrane.
(D) they are derived from the otic placode of the rhombencephalon.
(E) they contain stereocilia that are embedded in the tectorial membrane.

Answers and Explanations

1–B. Conduction deafness is produced by interruption of the passage of sound waves through the external or middle ear. An acoustic neuroma is a tumor of the vestibulocochlear nerve located in the internal auditory meatus or in the cerebellopontine angle of the posterior cerebral fossa. This tumor causes unilateral nerve deafness. In conduction deafness, a vibrating tuning fork placed on the vertex of the skull would be heard best in the deaf ear; this is the Weber test.

2–B. Sensorineural or nerve deafness results from damage to the organ of Corti, the cochlear nerve, or the central neural pathway. Middle ear infection (otitis media) results in conduction deafness. In patients with partial nerve deafness, air conduction is greater than bone conduction.

3–C. The inferior olivary nucleus is a cerebellar relay nucleus found in the medulla. The superior olivary nucleus is an important way station in the auditory pathway; it is found in the pons at the level of the facial nucleus.

4–D. The auditory system detects sound frequencies from 20 Hz to 20,000 Hz. The membranous labyrinth is perfused by the labyrinthine artery; this is usually a branch of the anterior inferior cerebellar artery (85%), but in some cases it is a direct branch of the basilar artery (15%).

5–E. The tympanic cavity contains the chorda tympani (of CN VII), which supplies taste to the anterior two-thirds of the tongue. The chorda tympani also contains parasympathetic input to the submandibular and sublingual glands. It contains two striated muscles, the tensor tympani (innervated by CN V) and the stapedius (innervated by CN VII). It communicates, via the auditory tube, with the nasopharynx. The tympanic branch of the glossopharyngeal nerve (CN IX) innervates the mucosa of the middle ear.

6–E. The organ of Corti, an inner ear structure, lies within the cochlear duct. It contains the peripheral receptor cells of the auditory system, the inner and outer hair cells. Hair cells are mechanoreceptors, receive input from the brainstem via the efferent cochlear bundle, and are innervated by bipolar neurons of the spiral ganglion (of CN VIII).

7–D. The basilar membrane supports the organ of Corti, separates the cochlear duct from the scala tympani, and is in contact with both endolymph and perilymph. The basilar membrane has a pitch localization along its length; high frequencies are registered at the base of the cochlea, low frequencies at the apex. The tectorial membrane is a projection of the spiral limbus that overlies the hair cells of the organ of Corti.

8–B. The hair cells of the spiral ganglion of Corti are mechanoreceptors. Vibrations of the basilar membrane force the stereocilia (microvilli) of the hair cells against the overlying tectorial membrane; this shearing force is the adequate stimulus. Hair cells stimulate the afferent bipolar neurons of the spiral ganglion, which project centrally to the cochlear nuclei of the brainstem. The inner ear is derived from the otic placode of the rhombencephalon.

12
Vestibular System

I. Introduction—The Vestibular System

–is a special somatic afferent (**SSA**) proprioceptive system.

–maintains **posture** and **equilibrium** and coordinates **head and eye movements**.

–functions in concert with the cerebellum and the visual system.

–contains receptors (hair cells) that are located in the labyrinth of the temporal bone.

II. Labyrinth (Figure 12.1)

–constitutes the inner ear **(auris interna)** of the temporal bone.

A. Structure

1. Bony labyrinth

–is a series of cavities (the cochlea, the vestibule, and the semicircular canals) that lodge the membranous labyrinth.

–contains **perilymph,** which fills the space between the bony labyrinth and the membranous labyrinth.

2. Membranous labyrinth

–is suspended within the bony labyrinth.

–is filled with **endolymph**.

–is a closed system; endolymph and perilymph do not mix.

–contains receptor (or hair) cells that are bathed in endolymph.

B. Function

1. Semicircular canal system (kinetic labyrinth)

–detects and responds to angular acceleration and deceleration of the head.

–consists of three **semicircular canals**.

–includes the following structures:

a. Three semicircular ducts

–consist of anterior, posterior, and lateral structures that lie in mutually perpendicular planes; each semicircular duct lies within a semicircular canal.

–contain hair cells.

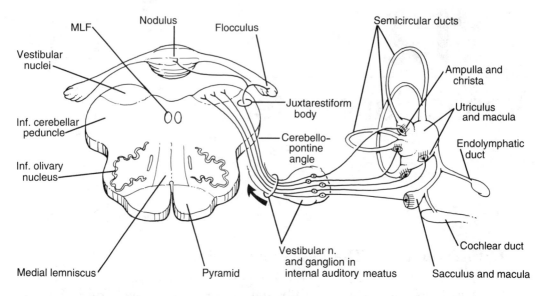

Figure 12.1. Peripheral connections of the vestibular system. Hair cells of the cristae ampullares and the macullae of the utricle and saccule project, via the vestibular nerve, to the vestibular nuclei of the medulla and pons and to the flocculonodular lobe of the cerebellum (vestibulocerebellum).

b. Hair cells

–are embedded in the **cupulae of the cristae ampullares**.
–are bathed in endolymph.
–contain one **kinocilium** and many **stereocilia**.
–are innervated by bipolar cells of the vestibular ganglion (Scarpa's ganglion).
–receive inhibitory input from vestibular nuclei.
–are stimulated by endolymphatic flow. Flow toward the kinocilium and the utricle is excitatory; flow away from the kinocilium is inhibitory.

2. Utricle and saccule (static labyrinth)

–detect and respond to the position of the head with respect to **linear acceleration** and the pull of **gravity**.
–are endolymph-containing dilatations of the membranous labyrinth.
–are located within the vestibule of the bony labyrinth.
–contain hair cells in the macula of the utricle and the macula of the saccule.

a. Maculae of the utricle and saccule

–are two patches of sensory epithelium.
–consist of supporting cells and hair cells.

b. Hair cells

–are structurally similar to those of the cristae ampullares.
–are embedded in the gelatinous **otolithic membrane,** which contains calcareous otolith crystals.
–are stimulated by the shearing effect of the otolithic membrane during head movements.
–receive an efferent innervation from the vestibular nuclei of the brainstem.

C. Fluids of the labyrinth

1. Perilymph

—resembles extracellular fluid and surrounds the membranous labyrinth (in the perilymphatic space).

—communicates with the subarachnoid space via the **perilymphatic duct of the cochlear canaliculus**.

—site of production and absorption is unknown.

2. Endolymph

—resembles intracellular fluid and is found within the membranous labyrinth (endolymphatic space).

—is secreted by the **stria vascularis** of the cochlear duct.

—is thought to be absorbed by the **endolymphatic sac**.

III. Vestibular Pathways (Figure 12.2; see Figure 12.1)

A. Hair cells

—see labyrinth, p 155.

B. Bipolar neurons of the vestibular ganglion (see Figure 12.1)

—are located in the fundus of the **internal auditory meatus**.

—project, via their peripheral processes, to hair cells.

—project their central processes, as the **vestibular nerve,** to the **vestibular nuclei** of the medulla and pons and, via the juxtarestiform body, to the **flocculonodular lobe** of the cerebellum (vestibulocerebellum).

C. Vestibular nuclei (see Figures 9.4–9.6)

—include the inferior, medial, superior, and lateral nuclei.

1. Receive input from:

a. Bipolar neurons of the vestibular ganglion

b. Flocculonodular lobe and uvula of the cerebellum

c. Vermis of the anterior lobe of the cerebellum

d. Vestibular nuclei of the contralateral side

e. Fastigial nuclei of the cerebellum

2. Project fibers to the:

a. Flocculonodular lobe and uvula of the cerebellum

b. Vestibular nuclei of the contralateral side

c. Inferior olivary nucleus

—receives input via the vestibulo-olivary tract.

—mediates vestibular influence to the caudal vermis of the cerebellum.

d. Abducent, trochlear, and oculomotor nuclei

—receive input via the medial longitudinal fasciculus (**MLF**).

e. Ventral horn motor neurons

—receive vestibular input from two descending pathways:

(1) MLF

—contains fibers from the medial vestibular nucleus that terminate in cervical and upper thoracic levels.

—coordinates head, neck, and eye movements.

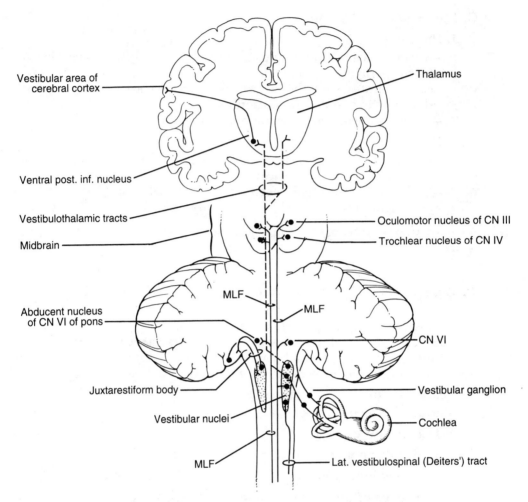

Figure 12.2. Major central connections of the vestibular system. Vestibular nuclei project via the ascending medial longitudinal fasciculi (MLFs) to the ocular motor nuclei and subserve vestibulo-ocular reflexes; they project, via the descending MLFs and the lateral vestibulospinal tracts, to the ventral horn motor neurons of the spinal cord and mediate postural reflexes.

(2) Vestibulospinal tract

–contains fibers from the ipsilateral lateral vestibular nucleus and is found at all spinal cord levels.

–facilitates extensor muscle tone in the antigravity muscles, thus maintaining upright posture.

f. Ventral posteroinferior (VPI) and ventral posterolateral (VPL) nuclei of the thalamus

–receive bilateral input from the vestibular nuclei.

D. VPI and VPL nuclei of the thalamus

–project to the primary vestibular cortex of the parietal lobe (VPI to area 2v; VPL to area 3a).

IV. Efferent Vestibular Connections

—arise from neurons found in the vestibular nuclei.

—exit the brainstem with the vestibular nerve and innervate hair cells in the cristae ampullares and maculae of the utricle and saccule.

—are thought to modulate the spontaneous firing rate of vestibular nerve fibers.

V. Medial Longitudinal Fasciculus

—extends from the spinal cord to the rostral midbrain.

—contains ascending vestibulo-ocular fibers to the ocular motor nuclei of CN III, CN IV, and CN VI.

—contains a descending medial vestibulospinal tract that coordinates head and eye movements.

—mediates adduction of the eyeball in lateral conjugate gaze on command.

—mediates vestibular nystagmus.

—transection results in medial rectus palsy on attempted lateral gaze; convergence is unaffected.

VI. Vestibulo-ocular Reflexes

—may be tested in conscious or unconscious subjects by stimulating the kinetic labyrinth.

A. Doll's head eye phenomenon (oculocephalic reflex)

—is not present in normal alert persons unless they voluntarily fix vision.

1. Test method

—consists of rapid movement of the patient's head in horizontal or vertical planes.

2. Test results

—with intact proprioception and brainstem (vestibular nuclei), the eyes move conjugately in the opposite direction.

—doll's head eye movements are absent or abnormal when lesions of the vestibular nuclei and MLFs are present.

B. Vestibular nystagmus

—consists of involuntary to and fro, up and down, or rotary movements of one or both eyes.

—consists of a slow component, opposite the direction of rotation, and a fast compensatory component, in the direction of rotation.

—is named after the fast component.

—results from the stimulation of hair cells within the semicircular ducts upon rotation, or after caloric irrigation of the external auditory meatus with hot or cold water.

C. Postrotational nystagmus

1. Test method

a. The subject sits in a Bárány chair with head erect and inclined 30° forward (to place horizontal canals in the plane of rotation).

b. The subject is rotated to the right 10 turns within 20 seconds, after which he is suddenly stopped.

2. Test results

a. The subject with normal labyrinths will have a horizontal nystagmus to the left (fast phase).

b. The subject will past-point (dysmetria), tend to fall to the right, and experience a sensation of turning (vertigo) to the left.

c. The induced nystagmus usually lasts 15–40 seconds.

D. Caloric nystagmus

—may be induced with cold or hot water irrigation of the external auditory meatus.

—may be used to stimulate each labyrinth separately.

—may be used to evaluate unconscious patients.

—may be used to stimulate individual semicircular canals.

1. Test method used to stimulate the horizontal semicircular canal

a. While sitting erect, the subject tilts his head back 60°, or the recumbent subject elevates his head 30° from a horizontal position.

b. Cold or hot water is syringed into the external ear canal.

2. Test results in normal subjects

a. Cold water irrigation results in nystagmus to the opposite side and past-pointing and falling to the same side.

b. Hot water irrigation results in the reverse reactions.

c. Remember the mnemonic **COWS = C**old, **O**pposite; **W**arm, **S**ame.

VII. Decerebrate and Decorticate Rigidity

—descending vestibulospinal and pontoreticulospinal pathways play an important role in the control of extensor muscle tone.

—transection of the brainstem or decortication results in a tremendous increase in antigravity tone.

A. Decerebrate rigidity (posturing)

—results from a lesion that transects the brainstem between the red nucleus and the vestibular nuclei.

—results in posture that is characterized by **opisthotonos,** which is extension, adduction, and hyperpronation of the arms, and extension of the feet with plantar flexion.

—in its classic form is also known as **gamma rigidity**.

—can be abolished by section of the vestibular nerve, destruction of vestibular nuclei or the vestibulospinal tract, and dorsal or ventral rhizotomy.

B. Decorticate rigidity (posturing)

—usually results from lesions of the internal capsule or the cerebral hemisphere.

—results in posture that consists of flexion of the arm, wrist, and fingers, with adduction in the upper extremity; and with extension, internal rotation, and plantar flexion in the lower extremity.

—is characterized by a motor pattern that is typical of chronic spastic hemiplegia.

–is known as **bilateral spastic hemiplegia,** in the form of bilateral decorticate rigidity.

VIII. Clinical Correlations

A. Vertigo

–is a sensation of irregular or whirling motion; it is an **illusion of movement**.

–is usually a result of vestibular or cerebellar disease.

B. Ménière's disease

–is an inner ear disease associated with an **increase in endolymphatic fluid pressure**.

–is characterized by episodic attacks of vertigo, tinnitus, hearing loss, nausea, vomiting, and a sensation of fullness and pressure in the ear.

–is characterized by the presence of horizontal nystagmus during the attack. The fast phase is to the opposite ear; past-pointing and falling are to the affected side.

C. Labyrinthitis

–is characterized by **inflammation of the labyrinth,** which may result from bacterial, viral, or toxic (e.g., alcohol, quinine, salicylates) causes.

–exhibits the same symptoms that are seen in Ménière's disease (see above).

D. Labyrinthectomy

1. Unilateral labyrinthectomy

–results in predominantly horizontal nystagmus directed to the opposite side.

2. Bilateral simultaneous labyrinthectomy

–does not give rise to nystagmus.

E. Benign positional vertigo

–is the most common cause of recurrent vertigo.

–is elicited by certain head positions; the paroxysm of vertigo is accompanied by nystagmus.

–is *not* associated with hearing loss or tinnitus.

–is due presumably to **cuprolithiasis** of the posterior semicircular duct (dislocation of the utricular macular otoliths).

F. MLF syndrome (internuclear ophthalmoplegia)

–consists of medial rectus paresis on attempted lateral gaze.

–is associated with monocular horizontal nystagmus in the abducting eye and intact convergence (this is diagnostically important).

–is usually the result of a demyelinating plaque.

–is most commonly seen in **multiple sclerosis**.

Review Test

Directions: Each of the numbered items or incomplete statements in this section is followed by answers or by completions of the statement. Select the **one** lettered answer or completion that is **best** in each case.

1. A patient sitting erect with his head inclined 30° forward was rotated to the right 10 turns in 20 seconds, after which he was suddenly stopped. All of the following signs and symptoms will be experienced EXCEPT

(A) the patient would have a vertical nystagmus.
(B) the fast phase of the nystagmus would be to the left.
(C) the slow phase of the nystagmus would be to the right.
(D) the patient would past-point to the right.
(E) the patient would experience a sensation of turning to the left.

2. Which of the following statements concerning caloric induced nystagmus is false?

(A) Cold water irrigation of the left ear results in nystagmus to the right (fast phase).
(B) Cold water irrigation of the left ear results in past-pointing to the left.
(C) Caloric testing permits the evaluation of the individual semicircular ducts.
(D) Caloric testing is contraindicated in comatose patients.
(E) Hot water irrigation results in the reverse reactions.

3. All of the following statements concerning decerebrate rigidity are correct EXCEPT

(A) it results from a lesion transecting the brainstem between the superior and inferior colliculi.
(B) it is considered to be alpha rigidity.
(C) it is characterized by opisthotonos with arms and legs extended and adducted.
(D) it can be abolished by dorsal root rhizotomy.
(E) it can be abolished by section of the vestibular nerve.

4. Which of the following statements concerning decorticate rigidity is false?

(A) Decorticate rigidity results from hemispheric lesions.
(B) Decorticate rigidity usually results from lesions of the internal capsule.
(C) Decorticate rigidity consists of extension and adduction of the arms and legs.
(D) Bilateral decorticate rigidity is bilateral spastic hemiplegia.
(E) Plantar responses are extensor on the affected side.

5. Vestibular nuclei project to all of the following structures EXCEPT the

(A) inferior olivary nucleus.
(B) ventral horn motor neurons.
(C) dentate nuclei of the cerebellum.
(D) VPI nucleus of the thalamus.
(E) VPL nucleus of the thalamus.

6. The membranous labyrinth contains all of the following EXCEPT

(A) the cristae ampullares.
(B) the semicircular ducts.
(C) the organ of Corti.
(D) the maculae of the sacculi and utriculi.
(E) the spiral ganglion.

7. Which of the following statements concerning the semicircular ducts is false?

(A) They are three in number.
(B) They contain endolymph.
(C) They contain hair cells.
(D) They are found within the vestibule.
(E) They comprise the kinetic labyrinth.

8. All of the following statements concerning the hair cells of the vestibular apparatus are correct EXCEPT

(A) hair cells contain one kinocilium and many stereocilia (microvilli).
(B) hair cells of the semicircular ducts are stimulated by perilymphatic flow.
(C) hair cells are innervated by bipolar cells found in the internal auditory meatus.
(D) hair cells are found in the cristae ampullares.
(E) hair cells are found in the maculae of the saccule and utricle.

9. All of the following statements concerning the static labyrinth are correct EXCEPT

(A) it responds to linear acceleration.
(B) it responds to the pull of gravity.
(C) it lies within the vestibule of the bony labyrinth.
(D) it includes the macula of the utricle.
(E) it is tested clinically by caloric stimulation.

10. All of the following statements concerning the vestibular ganglion are correct EXCEPT

(A) it lies within the bony modiolus.
(B) it innervates the hair cells of the cristae ampullares.
(C) it innervates the hair cells of the utricle and saccule.
(D) it contains bipolar ganglion cells.
(E) it projects directly to the cerebellar cortex.

11. All of the following statements concerning the vestibular nuclei are correct EXCEPT they

(A) are three in number.
(B) receive input from the fastigial nuclei.
(C) project to the MLF.
(D) project to the nuclei of the extraocular muscles.
(E) are found in the medulla and pons.

12. All of the following statements concerning the lateral vestibulospinal tract are correct EXCEPT

(A) it arises from the lateral vestibular nucleus.
(B) it is located in the ventral funiculus of the spinal cord.
(C) it is found at all spinal cord levels.
(D) it facilitates extensor muscle tone in antigravity muscles.
(E) it is a crossed pathway.

13. All of the following statements concerning the MLF are correct EXCEPT

(A) it is located in the midbrain.
(B) it is located in the spinal cord.
(C) it contains vestibulo-oculomotor fibers.
(D) it mediates adduction in lateral conjugate gaze on command.
(E) transection results in paralysis of convergence.

14. All of the following statements concerning vestibular nystagmus are correct EXCEPT

(A) it is named after the fast component.
(B) it has a slow component that is opposite the direction of rotation.
(C) it may be horizontal, vertical, or rotatory.
(D) it is frequently associated with nausea and vertigo.
(E) irrigation of the external auditory meatus with ice water results in nystagmus to the same side.

15. All of the following statements concerning the primary vestibular cortex are correct EXCEPT

(A) it receives input from the ventral posterior inferior nucleus.
(B) it receives input from the VPL nucleus.
(C) it is located in areas 2 and 3.
(D) it is located in the somesthetic cortex.
(E) it is located in the paracentral lobule.

Directions: Each group of items in this section consists of lettered options followed by a set of numbered items. For each item, select the **one** lettered option that is most closely associated with it. Each lettered option may be selected once, more than once, or not at all.

Questions 16–20

Match each characteristic with the condition it best describes.

(A) Ménière's disease
(B) Benign positional vertigo
(C) Labyrinthitis
(D) MLF syndrome
(E) Multiple sclerosis

16. Is the most common cause of recurrent vertigo

17. Is an inner ear disease associated with increased endolymphatic fluid pressure

18. Presumably is due to cuprolithiasis of a semicircular canal

19. Is the most common cause of internuclear ophthalmoplegia

20. Consists of lateral gaze palsy and monocular nystagmus

Answers and Explanations

1–A. Forward 30° inclination of the erect head would result in maximal stimulation of the cristae ampullares of the lateral (horizontal) semicircular ducts. Rotation of this plane would result in horizontal nystagmus.

2–D. One of the advantages of caloric stimulation is that it can be used safely in all states of consciousness. Caloric testing enables the examiner to evaluate the individual semicircular canals separately. Past-pointing and falling is to the side of irrigation. Remember the mnemonic for calorics: COWS = Cold, Opposite; Warm, Same.

3–B. Classic decerebrate (posturing) rigidity is considered to be gamma rigidity. Alpha rigidity is seen when the anterior cerebellum of a decerebrate preparation is infarcted.

4–C. Decorticate posturing consists of flexion of the arm, wrist, and fingers, with adduction in the upper extremity, and extension, internal rotation, and plantar flexion in the lower extremity (e.g., the hemiparetic gait and posture of a stroke victim). The plantar reflex in the affected extremity would be extensor (i.e., Babinski's sign).

5–C. Vestibular nuclei do not project to the dentate nucleus. Major vestibular projections are to the flocculonodular lobe of the cerebellum, ocular motor nuclei via the MLF, spinal cord, inferior olivary nucleus, and VPI and VPL nuclei of the thalamus.

6–E. The membranous labyrinth contains endolymph and includes the three semicircular ducts, the utricle and saccule, the endolymphatic duct and sac, and the cochlear duct. The organ of Corti lies within the cochlear duct; the maculae lie within the saccule and utricle. The spiral (cochlear) ganglion lies in the modiolus of the temporal bone.

7–D. The three semicircular (membranous) ducts lie within the three semicircular (osseus) canals of the petrous part of the temporal bone. They contain endolymph and have hair cells within the cristae ampullares. The kinetic labyrinth consists of the semicircular ducts; the static labyrinth consists of the utricle and saccule. The vestibule is a central cavity of the inner ear that contains the saccule and the utricle.

8–B. The hair cells of the vestibular apparatus contain one kinocilium and many stereocilia (microvilli). Hair cells of the semicircular ducts are stimulated by endolymphatic flow (not perilymphatic flow); they are innervated by bipolar cells found in the fundus of the internal auditory meatus. Hair cells are found in the cristae ampullares and in the maculae of the utricle and saccule.

9–E. The static labyrinth consists of the utricle and saccule, which are found in the vestibule of the bony labyrinth. The hair cells of the maculae of the utricule and saccule respond to linear acceleration and deceleration and gravitational pull. Introduction of warm or cold water into the external auditory meatus stimulates the hair cells of the semicircular ducts (i.e., the kinetic labyrinth).

10–A. The vestibular ganglion of Scarpa lies in the fundus of the internal auditory meatus. It contains bipolar neurons that innervate the hair cells of the cristae ampullares and the maculae of the utricle and the sacculus. Bipolar neurons project centrally to the vestibular nuclei of the brainstem and the flocculonodular lobe of the cerebellum. The spiral (cochlear) ganglion of the cochlear nerve lies in the modiolus of the petrosal bone.

11–A. There are four vestibular nuclei: lateral, medial, inferior, and superior. They receive input from the fastigial nuclei via the uncinate fasciculus and the juxtarestiform body. Vestibulocerebellar fibers project to the nodulus, flocculus, and uvula but not to the fastigial nucleus. They project via the MLF to the ocular motor nuclei (of CN III, CN IV, and CN VI). Vestibular nuclei are found in the medulla and pons.

12–E. The lateral vestibulospinal tract arises from the ipsilateral lateral vestibular nucleus of Deiters, located in the lateral pontine tegmentum, and descends to all spinal cord levels in the ventral funiculus. It facilitates extensor muscle tone in the antigravity muscles. It is an uncrossed tract.

13–E. Transection of the MLF results in a medial rectus palsy on attempted lateral gaze; convergence remains intact. The MLF extends from the spinal cord to the rostral midbrain; it contains vestibulo-oculomotor fibers that mediate eye movements in response to head and neck posture. It carries fibers to the medial rectus subnucleus from the pontine lateral conjugate gaze center.

14–E. Nystagmus is named after the fast component; the slow component is opposite the direction of rotation, thus maintaining visual fixation. Nystagmus may be horizontal, vertical, or rotatory and is frequently associated with nausea, vomiting, and vertigo. Irrigation of the external auditory meatus (with the head tilted back 60°) with ice water results in nystagmus to the opposite side. Remember the mnemonic COWS = Cold, Opposite; Warm, Same.

15–E. The primary vestibular cortex (areas 2v and 3a) is located in the postcentral gyrus, the somesthetic cortex of the parietal lobe. The vestibular cortex receives input from the VPI, VPL, and the ventral lateral nuclei of the thalamus. The paracentral lobule is a continuation of the motor and sensory strips onto the medial surface of the hemisphere; it receives no vestibular input.

16–B Benign positional vertigo is the most common cause of vertigo.

17–A. Ménière's disease is an inner ear disease associated with increased endolymphatic fluid pressure.

18–B. Benign positional vertigo is presumably due to cuprolithiasis of the posterior semicircular duct (dislocation of the utricular macular otoliths).

19–E. Multiple sclerosis is the most common cause of MLF syndrome (internuclear ophthalmoplegia).

20–D. MLF syndrome consists of a medial rectus palsy on attempted lateral gaze and uniocular horizontal nystagmus in the adducting eye. Convergence is intact.

13

Cranial Nerves

I. Introduction—Cranial Nerves

—are the 12 peripheral nerves of the brain that supply the structures of the head and neck (Figures 13.1 and 13.2; see Figures 1.1 and 1.7).

II. Olfactory Nerve (CN I) [see Chapter 20]

A. General characteristics—CN I

—is a special visceral afferent **(SVA)** nerve that mediates the **sense of smell** (olfaction).

—consists of unmyelinated axons of bipolar neurons located in the nasal mucosa, the olfactory epithelium.

—enters the skull via the foramina of the cribriform plate of the ethmoid bone.

—projects directly to the telencephalon.

—synapses with mitral cells found in the olfactory bulb, an outgrowth of the telencephalon.

—is the only cranial nerve that projects directly to the forebrain.

B. Clinical correlation—CN I

—when damaged (e.g., ethmoid bone fracture), results in **anosmia,** loss of olfactory sensation.

III. Optic Nerve (CN II) [see Figures 1.2, 17.1, and 17.3; see Chapter 17]

A. General characteristics—CN II

—is a special somatic afferent **(SSA)** nerve that subserves **vision** and **pupillary light reflexes** (the afferent limb).

—consists of axons of neurons located in the ganglion cell layer of the retina.

—enters the skull via the optic canal of the sphenoid bone.

—projects, via the optic chiasm and optic tract, to the lateral geniculate body, a thalamic relay nucleus that projects to the visual cortex (area 17) of the occipital lobe.

—is **not a true peripheral nerve** but a tract of the diencephalon.

—contains fibers from the nasal retina that decussate in the optic chiasm.

—contains fibers from the temporal retina that pass ipsilaterally through the optic chiasm.

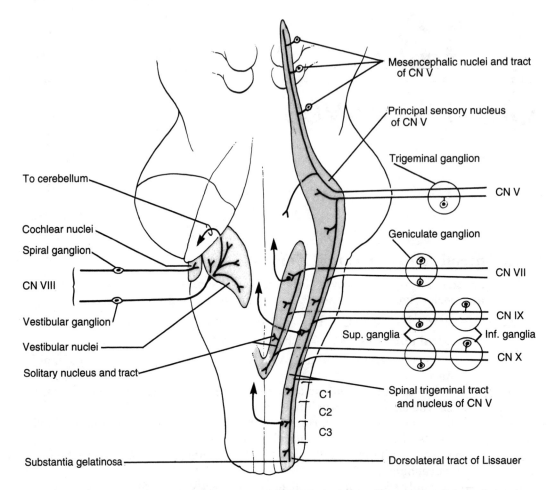

Figure 13.1. Location of the sensory cranial nerve nuclei within the brainstem. Phantom view of the brainstem from the dorsal aspect. Note that the spinal trigeminal tract and nucleus extends into the cervical cord (*C3*). Three sensory areas are prominent: the SSA area, including the cochlear and vestibular nuclei of CN VIII; the combined GVA and SVA column, the solitary nucleus of CN VII, CN IX, and CN X; and the GSA column, including the spinal trigeminal, principal sensory, and mesencephalic nuclei of CN V, CN VII, CN IX, and CN X. (Modified with permission from Noback CR and Demarest RJ: *The Human Nervous System*. Malvern, Pa, Lea & Febiger, 1991, p 222.)

    —contains axons that are myelinated by oligodendrocytes.
    —is invested by the dura and pia–arachnoid membranes and lies within the
      subarachnoid space.

B. Clinical correlations—CN II
    —when transected, **ipsilateral blindness** and **loss of direct pupillary
      light reflex** result; regeneration of the optic nerve does not occur.
    —when subjected to increased intracranial pressure (e.g., tumor), **papille-
      dema,** a "choked" optic disk results.
    —when constricted, **optic atrophy** (i.e., axonal degeneration) results.

IV. Oculomotor Nerve (CN III) [see Figures 1.1, 1.7, and 13.2; see Chapter 17)

A. General characteristics—CN III
    —contains general somatic efferent **(GSE)** and general visceral efferent
      (GVE) fibers.

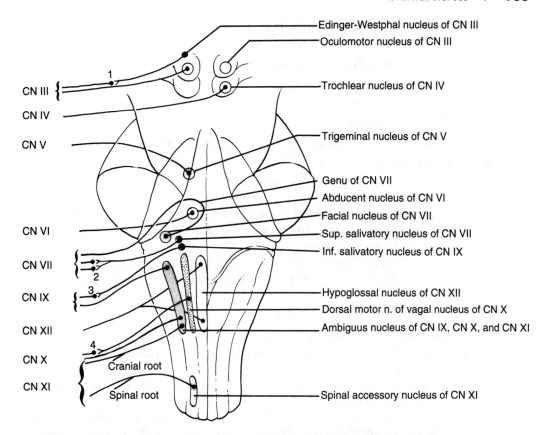

Figure 13.2. Location of motor cranial nerve nuclei within the brainstem. Three functional cell columns are visible from medial to lateral: the GSE column of CN III, CN IV, CN VI, and CN XII; the GVE column of CN III, CN VII, CN IX, and CN X; and the SVE column of CN V, CN VII, CN IX, CN X, and CN XI. Parasympathetic ganglia are indicated as *1* = ciliary ganglion; *2* = pterygopalatine and submandibular ganglia; *3* = otic ganglion; and *4* = terminal (intramural) ganglia. (Modified with permission from Noback CR and Demarest RJ: *The Human Nervous System.* Malvern, Pa, Lea & Febiger, 1991, p 223.)

—is a pure motor nerve that **moves the eye, constricts the pupil, accommodates,** and **converges**.

—exits the brainstem from the interpeduncular fossa of the midbrain, passes through the lateral wall of the cavernous sinus, and enters the orbit via the superior orbital fissure.

1. GSE component

—arises from the oculomotor nucleus of the midbrain.

—innervates four extraocular muscles and the levator palpebrae muscle. (Remember the mnemonic: **SIN** = **S**uperior muscles are **IN**torters of the globe.)

a. Medial rectus muscle

—adducts the eye.

—with its opposite partner, converges the eyes.

b. Superior rectus muscle

—elevates, intorts, and adducts the eye.

c. Inferior rectus muscle

—depresses, extorts, and adducts the eye.

d. Inferior oblique muscle
—elevates, extorts, and abducts the eye.

e. Levator palpebrae muscle
—elevates the upper lid.

2. GVE component

a. Composition
—consists of preganglionic parasympathetic fibers.

b. Pathway
—arises from the Edinger-Westphal nucleus (accessory oculomotor nucleus) of the midbrain.

(1) Edinger-Westphal nucleus
—projects to the ciliary ganglion of the orbit via CN III.

(2) Ciliary ganglion
—projects postganglionic parasympathetic fibers to the sphincter muscle of the iris (miosis) and to the ciliary muscle (accommodation).

B. Clinical correlations—CN III

1. Oculomotor paralysis
—is seen frequently with **transtentorial herniation** (subdural or epidural hematoma).

—denervation of the levator palpebrae muscle results in **ptosis** (drooping of the upper eyelid).

—denervation of the extraocular muscles causes the affected eye to **"look down and out"** due to the unopposed action of the lateral rectus and superior oblique muscles. The superior oblique and lateral rectus muscles are innervated by CN IV and CN VI.

—results in **diplopia** (double vision) when the patient looks in the direction of the paretic muscle.

—interruption of parasympathetic innervation results in a **dilated and fixed pupil** and **paralysis of accommodation (cycloplegia)**.

2. Other conditions associated with CN III impairment

a. Transtentorial (uncal) herniation
—increased supratentorial pressure (tumor) forces the hippocampal uncus through the tentorial notch and compresses the oculomotor nerve. Pupilloconstrictor fibers are affected first, resulting in a dilated and fixed pupil; somatic efferent fibers are affected later, resulting in a convergent strabismus.

b. Aneurysms (carotid and posterior communicating arteries)
—frequently compress the oculomotor nerve within the cavernous sinus or the interpeduncular cistern.

—usually affect the peripheral pupilloconstrictor fibers first, as in uncal herniation.

c. Diabetes mellitus (diabetic oculomotor palsy)
—frequently affects the oculomotor nerve, damaging the central fibers and sparing the pupilloconstrictor fibers.

V. Trochlear nerve (CN IV) [see Figures 1.7 and 13.2]

A. General characteristics—CN IV

–is a pure **GSE** nerve that **innervates** the superior oblique muscle, which **depresses, intorts,** and **abducts** the eye.

–arises from the contralateral trochlear nucleus of the midbrain.

–decussates within the midbrain and exits the brainstem on its dorsal surface, caudal to the inferior colliculus.

–encircles the midbrain in the subarachnoid space, passes through the lateral wall of the cavernous sinus, and enters the orbit via the superior orbital fissure.

B. Clinical correlations—CN IV paralysis

–results in the following conditions:

1. Extorsion of the eye and weakness of downward gaze

2. Vertical diplopia, which increases when looking down

3. Head tilting, to compensate for extorsion

VI. Trigeminal Nerve (CN V) [see Figures 1.1, 1.7, 13.1, and 13.2; see Chapter 10]

A. General characteristics—CN V

–contains general somatic afferent **(GSA)** and special visceral efferent **(SVE)** fibers.

–innervates the **muscles of mastication** and mediates **general sensation** from the face, eye, and nasal and oral cavities.

–is the nerve of the first branchial arch (mandibular).

–exits the brainstem from the pons.

–contains first-order sensory neurons in the trigeminal ganglion and in the mesencephalic nucleus.

–contains motor neurons in the motor trigeminal nucleus of the rostral pons.

–has three divisions: **ophthalmic** (CN V-1); **maxillary** (CN VI-2); and **mandibular** (CN V-3) [see Figures 10.1 and 10.2; Chapter 10].

1. GSA component (see Figure 10.1)

–provides **sensory innervation** to the face, mucous membranes of the nasal and oral cavities and frontal sinus, teeth, hard palate, and deep structures of the head (proprioception from muscles and the temporomandibular joint).

–innervates the dura of the anterior and middle cranial fossae.

2. SVE component

–innervates the **muscles of mastication** (temporalis, masseter, lateral and medial pterygoids), the **tensores tympani** and **veli palatini,** the **mylohyoid,** and the **anterior belly of the digastric muscles**.

B. Clinical correlations—lesions of CN V

–result in the following conditions:

1. Loss of general sensation from the face and mucous membranes of the oral and nasal cavities

2. Loss of the corneal reflex (afferent limb, CN V-1)

3. Flaccid paralysis of the muscles of mastication

4. Deviation of the patient's jaw to the weak side, due to the unopposed action of the opposite lateral pterygoid muscle

5. Paralysis of the tensor tympani, leading to hypacusis (partial deafness to low-pitched sounds)

VII. Abducent Nerve (CN VI) [see Figures 1.1, 1.7, and 13.2]

A. General characteristics—CN VI

−is a pure **GSE** nerve that innervates the lateral rectus muscle, which **abducts the eye**.

−arises from the abducent nucleus of the caudal pons.

−exits the brainstem from the inferior pontine sulcus.

−passes through the cavernous sinus and enters the orbit via the superior orbital fissure.

B. Clinical correlations—CN VI paralysis

−is the most common isolated muscle palsy.

−results in the following conditions:

1. Convergent strabismus (esotropia), with the inability to abduct the eye due to the unopposed action of the medial rectus muscle

2. Horizontal diplopia, with maximum separation of the double images when looking toward the paretic lateral rectus muscle

VIII. Facial Nerve (CN VII) [see Figures 1.1, 1.7, and 13.1, and 13.2]

A. General characteristics—CN VII

−contains **GSA, SVA, SVE,** and **GVE** fibers.

−mediates **facial movements, taste, salivation, and lacrimation**.

−is the nerve of the second branchial arch (hyoid).

−includes the **facial nerve proper** (motor division), which contains the SVE fibers that innervate the muscles of facial expression.

−includes the **intermediate nerve** (sensory division), which contains GSA, SVA, and GVE fibers. All first-order sensory neurons are found in the geniculate ganglion within the temporal bone.

−exits the brainstem at the cerebellopontine angle.

−enters the internal auditory meatus and facial canal.

−exits the facial canal and skull via the **stylomastoid foramen**.

1. GSA component

−has cell bodies located in the geniculate ganglion.

−innervates the **posterior surface of the external ear** via the posterior auricular branch of the facial nerve.

−projects centrally to the spinal trigeminal tract and nucleus.

2. SVA component

−has cell bodies located in the geniculate ganglion.

−projects centrally to the solitary tract and nucleus.

−innervates the **taste buds** from the anterior two-thirds of the tongue via:

a. Intermediate nerve

b. Chorda tympani (Figure 13.3)

–is located in the tympanic cavity medial to the tympanic membrane and malleus.

–contains **SVA** and **GVE** fibers.

c. Lingual nerve (a branch of CN V-3)

3. GVE component

–is a parasympathetic component that innervates the **lacrimal, submandibular, and sublingual glands**.

–contains preganglionic neurons located in the superior salivatory nucleus of the caudal pons.

a. Lacrimal pathway (see Figure 13.3)

–begins in the superior salivatory nucleus, which projects via the intermediate nerve, the greater petrosal nerve, and the nerve of the pterygoid canal to the pterygopalatine ganglion.

–continues, as the postganglionic neurons of the pterygopalatine ganglion project through the inferior orbital fissure and via the zygomatic nerve (a branch of CN V-2) and the lacrimal nerve (a branch of CN V-1) to innervate the lacrimal gland.

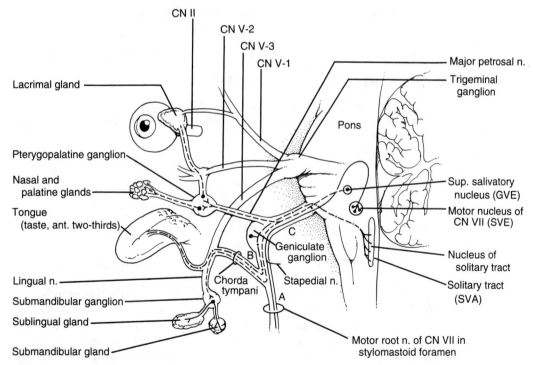

Figure 13.3. The functional components of the facial nerve (CN VII). The intermediate nerve is the sensory and visceromotor division of the seventh nerve. *A, B,* and *C* indicate three lesions of the nerve. Lesion *A* is at the stylomastoid foramen and spares lacrimation, nasal and palatine secretion, taste to the anterior two-thirds of the tongue, salivation, and the stapedial reflex; the patient has a lower motor neuron lesion involving the muscles of facial expression. Lesion *B* is between the geniculate ganglion and the chorda tympani and spares lacrimation and secretion from the nasal and palatine glands. Lesion *C* is proximal to the geniculate ganglion and is total.

  b. Submandibular pathway (see Figure 13.3)

   –begins in the superior salivatory nucleus, which projects via the intermediate nerve and chorda tympani to the submandibular ganglion.

   –continues as the postganglionic neurons of the submandibular ganglion project to and innervate the submandibular and sublingual glands.

 4. SVE component

  –arises from the facial nucleus of the caudal pons and exits the brainstem at the cerebellopontine angle.

  –enters the internal auditory meatus, traverses the facial canal, sends a branch to the stapedius muscle of the middle ear, and exits the skull via the stylomastoid foramen.

  –innervates the **muscles of facial expression,** the **stylohyoid muscle,** the **posterior belly of the digastric muscle,** and the **stapedius muscles**.

B. Clinical correlations—lesions of CN VII (see Figures 9.11 and 13.3)

 –result in the following conditions:

 1. Flaccid paralysis of the muscles of facial expression (upper and lower face)

 2. Loss of the corneal (blink) reflex (efferent limb), which may lead to corneal ulceration

 3. Loss of taste from the anterior two-thirds of the tongue

 4. Hyperacusis (increased acuity to sounds), due to stapedius paralysis

 5. Bell's palsy, caused by trauma to the nerve within the facial canal

IX. Vestibulocochlear Nerve (CN VIII) [see Figures 1.1, 1.7, and 13.1]

–serves to **maintain balance** and **mediates hearing**.

–consists of two functional divisions: the **vestibular nerve** and the **cochlear nerve** (see Chapter 11).

–is a pure **SSA** nerve.

–exits the brainstem at the cerebellopontine angle.

–enters the internal auditory meatus and is confined to the temporal bone.

A. Vestibular nerve (see Chapters 11 and 12)

 1. General characteristics—vestibular nerve

  –serves **equilibrium** and **balance**.

  –is associated functionally with the cerebellum (flocculonodular lobe).

  –regulates **compensatory eye movements.**

  –has its first-order sensory bipolar neurons in the vestibular ganglion of the internal auditory meatus.

  –projects its peripheral processes to the hair cells of the cristae of the semicircular ducts and to hair cells of the utricular and saccular maculae.

  –projects its central processes to the four vestibular nuclei of the brainstem and to the flocculonodular lobe of the cerebellum.

  –conducts efferent fibers to hair cells from the brainstem.

 2. Clinical correlation—lesions of the vestibular nerve

  –result in **disequilibrium, vertigo,** and **nystagmus.**

B. **Cochlear nerve** (see Chapter 11)

1. **General characteristics—cochlear nerve**
   —serves **audition** (hearing).
   —has its first-order sensory bipolar neurons in the spiral (cochlear) ganglion of the modiolus of the cochlea, within the temporal bone.
   —projects its peripheral processes to the hair cells of the organ of Corti.
   —projects its central processes to the dorsal and ventral cochlear nuclei of the brainstem.
   —conducts efferent fibers to the hair cells from the brainstem.

2. **Clinical correlations—lesions of the cochlear nerve**
   —result in **hearing loss** (sensorineural deafness) [destructive lesions].
   —cause **tinnitus** (ear ringing) [irritative lesions].

X. Glossopharyngeal Nerve (CN IX) [see Figures 1.1, 1.7, 13.1, and 13.2]

A. **General characteristics—CN IX**
   —contains **GSA, GVA** (general visceral afferent), **SVA, SVE,** and **GVE** components.
   —mediates **taste, salivation,** and **swallowing**.
   —mediates **input from the carotid sinus,** which contains baroreceptors that monitor arterial blood pressure.
   —mediates **input from the carotid body,** which contains chemoreceptors that monitor the CO_2 and O_2 concentration of the blood.
   —is the nerve of the third branchial arch.
   —is predominantly a sensory nerve.
   —exits the brainstem (medulla) from the postolivary sulcus with CN X and CN XI.
   —exits the skull via the jugular foramen with CN X and CN XI.

1. **GSA component**
   —innervates **part of the external ear** and the **external auditory meatus** via the auricular branch of the vagus nerve.
   —has cell bodies in the superior ganglion.
   —projects its central processes to the spinal trigeminal tract and nucleus.

2. **GVA component**
   —innervates **structures derived from the endoderm** (e.g., the pharynx [foregut]).
   —innervates the **mucous membranes of the posterior third of the tongue, tonsil, upper pharynx, tympanic cavity, and auditory tube**.
   —innervates the **carotid sinus** (baroreceptors) and the **carotid body** (chemoreceptors) via the sinus nerve.
   —has cell bodies in the inferior (petrosal) ganglion.
   —is the afferent limb of the gag reflex and the carotid sinus reflex.

3. **SVA component**
   —innervates the **taste buds** of the posterior third of the tongue.
   —has cell bodies in the inferior (petrosal) ganglion.
   —projects its central processes to the solitary tract and nucleus.

4. SVE component

–innervates the **stylopharyngeus muscle**.

–arises from the nucleus ambiguus of the lateral medulla.

5. GVE component

–is a parasympathetic component that innervates the **parotid gland**.

–consists of preganglionic neurons located in the inferior salivatory nucleus of the medulla that project, via the tympanic nerve and via the lesser petrosal nerve, to the otic ganglion; postganglionic fibers from the otic ganglion project to the parotid gland via the auriculotemporal nerve (CN V-3).

B. Clinical correlations—lesions of CN IX

–result in the following conditions:

1. Loss of the gag (pharyngeal) reflex (interruption of afferent limb)

2. Loss of the carotid sinus reflex (interruption of the sinus nerve)

3. Loss of taste from the posterior third of the tongue

4. Glossopharyngeal neuralgia

XI. Vagal Nerve (CN X) [see Figures 1.1, 1.7, 13.1, and 13.2]

A. General characteristics—CN X

–contains **GSA, GVA, SVA, SVE,** and **GVE** components.

–mediates **phonation, swallowing, elevation of the palate, and taste**.

–innervates **viscera of the neck, thorax,** and **abdomen**.

–is the nerve of the fourth and sixth branchial arches.

–exits the brainstem (medulla) from the postolivary sulcus.

–exits the skull via the jugular foramen with CN IX and CN XI.

1. GSA component

–innervates the **infratentorial dura, posterior surface of the external ear, external auditory meatus,** and **tympanic membrane**.

–has cell bodies in the superior (jugular) ganglion.

–projects its central processes to the spinal trigeminal tract and nucleus.

2. GVA component

–innervates the **mucous membranes** of the **pharynx, larynx, esophagus, trachea,** and **thoracic and abdominal viscera** (to the left colic flexure).

–has cell bodies in the inferior (nodose) ganglion.

–projects its central processes to the solitary tract and nucleus.

3. SVA component

–innervates the **taste buds** in the **epiglottis**.

–has cell bodies located in the inferior (nodose) ganglion.

–projects its central processes to the solitary tract and nucleus.

4. SVE component

–innervates the **branchial arch muscles of the larynx and pharynx, striated muscle of the upper esophagus, muscle of the uvula,** and the **levator veli palatini and palatoglossus muscles**.

–receives SVE input from the cranial division of the spinal accessory nerve (CN XI).

–arises from the nucleus ambiguus in the lateral medulla.

–provides the efferent limb of the gag reflex.

5. **GVE component** (see Figure 18.2)

–innervates the **viscera of the neck** and of the **thoracic and abdominal cavities** as far as the left colic flexure.

–consists of preganglionic parasympathetic neurons located in the dorsal motor nucleus of the medulla, which project to the intramural ganglia of the visceral organs.

–consists of postganglionic parasympathetic neurons located in the **nucleus ambiguus** of the medulla, which project to the intramural ganglia of the heart.

B. **Clinical correlations—lesions of CN X**

–result in the following conditions:

1. **Ipsilateral paralysis** of the soft palate, pharynx, and larynx leading to **dysphonia** (hoarseness), **dyspnea, dysarthria,** and **dysphagia**

2. **Loss of the gag (palatal) reflex** (efferent limb)

3. **Anesthesia of the pharynx and larynx,** leading to unilateral **loss of the cough reflex**

4. **Aortic aneurysms and tumors of the neck and thorax**

–frequently compress the vagal nerve.

XII. Accessory Nerve (CN XI) [see Figures 1.1, 1.7, and 13.2]

A. **General characteristics—CN XI**

–contains the **SVE** component.

–mediates **head and shoulder movement** and innervates **laryngeal muscles.**

–includes the following divisions:

1. **Cranial division**

–arises from the **nucleus ambiguus** of the medulla.

–exits the medulla from the postolivary sulcus and joins the vagal nerve (CN X).

–exits the skull via the jugular foramen with CN IX and CN X.

–innervates the **intrinsic muscles of the larynx** via the inferior (recurrent) laryngeal nerve, with the exception of the cricothyroid muscle.

2. **Spinal division**

–arises from the ventral horn of cervical segments C1–C6.

–spinal roots exit the spinal cord laterally between the ventral and dorsal spinal roots, ascend through the foramen magnum, and exit the skull via the jugular foramen.

–innervates the **sternocleidomastoid** (with C2) and **trapezius muscles** (with C3 and C4).

B. **Clinical correlations—lesions of CN XI**

–result in the following conditions:

1. **Paralysis of the sternocleidomastoid muscle**

–results in difficulty in turning the head to the side opposite the lesion.

2. Paralysis of the trapezius muscle

−results in a shoulder droop and winging of the scapula.

3. Paralysis of the larynx, if the cranial root is involved

XIII. Hypoglossal Nerve (CN XII) [see Figures 1.1, 1.7, and 13.2]

A. General characteristics—CN XII

−mediates **tongue movement.**
−is a pure **GSE** nerve.
−arises from the hypoglossal nucleus of the medulla.
−exits the medulla in the preolivary sulcus.
−exits the skull via the hypoglossal canal.
−innervates **intrinsic and extrinsic muscles of the tongue.**

B. Clinical correlations—CN XII

−when transected, **hemiparalysis of the tongue** results.
−when protruded, the tongue points toward the weak side due to the unopposed action of the opposite genioglossus muscle.

Review Test

Directions: Each of the numbered items or incomplete statements in this section is followed by answers or by completions of the statement. Select the **one** lettered answer or completion that is **best** in each case.

1. The cavernous sinus contains all of the following structures EXCEPT the

(A) ophthalmic nerve.
(B) mandibular nerve.
(C) abducent and trochlear nerves.
(D) postganglionic sympathetic fibers.
(E) preganglionic parasympathetic fibers.

2. Parasympathetic fibers are found in all of the following cranial nerves EXCEPT the

(A) oculomotor nerve.
(B) trigeminal nerve.
(C) facial nerve.
(D) glossopharyngeal nerve.
(E) vagal nerve.

3. The superior orbital fissure contains all of the following structures EXCEPT the

(A) ophthalmic veins.
(B) ophthalmic nerve.
(C) trochlear nerve.
(D) abducent nerve.
(E) optic nerve.

4. Transection of the left oculomotor nerve results in all of the following conditions EXCEPT

(A) diplopia when attempting to adduct the left eye.
(B) a fixed dilated pupil on the left side.
(C) no consensual reaction when light is shone in the left eye.
(D) a normal bilateral corneal reflex.
(E) a left eye that "looks down and out."

5. A glioma destroying the right trochlear nucleus would result in all of the following conditions EXCEPT

(A) extorsion of the affected eye.
(B) diplopia when looking down.
(C) a head tilt.
(D) paralysis of the right superior oblique muscle.
(E) unaffected pupillary light reflexes.

6. Which of the following statements concerning the vestibulocochlear nerve is false?

(A) It exits the brainstem in the cerebellopontine angle.
(B) The vestibular ganglion is located in the internal auditory meatus.
(C) Irritative lesions cause tinnitus and nystagmus.
(D) Destructive lesions cause unilateral deafness.
(E) It is a SVA nerve.

7. All of the following statements concerning the vagal nerve are correct EXCEPT

(A) its dorsal motor nucleus lies in the medulla.
(B) it contains parasympathetic fibers from the nucleus ambiguus.
(C) it emerges from the postolivary sulcus.
(D) it exits the skull via the foramen magnum.
(E) it innervates the levator veli palatini muscle.

8. All of the following statements concerning the geniculate ganglion are correct EXCEPT

(A) it is found within the temporal bone.
(B) it receives taste fibers from the anterior two-thirds of the tongue.
(C) it gives rise to the greater petrosal nerve.
(D) it contains postganglionic parasympathetic neurons.
(E) it contains sensory neurons that innervate the outer ear.

9. All of the following statements concerning the olfactory nerve are correct EXCEPT

(A) it projects directly to the forebrain.
(B) it synapses with mitral cells.
(C) its cells of origin are found in the nasal mucosa.
(D) it is a SSA nerve.
(E) it enters the skull via the cribriform plate of the ethmoid bone.

10. All of the following statements concerning the optic nerve are correct EXCEPT

(A) it enters the skull via the superior orbital fissure.
(B) it is the afferent limb of the pupillary light reflex.
(C) there is no regeneration after injury.
(D) it lies within the subarachnoid space.
(E) its axons are myelinated by oligodendrocytes.

11. All of the following statements concerning the oculomotor nerve are correct EXCEPT

(A) it originates in the rostral midbrain.
(B) it traverses the cavernous sinus.
(C) it exits the cranial vault via the superior orbital fissure.
(D) it has a sympathetic component.
(E) transection results in ptosis.

12. All of the following statements concerning the accessory nerve are correct EXCEPT

(A) it exits the skull via the jugular foramen.
(B) it contains fibers from the nucleus ambiguus.
(C) it contains fibers from the dorsal motor nucleus.
(D) it contains fibers from cervical spinal cord levels.
(E) it innervates two muscles of branchiomeric origin.

13. All of the following statements concerning the facial nerve are correct EXCEPT

(A) it innervates the lacrimal gland.
(B) it innervates the stapedius muscle.
(C) it innervates the posterior belly of the digastric muscle.
(D) it provides the efferent limb for the corneal reflex.
(E) it projects to the otic ganglion.

14. All of the following statements concerning the trigeminal nerve are correct EXCEPT

(A) it contains SVE and GSA fibers.
(B) it innervates the tensor tympani muscle.
(C) it innervates the anterior belly of the digastric muscle.
(D) it innervates the supratentorial dura.
(E) it innervates the skin over the angle of the jaw.

15. Transection of the glossopharyngeal nerve results in all of the following deficits EXCEPT

(A) loss of the gag reflex.
(B) loss of neurons in the superior salivatory nucleus.
(C) loss of taste and pain sensation from the posterior third of the tongue.
(D) loss of the carotid sinus reflex.
(E) loss of neurons in the nucleus ambiguus.

Directions: Each group of items in this section consists of lettered options followed by a set of numbered items. For each item, select the **one** lettered option that is most closely associated with it. Each lettered option may be selected once, more than once, or not at all.

Questions 16–20

Match each description with the appropriate nerve.

(A) Glossopharyngeal nerve
(B) Accessory nerve
(C) Trigeminal nerve
(D) Facial nerve
(E) Vagal nerve

16. Innervates the parotid gland

17. Is the efferent limb of the corneal reflex

18. Is the efferent limb of the gag reflex

19. Innervates the infratentorial dura

20. Is a pure motor nerve

Answers and Explanations

1–B. The mandibular nerve (CN V-3) does not pass through the cavernous sinus; it exits the skull via the foramen ovale.

2–B. The trigeminal nerve (CN V) contains only SVE and GSA fibers.

3–E. The optic nerve (CN II) enters the skull via the optic canal. The optic canal also contains the ophthalmic artery.

4–C. Transection of the oculomotor nerve (CN III) does not interrupt the afferent limb of the pupillary reflex, which is bilateral. Light shone into the left eye results in constriction of the contralateral pupil, the consensual reaction.

5–D. The right trochlear nucleus of CN IV projects to the left superior oblique muscle. Diplopia occurs when an image falls on disparate parts of the retina. The pupillary light reflex is mediated by the parasympathetic fibers of the oculomotor nerve.

6–E. The vestibulocochlear nerve (CN VIII) is classified as a SSA nerve, as is the optic nerve (CN II).

7–D. The vagal nerve (CN X) emerges from the brainstem in the postolivary sulcus of the medulla and exits the skull via the jugular foramen with CN IX and CN XI. It contains preganglionic parasympathetic fibers from the nucleus ambiguus that project to the cardiac ganglia of the heart. The vagal nerve innervates the levator veli palatini muscle, which raises and retracts the soft palate. The dorsal motor nucleus of the vagal nerve lies in the medulla.

8–D. The geniculate ganglion contains all of the first-order sensory neurons of the facial nerve (CN VII) [GSA and SVA]. It is found within the temporal bone and gives rise to the greater petrosal nerve. Sensory neurons in the geniculate ganglion innervate taste buds from the anterior two-thirds of the tongue. Taste fibers from the posterior third of the tongue belong to the glossopharyngeal nerve (CN IX). Pseudounipolar ganglion cells of the geniculate ganglion innervate part of the outer ear.

9–D. The olfactory nerve (CN I), a SVA nerve, consists of the unmyelinated axons of bipolar neurons found in the olfactory epithelium of the upper nasal cavity. There are 25 million neurosensory cells on each side. These axons synapse with mitral cells in the olfactory bulb, a rhinencephalic structure of the forebrain. Mitral cells project directly via the olfactory tract to the primary olfactory cortex of the uncus.

10–A. The optic nerve (CN II) enters the skull via the optic canal of the sphenoid bone (the ophthalmic artery is also found in the optic canal). Efferent retinal fibers are the afferent limb of the pupillary light reflex. The efferent limb is the oculomotor nerve (CN III). The optic nerve is invested with meninges and lies in the subarachnoid space. The optic nerve is a tract of the CNS and not a peripheral nerve. There is no regeneration after transection. The axons of the optic nerve are myelinated by oligodendrocytes; peripheral nerve axons are myelinated by Schwann cells.

11–D. The oculomotor nucleus is found in the rostral midbrain at the level of the superior colliculus. Ptosis results after transection of the fibers to the levator palpebrae muscle. The oculomotor nerve (CN III) traverses the wall of the cavernous sinus with CN IV, CN VI, CN V-1, and CN V-2. The oculomotor nerve has a GVE parasympathetic component, which arises from the Edinger-Westphal nucleus. CN III exits the cranium via the superior orbital fissure.

12–C. The accessory (spinal) nerve (CN XI) exits the skull via the jugular foramen (with CN IX and CN X). The spinal part of the spinal accessory nerve enters the skull via the foramen magnum. CN XI contains SVE fibers from the nucleus ambiguus that innervate intrinsic muscles of the larynx; CN XI contains SVE fibers from the cervical spinal cord that innervate two muscles of branchiomeric origin, the trapezius and the sternocleidomastoid. The dorsal motor nucleus is the GVE nucleus of the vagal nerve (CN X).

13–E. The facial nerve (CN VII) provides the preganglionic parasympathetic innervation for the lacrimal, sublingual, and submandibular glands and innervates the stapedius muscle of the tympanic cavity and the posterior belly of the digastric muscle. The otic ganglion receives preganglionic parasympathetic input from the glossopharyngeal nerve (CN IX) and projects postganglionic parasympathetic fibers to the parotid gland.

14–E. The trigeminal nerve (CN V) [GSA and SVE] innervates the tensor tympani muscle and the anterior belly of the digastric muscle. It innervates the supratentorial dura. The skin over the angle of the jaw and the scalp of the back of the head is innervated by the second and third cervical nerves.

15–B. Transection of the glossopharyngeal nerve (CN IX) results in degeneration of neurons in the rostral part of the nucleus ambiguus and in the inferior salivatory nucleus, loss of the gag reflex, loss of sensation from the tonsilar bed, loss of taste and pain sensation from the posterior third of the tongue, and loss of the carotid sinus reflex. The superior salivatory nucleus is a GVE nucleus of CN VII.

16–A. The glossopharyngeal nerve (CN IX) innervates the parotid gland via the tympanic and lesser petrosal nerves, the otic ganglion, and the auriculotemporal nerve.

17–D. The facial nerve (CN VII) provides the efferent limb of the corneal reflex (orbicularis oculi muscle).

18–E. The vagal nerve (CN X) provides the efferent limb of the gag reflex (muscles of the soft palate). The glossopharyngeal nerve provides the afferent limb of the gag reflex.

19–E. The vagal nerve (CN X) innervates, via the recurrent meningeal ramus, the infratentorial dura (the dura of the posterior cranial fossa).

20–B. The accessory nerve (CN XI) is a pure SVE motor nerve. The cranial division innervates, via the recurrent laryngeal nerve, the intrinsic muscles of the larynx; the spinal division innervates, via motor branches, the sternocleidomastoid muscle and upper parts of the trapezius muscle.

14

Lesions of the Brainstem

I. Introduction—Lesions of the Brainstem

—are most frequently syndromes of arterial occlusion or circulatory insufficiency that involve the vertebrobasilar system.

II. Vascular Lesions of the Medulla

—result from occlusion of the vertebral artery or its branches (i.e., the anterior and posterior spinal arteries and the posterior inferior cerebellar artery [PICA]).

A. Medial medullary syndrome (Figure 14.1A)

—results from occlusion of the anterior spinal artery.
—includes the following affected **structures** and resultant **deficits:**

1. Corticospinal tract

—contralateral hemiparesis of the trunk and extremities

2. Medial lemniscus

—contralateral loss of proprioception, discriminative tactile sensation, and vibration sensation from the trunk and extremities

3. Hypoglossal nerve roots (intra-axial fibers)

—ipsilateral flaccid paralysis of the tongue

B. Lateral medullary syndrome (PICA syndrome) [see Figure 14.1B]

—results from occlusion of the vertebral artery or one of its medullary branches (e.g., PICA).
—includes the following affected **structures** and resultant **deficits:**

1. Vestibular nuclei (medial and inferior)

—nystagmus, nausea, vomiting, and vertigo

2. Inferior cerebellar peduncle

—ipsilateral cerebellar signs (dystaxia, dysmetria, dysdiadochokinesia)

183

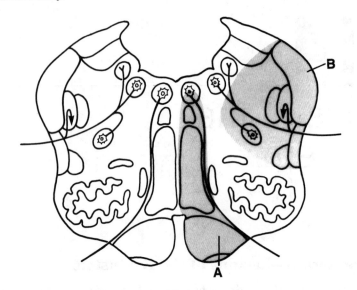

Figure 14.1. Vascular lesions of the caudal medulla at the level of the hypoglossal nucleus of CN XII and the dorsal motor nucleus of CN X. (*A*) Medial medullary syndrome (anterior spinal artery). (*B*) Lateral medullary syndrome (PICA syndrome).

3. Nucleus ambiguus of CN IX, CN X, and CN XI (SVE)

–ipsilateral laryngeal, pharyngeal, and palatal paralysis (loss of the gag reflex [efferent limb], dysarthria, dysphagia, and dysphonia [hoarseness])

4. Glossopharyngeal nerve roots (intra-axial fibers)

–loss of the gag reflex (afferent limb)

5. Vagal nerve roots (intra-axial fibers)

–neurologic deficits same as those seen in lesion of the nucleus ambiguus

6. Spinothalamic tracts

–contralateral loss of pain and temperature sensation from the trunk and extremities

7. Spinal trigeminal nucleus and tract

–ipsilateral loss of pain and temperature sensation from the face

8. Descending sympathetic tract

–ipsilateral Horner's syndrome (ptosis, miosis, hemianhydrosis, and apparent enophthalmos)

III. Vascular Lesions of the Pons

–result from occlusion of the basilar artery or its branches (the anterior inferior cerebellar artery [AICA], transverse pontine arteries, and superior cerebellar artery).

A. Medial inferior pontine syndrome (Figure 14.2A)

–results from occlusion of the paramedian branches of the basilar artery.
–includes the following affected **structures** and resultant **deficits:**

1. Abducent nerve roots (intra-axial fibers)

–ipsilateral lateral rectus paralysis

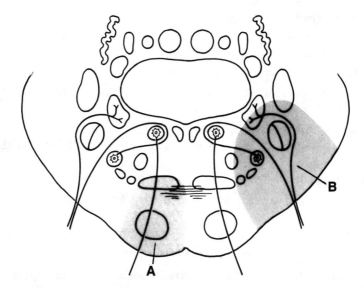

Figure 14.2. Vascular lesions of the caudal pons at the level of the abducent nucleus of CN VI and the facial nucleus of CN VII. (*A*) Medial inferior pontine syndrome. (*B*) Lateral inferior pontine syndrome (AICA syndrome).

2. Corticobulbar tracts
–contralateral weakness of the lower face

3. Corticospinal tracts
–contralateral hemiparesis of the trunk and extremities

4. Base of the pons (middle cerebellar peduncle)
–ipsilateral limb and gait ataxia

5. Medial lemniscus
–contralateral loss of proprioception, discriminative tactile sensation, and vibration sensation from the trunk and extremities

B. Lateral inferior pontine syndrome (AICA syndrome) [see Figure 14.2*B*]
–results from occlusion of a long circumferential branch of the basilar artery, AICA.
–includes the following affected **structures** and resultant **deficits:**

1. Facial nucleus and intra-axial nerve fibers
–ipsilateral facial nerve paralysis
–loss of taste from the anterior two-thirds of the tongue
–loss of the corneal and stapedial reflexes

2. Cochlear nuclei and intra-axial nerve fibers
–unilateral central nerve deafness

3. Vestibular nuclei and intra-axial nerve fibers
–nystagmus, nausea, vomiting, and vertigo

4. Spinal trigeminal nucleus and tract
–ipsilateral loss of pain and temperature sensation from the face

5. Middle and inferior cerebellar peduncles
–ipsilateral limb and gait dystaxia

6. Spinothalamic tracts

—contralateral loss of pain and temperature sensation from the trunk and extremities

7. Descending sympathetic tract

—ipsilateral Horner's syndrome (ptosis, miosis, hemianhydrosis, and apparent enophthalmos)

C. Lateral midpontine syndrome

—results from occlusion of a short circumferential branch of the basilar artery.

—includes the following affected **structures** and resultant **deficits:**

1. Trigeminal nuclei and nerve root (motor and principal sensory nuclei)

—results in complete ipsilateral trigeminal paralysis including:

a. Paralysis of the muscles of mastication

b. Jaw deviation to the paretic side (due to unopposed action of the intact lateral pterygoid muscle)

c. Facial hemianesthesia (pain, temperature, touch, and proprioception)

d. Loss of the corneal reflex (afferent limb of CN V-1)

2. Middle cerebellar peduncle (base of the pons)

—ipsilateral limb and gait dystaxia

D. Lateral superior pontine syndrome

—results from occlusion of a long circumferential branch of the basilar artery, the **superior cerebellar artery.**

—includes the following affected **structures** and resultant **deficits**:

1. Superior and middle cerebellar peduncles

—ipsilateral limb and trunk dystaxia

2. Dentate nucleus

—signs similar to those seen with damage to the superior cerebellar peduncle (dystaxia, dysmetria, and intention tremor)

3. Spinothalamic and trigeminothalamic tracts

—contralateral loss of pain and temperature sensation from the trunk, extremities, and face

4. Descending sympathetic tract

—ipsilateral Horner's syndrome (ptosis, miosis, hemianhydrosis, and apparent enophthalmos)

5. Medial lemniscus (lateral division [gracilis])

—contralateral loss of proprioception, discriminative tactile sensation, and vibration sensation from the trunk and lower extremity

IV. Lesions of the Midbrain

—result from vascular occlusion of the mesencephalic branches of the posterior cerebral artery (PCA).

—may result from aneurysms of the posterior circle of Willis.

—may result from tumors of the pineal region.

—may result from hydrocephalus.

A. Dorsal midbrain (Parinaud's) syndrome (Figure 14.3*A*)

—is frequently the result of a **pinealoma or germinoma** of the pineal region.

—includes the following affected **structures** and resultant **deficits**:

1. Superior colliculus and pretectal area

—paralysis of upward and downward gaze, pupillary disturbances, and absence of convergence

2. Cerebral aqueduct

—compression from a pineal tumor results in a noncommunicating hydrocephalus

B. Paramedian midbrain (Benedikt's) syndrome (see Figure 14.3*B*)

—results from occlusion or hemorrhage of the paramedian midbrain branches of the posterior cerebral artery.

—includes the following affected **structures** and resultant **deficits**:

1. Oculomotor nerve roots (intra-axial fibers)

—complete **ipsilateral oculomotor nerve paralysis**

—**eye abduction and depression,** due to the unopposed action of the lateral rectus (CN VI) and the superior oblique (CN IV) muscles

—severe **ptosis** (paralysis of the levator palpebrae muscle)

—ipsilateral **fixed and dilated pupil** (complete internal ophthalmoplegia)

2. Red nucleus and dentatorubrothalamic tract

—contralateral cerebellar dystaxia with intention tremor

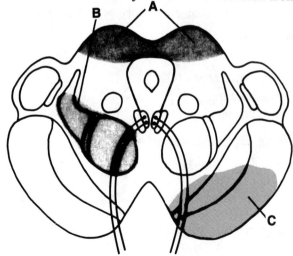

Figure 14.3. Lesions of the rostral midbrain at the level of the superior colliculus and oculomotor nucleus of CN III. (*A*) Dorsal midbrain (Parinaud's) syndrome. (*B*) Paramedian midbrain (Benedikt's) syndrome. (*C*) Medial midbrain (Weber's) syndrome.

3. Medial lemniscus

–contralateral loss of proprioception, discriminative tactile sensation, and vibration sensation from trunk and extremities

C. Medial midbrain (Weber's) syndrome (see Figure 14.3*C*)

–results from occlusion of midbrain branches of the posterior cerebral artery and aneurysms of the circle of Willis.

–includes the following **structures** and resultant **deficits**:

1. Oculomotor nerve roots (intra-axial fibers)

–see paramedian midbrain (Benedikt's) syndrome

2. Cortocobulbar tracts

–contralateral weakness of the lower face (CN VII), tongue (CN XII), and palate (CN X)

3. Corticospinal tracts

–contralateral hemiparesis of the trunk and extremities

V. Acoustic Neuroma (Schwannoma)

–is a benign tumor of the Schwann cells affecting the vestibulocochlear nerve (CN VIII).

–is a posterior fossa tumor of the internal auditory meatus and the cerebello-pontine (CP) angle.

–frequently compresses the facial nerve (CN VII), which accompanies CN VIII in the cerebellopontine angle and internal auditory meatus.

–may impinge on the pons and affect the spinal trigeminal tract (CN V).

–includes the following affected **structures** and resultant **deficits:**

A. Cochlear nerve of CN VIII

–unilateral nerve deafness and tinnitus (ear ringing)

B. Vestibular nerve of CN VIII

–vertigo, nystagmus, nausea, vomiting, and unsteadiness of gait

C. Facial nerve (CN VII)

–facial weakness and loss of corneal reflex (efferent limb)

D. Spinal trigeminal tract (CN V)

–paresthesias and anesthesia of ipsilateral face
–loss of the corneal reflex (afferent limb)

VI. Internuclear Ophthalmoplegia

–is also known as medial longitudinal fasciculus (MLF) syndrome, which results from a lesion of the MLF.

–lesions occur in the dorsomedial pontine tegmentum and may affect one or both MLFs.

–is a frequent sign of multiple sclerosis.

–results in medial rectus palsy on attempted lateral gaze and monocular nystagmus in the abducting eye with normal convergence.

–lesions of the abducent nucleus of CN VI result in all MLF signs and a lateral rectus paralysis with internal strabismus.

VII. Jugular Foramen (Vernet's) Syndrome

–affects CN IX, CN X, and CN XI.
–includes the following affected **structures** and resultant **deficits:**

A. Glossopharyngeal nerve (CN IX)

–loss of the gag reflex (afferent limb)
–loss of taste sensation in the posterior third of the tongue
–unilateral loss of the carotid sinus reflex

B. Vagal nerve (CN X)

–laryngeal paralysis with dysarthria, dysphagia, and dysphonia (hoarseness)
–palatal paralysis with loss of the gag reflex (efferent limb)

C. Accessory nerve (CN XI)

–weakness of the sternocleidomastoid and upper trapezius muscles (the shoulder droops and the scapula is winged)

Review Test

Directions: Each of the numbered items or incomplete statements in this section is followed by answers or by completions of the statement. Select the **one** lettered answer or completion that is **best** in each case.

Questions 1–8

For each of the following questions, select the appropriate site of the lesion responsible for the neurologic deficits revealed in the examination.

1. Neurologic examination revealed:
   —miosis, ptosis, hemianhydrosis, left side
   —laryngeal and palatal paralysis, left side
   —facial anesthesia, left side
   —loss of pain and temperature sensation from the trunk and extremities, right side

The lesion site responsible is in the

(A) caudal medulla, ventral median zone, right side.
(B) rostral medulla, lateral zone, left side.
(C) rostral pontine base, left side.
(D) caudal pontine tegmentum, lateral zone, right side.
(E) rostral pontine tegmentum, dorsal median zone, left side.

2. Neurologic examination revealed:
   —severe ptosis, eye "looks down and out," right side
   —fixed dilated pupil, right side
   —spastic hemiparesis, left side
   —lower facial weakness, left side

The lesion site responsible is in the

(A) caudal pontine tegmentum, dorsal median zone, left side.
(B) rostral pontine tegmentum, dorsal lateral zone, right side.
(C) pontine isthmus, dorsal lateral tegmentum, left side.
(D) rostral midbrain, medial basis pedunculi, right side.
(E) rostral midbrain, medial tegmentum, left side.

3. Neurologic examination revealed:
   —sixth nerve palsy, right side
   —facial weakness, left side
   —hemiparesis, left side
   —limb and gait dystaxia, right side

The lesion site responsible is in the

(A) caudal pontine tegmentum, lateral zone, right side.
(B) caudal pontine tegmentum, dorsal median zone, left side.
(C) caudal medulla, ventral median zone, right side.
(D) rostral pontine tegmentum, lateral zone, left side.
(E) caudal pontine base, median zone, right side.

4. Neurologic examination revealed:
   —paralysis of upward and downward gaze
   —absence of convergence
   —absence of pupillary reaction to light

The lesion site responsible is in the

(A) rostral midbrain tectum.
(B) caudal midbrain tectum.
(C) rostral pontine tegmentum.
(D) caudal pontine tegmentum.
(E) caudal midbrain tegmentum.

5. Neurologic examination revealed:
   —bilateral medial rectus paresis on attempted lateral gaze
   —monocular horizontal nystagmus in the abducting eye
   —unimpaired convergence

The lesion site responsible is in the

(A) midpontine tegmentum, dorsomedial zones, bilateral.
(B) rostral midbrain tectum.
(C) caudal midbrain tectum.
(D) caudal pontine base.
(E) rostral midbrain, bases pedunculorum.

6. Neurologic examination revealed:
—ptosis, miosis, and hemianhydrosis, left side
—loss of vibration sensation in the right leg
—loss of pain and temperature sensation from the trunk, extremities, and face, right side
—severe dystaxia and intention tremor, left arm

The lesion site responsible is in the

(A) rostral midbrain tegmentum, right side.
(B) rostral pontine tegmentum, dorsal medial zone, left side.
(C) pontine isthmus, dorsal lateral zone, left side.
(D) rostral medulla, lateral zone, left side.
(E) caudal medulla, lateral zone, right side.

7. Neurologic examination revealed:
—weakness of the pterygoid and masseter muscles, left side
—corneal reflex absent on left side
—left facial hemianesthesia

The lesion site responsible is in the

(A) midpontine tegmentum, lateral zone, left side.
(B) midpontine base, medial zone, left side.
(C) caudal pontine tegmentum, lateral zone, left side.
(D) caudal pontine tegmentum, dorsal medial zone, left side.
(E) foramen ovale, left side.

8. Neurologic examination revealed:
—loss of the stapedial reflex
—loss of the corneal reflex
—inability to purse the lips
—loss of taste sensation on the apex of the tongue

The lesion site responsible is in the

(A) stylomastoid foramen.
(B) basis pedunculi of the midbrain.
(C) rostral lateral pontine tegmentum.
(D) caudal lateral pontine tegmentum.
(E) rostral medulla.

9. All of the following statements concerning the anterior spinal artery are correct EXCEPT

(A) it is a branch of the vertebral artery.
(B) it irrigates the medullary pyramid.
(C) it irrigates the root fibers of the hypoglossal nerve.
(D) it irrigates the inferior olivary nucleus.
(E) it irrigates the medial lemniscus.

10. All of the following statements concerning the posterior inferior cerebellar artery (PICA) are correct EXCEPT

(A) it is a branch of the vertebral artery.
(B) it supplies the vestibular nuclei in the medulla.
(C) it supplies the medial lemniscus in the medulla.
(D) it supplies the inferior cerebellar peduncle.
(E) it supplies the lateral spinothalamic tract.

11. All of the following statements concerning the anterior inferior cerebellar artery (AICA) are correct EXCEPT

(A) it gives rise, in most cases, to the labyrinthine artery.
(B) it supplies the cochlear nuclei.
(C) it supplies the facial nucleus.
(D) it supplies the MLF.
(E) it supplies the spinal trigeminal tract and nucleus.

12. All of the following statements concerning internuclear ophthalmoplegia are correct EXCEPT

(A) it results from a lesion in the dorsal pontine tegmentum.
(B) it has no affect on convergence.
(C) it is frequently seen in multiple sclerosis.
(D) it results in monocular horizontal nystagmus.
(E) it results in a lateral rectus palsy on attempted lateral conjugate gaze.

13. Paramedian infarction of the base of the pons involves which one of the following structures?

(A) Trapezoid body
(B) Descending trigeminal tract
(C) Rubrospinal tract
(D) Pyramidal tract
(E) Ventral spinocerebellar tract

Answers and Explanations

1–B. The lesion is a classic Wallenberg's syndrome (PICA syndrome) of the lateral medullary zone. Interruption of the descending sympathetic tract produces ipsilateral Horner's syndrome. Involvement of the nucleus ambiguus or its exiting intra-axial fibers accounts for lower motor neuron (LMN) paralysis of the larynx and soft palate. The ipsilateral facial anesthesia is due to interruption of the spinal trigeminal tract; the contralateral loss of pain and temperature sensation from the trunk and extremities is due to transection of the spinothalamic tracts. The combination of ipsilateral and contralateral sensory loss is called alternating hemianesthesia. Singultus (hiccup) is frequently seen in this syndrome and is thought to result from irritation of the reticulophrenic pathway.

2–D. This constellation of deficits constitutes Weber's syndrome, which affects the basis pedunculi and the exiting intra-axial oculomotor fibers. Severe ptosis (compare mild ptosis of Horner's syndrome), the abducted and depressed eyeball, and the internal ophthalmoplegia (fixed dilated pupil) are third nerve signs. The contralateral hemiparesis results from interruption of the corticospinal tracts; lower facial weakness is due to interruption of the corticobulbar tracts. The combination of ipsilateral and contralateral motor deficits is called alternating hemiplegia. In cases of sensory or motor long tract involvement, the involved cranial nerve indicates the rostrocaudal site of the lesion; the cranial nerve signs are ipsilateral and lateralize the lesion (the trochlear nerve is the exception).

3–E. These signs point to the base of the pons (medial inferior pontine syndrome) on the right side and include involvement of the exiting intra-axial abducent fibers that pass through the uncrossed corticospinal fibers; this results in an ipsilateral lateral rectus paralysis (LMN lesion) and contralateral hemiparesis. Contralateral facial weakness results from damage to the corticobulbar fibers prior to their decussation. Involvement of the transverse pontine fibers destined for the middle cerebellar peduncle results in cerebellar signs. Again, the involved cranial nerve and pyramidal tract indicate where the lesion must be to account for the deficits. An ipsilateral sixth nerve paralysis and crossed hemiplegia is called the Millard-Gubler syndrome.

4–A. These deficits indicate Parinaud's syndrome, dorsal midbrain syndrome. This condition frequently is the result of a pinealoma, which compresses the superior colliculus and the underlying accessory oculomotor nuclei that are responsible for upward and downward vertical conjugate gaze. Patients usually have pupillary disturbances and absence of convergence.

5–A. This lesion site indicates MLF syndrome, internuclear ophthalmoplegia. The lesion is located in the dorsomedial tegmentum and is found between the abducent nucleus and the oculomotor nucleus.

6–C. These deficits correspond to a lesion in the dorsolateral zone of the pontine isthmus, lateral superior pontine syndrome. Interruption of the descending sympathetic pathway to the ciliospinal center of Budge (T1–T2) results in Horner's syndrome (always ipsilateral). Involvement of the lateral aspect (includes the leg fibers) of the medial lemniscus results in a loss of vibration sensation and other dorsal column modalities. Damage to the trigeminothalamic and spinothalamic tracts at this level results in contralateral hemianesthesia of the face and body. Infarction of the superior cerebellar peduncle leads to severe cerebellar dystaxia on the same side.

7–A. These signs indicate lateral midpontine syndrome. This lesion involves the motor and principal trigeminal nuclei and the intra-axial root fibers of the trigeminal nerve as it passes through the base of the pons. All signs are ipsilateral and refer to CN V. The afferent limb of the corneal reflex has been interrupted. This syndrome results from occlusion of the trigeminal artery, a short circumferential branch of the basilar artery.

8–D. These signs constitute lateral inferior pontine syndrome (AICA syndrome). The neurologic findings are all signs of a lesion involving the facial nerve (CN VII). The facial nerve nucleus and intra-axial fibers are found in the caudal lateral pontine tegmentum. A lesion of the stylomastoid foramen would not include the absence of the stapedial reflex or the loss of taste sensation from the anterior two-thirds of the tongue. The stapedial nerve and the chorda tympani exit the facial canal proximal to the stylomastoid foramen.

9–D. The anterior (ventral) spinal artery, a branch of the vertebral artery, irrigates the ventral median zone of the medulla, which includes the pyramid (corticospinal tracts), the medial lemniscus, and the exiting intra-axial root fibers of the hypoglossal nerve (CN XII). The inferior olivary nucleus lies in the paramedian zone of the medulla and is supplied by the short lateral branches of the vertebral artery.

10–C. The PICA, a branch of the vertebral artery, perfuses the lateral zone of the medulla, which includes the medial and inferior vestibular nuclei, the inferior cerebellar peduncle, and the lateral spinothalamic tract.

11–D. The AICA usually (in 85% of cases) gives rise to the labyrinthine artery. The AICA supplies the lateral zone of the caudal pontine tegmentum (including the cochlear nuclei, the facial nucleus, and intra-axial fibers) and the spinal trigeminal nucleus and tract. The MLF is irrigated by paramedian penetrating branches of the basilar artery.

12–E. Internuclear ophthalmoplegia results from a lesion of the MLF, which extends in the dorsomedial tegmentum from the abducent nucleus of CN VI to the oculomotor nucleus of CN III. Transection of the MLF results in medial rectus palsy on attempted lateral gaze and monocular nystagmus in the abducting eye. Convergence is normal. Bilateral MLF syndrome is a common ocular motor manifestation of multiple sclerosis.

13–D. The base of the pons includes corticospinal (pyramidal), corticobulbar, and corticopontine tracts, pontine nuclei, and transverse pontine fibers. At caudal levels, intra-axial abducent fibers of CN VI pass through the lateral pyramidal fascicles.

15

Cerebellum

I. Overview—The Cerebellum

    —develops from the alar plates (rhombic lips) of the metencephalon.

    —is located infratentorially within the posterior fossa and lies between the temporal and occipital lobes and the brainstem.

    —has three primary functions: the **maintenance of posture and balance,** the **maintenance of muscle tone,** and the **coordination of voluntary motor activity**.

II. Major Divisions—The Cerebellum

    —consists of a midline **vermis** and two lateral **hemispheres**.

    —is covered by a three-layered **cortex,** which contains folia and fissures.

    —contains a central medullary core, which is the **white matter** that contains myelinated axons and the four cerebellar nuclei (dentate, emboliform, globose, and fastigial nuclei). The emboliform and globose nuclei are called the interposed nucleus.

A. Cerebellar lobes (Figure 15.1)

    —are phylogenetic and functional divisions.

1. Anterior lobe

    —lies anterior to the primary fissure.

    —receives input from stretch receptors (muscle spindles) and Golgi tendon organs via the spinocerebellar tracts.

    —plays a role in the regulation of muscle tone.

2. Posterior lobe

    —lies between the primary fissure and the posterolateral fissure.

    —receives massive input from the neocortex via the corticopontocerebellar fibers.

    —serves the coordination of voluntary motor activity.

3. Flocculonodular lobe (vestibulocerebellum)

    —consists of the nodulus (of the vermis) and the flocculus.

    —receives input from the vestibular system.

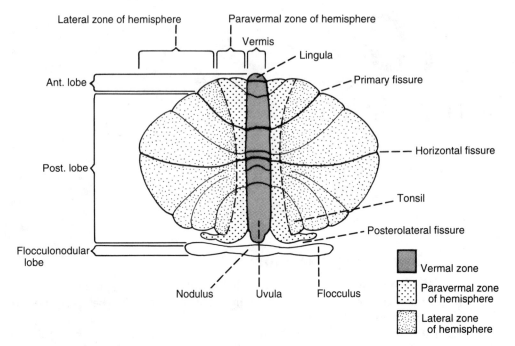

Figure 15.1. Schematic diagram of the fissures, lobules, and lobes of the cerebellum. Functional longitudinal zones of the cerebellum are associated with cerebellar nuclei. The vermal (median) zone projects to the fastigial nucleus; the paravermal (paramedian) zone projects to the interposed nucleus; the lateral zone projects to the dentate nucleus.

　　　　–subserves the maintenance of posture and balance.

  B. Longitudinal organization of the cerebellum (see Figure 15.1)

    –includes three functional longitudinal zones that are associated with specific cerebellar nuclei and pathways.

    1. Median (vermal) zone of the hemisphere

      –contains the vermal cortex, which projects to the fastigial nucleus.

    2. Paramedian (paravermal) zone of the hemisphere

      –contains the paravermal cortex, which projects to the interposed nuclei (emboliform and globose nuclei).

    3. Lateral zone of the hemisphere

      –contains the hemispheric cortex, which projects to the dentate nucleus.

  C. Cerebellar peduncles (see Figure 1.7)

    1. Inferior cerebellar peduncle

      –connects the cerebellum to the medulla.

      –consists of two divisions:

      a. Restiform body

        –is an afferent fiber system containing:

        (1) Dorsal spinocerebellar tract

        (2) Cuneocerebellar tract

        (3) Olivocerebellar tract

b. Juxtarestiform body
–contains afferent and efferent fibers:
(1) Vestibulocerebellar fibers (afferent)
(2) Cerebellovestibular fibers (efferent)

2. Middle cerebellar peduncle
–connects the cerebellum to the pons.
–is an afferent fiber system containing **pontocerebellar fibers** to the neocerebellum.

3. Superior cerebellar peduncle
–connects the cerebellum to the pons and midbrain.
–represents the major output from the cerebellum.

a. Efferent pathways
(1) Dentatorubrothalamic tract
(2) Interpositorubrothalamic tract
(3) Fastigiothalamic tract
(4) Fastigiovestibular tract

b. Afferent pathways
(1) Ventral spinocerebellar tract
(2) Trigeminocerebellar fibers
(3) Ceruleocerebellar fibers

III. Cerebellar Cortex

A. Three-layered cerebellar cortex (Figure 15.2)

1. Molecular layer
–is the outer cell-sparse layer that underlies the pia mater.
–consists of dendritic arborizations of Purkinje cells.
–contains stellate (outer) cells and basket cells.

2. Purkinje cell layer
–is found between the molecular layer and the granule cell layer.

3. Granule cell layer
–is found between the Purkinje cell layer and the white matter.
–contains granule cells, Golgi cells, and cerebellar glomeruli.

B. Neurons and fibers of the cerebellum (Figure 15.3; see Figure 15.2)

1. Purkinje cell
–conveys the only output from the cerebellar cortex.
–projects inhibitory output (γ-aminobutyric acid [GABA]) to the cerebellar and vestibular nuclei.
–is excited by parallel and climbing fibers.
–is inhibited (by GABA) by basket and stellate cells.

2. Granule cell
–excites (by glutamate) Purkinje, basket, stellate, and Golgi cells via parallel fibers.
–is inhibited by Golgi cells.
–is excited by mossy fibers.

Cerebellar cortex

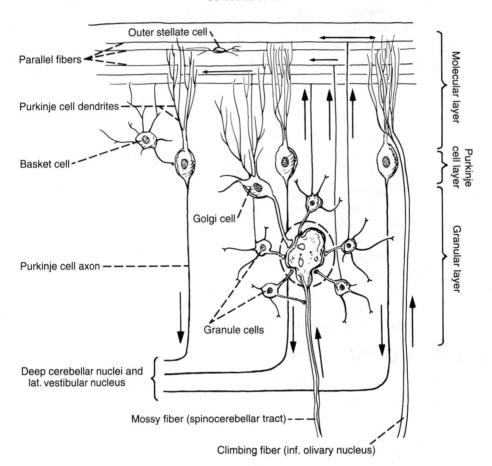

Figure 15.2. Schematic diagram of the three-layered cerebellar cortex, showing the neuronal elements and their connections. The *circular broken line* contains a cerebellar glomerulus. Climbing and mossy fibers represent excitatory input. Purkinje cell axons provide the sole output from the cerebellar cortex, which is inhibitory.

3. Mossy fibers
–are the afferent excitatory fibers of the **spinocerebellar and pontocerebellar tracts**.
–terminate as mossy fiber rosettes on granule cells.
–excite granule cells to discharge via their parallel fibers.

4. Climbing fibers
–are the afferent excitatory fibers of the **olivocerebellar tract**.
–terminate on neurons of the cerebellar nuclei and on dendrites of Purkinje cells.

IV. Major Cerebellar Pathways (Figure 15.4)
A. Vestibulocerebellar pathway
–plays a role in the maintenance of posture, balance, and the coordination of eye movements.

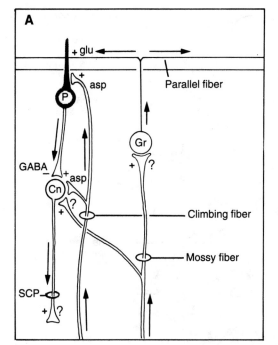
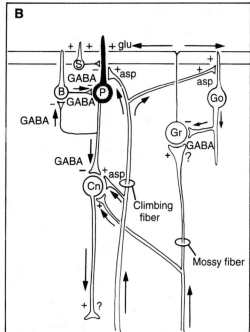

Figure 15.3. The basic connections of the cerebellar cortex. (*A*) The basic input and output circuit. (*B*) Connections of the inhibitory interneurons of the cerebellar cortex. *asp* = aspartate; *B* = basket cell; *Cn* = neuron of the cerebellar nuclei; *Gr* = granule cell; *GABA* = γ-aminobutyric acid; *glu* = glutamate; *Go* = Golgi cell; *P* = Purkinje cell; *S* = stellate cell; *SCP* = superior cerebellar peduncle. Inhibitory neurons of the cerebellum use GABA. Glutamate is the transmitter for granule cells. Aspartate is thought to be the transmitter of the climbing fibers. Excitatory synapses are indicated by plus sign (+); inhibitory synapses are indicated by a minus sign (−); the question mark (*?*) indicates that the neurotransmitter is not known.

–receives its major input from the vestibular receptors of the kinetic and static labyrinths.

1. Semicircular ducts and otolith organs

–project to the flocculonodular lobe and the vestibular nuclei.

2. Flocculonodular lobe

–receives visual input from the superior colliculus and the striate cortex.
–projects to the vestibular nuclei.

3. Vestibular nuclei

–project via the medial longitudinal fasciculi (MLFs) to the ocular motor nuclei of CN III, CN IV, and CN VI to coordinate eye movements.
–project via the medial and lateral vestibulospinal tracts to the spinal cord to regulate antigravity muscles.

B. Vermal spinocerebellar pathway

–maintains muscle tone and postural control over truncal (axial) and proximal (limb girdle) muscles.

1. Vermis

–receives spinocerebellar and labyrinthine input.
–projects to the fastigial nucleus.

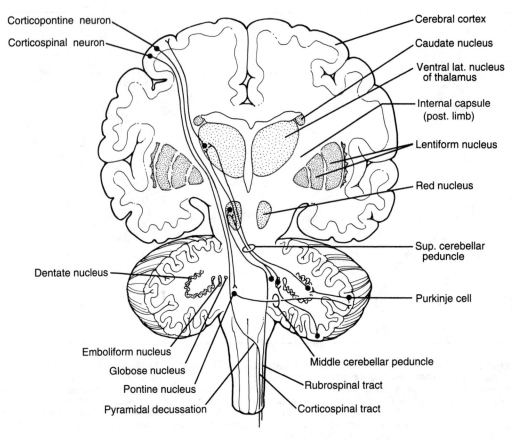

Figure 15.4. Principal cerebellar connections. The major efferent pathway is the dentatothalamocortical tract. The cerebellum receives input from the cerebral cortex via the corticopontocerebellar tract.

2. Fastigial nucleus

–projects via the vestibular nuclei to the spinal cord.

–projects to the ventral lateral nucleus of the thalamus.

3. Ventral lateral nucleus of the thalamus

–receives input from the fastigial nucleus.

–projects to the trunk area of the precentral gyrus.

4. Precentral gyrus

–gives rise to the **ventral corticospinal tract,** which regulates muscle tone of the truncal and proximal muscles.

C. Paravermal spinocerebellar pathway

–maintains muscle tone and postural control over distal muscle groups.

1. Paravermis

–receives spinocerebellar input from distal muscles.

–projects to the interposed nuclei.

2. Interposed nuclei

–project to:

a. Ventral lateral nucleus

–projects to the extremities area of the precentral gyrus. The precentral gyrus gives rise to the **lateral corticospinal tract,** which regulates the distal muscle groups.

b. Red nucleus

–gives rise to the crossed **rubrospinal tract,** which mediates control over distal muscles.

–receives input from the contralateral nucleus interpositus and bilateral input from the motor and premotor cortices.

D. Lateral hemispheric cerebellar pathway (see Figure 15.4)

–is also called the **neocerebellar or pontocerebellar pathway.**

–regulates the initiation, planning, and timing of volitional motor activity.

1. Cerebellar hemisphere

–receives input from the contralateral motor and sensory cortex via the **corticopontocerebellar tract.**

–projects via Purkinje cell axons to the dentate nucleus.

2. Dentate nucleus

–projects via the superior cerebellar peduncle to the contralateral red nucleus, ventral lateral nucleus of the thalamus, and the inferior olivary nucleus.

a. Red nucleus pathway

(1) The **red nucleus** projects to the inferior olivary nucleus.

(2) The **inferior olivary nucleus** projects via the contralateral inferior cerebellar peduncle to the cerebellum.

b. Ventral lateral nucleus pathway

(1) The **ventral lateral nucleus of the thalamus** projects to the precentral gyrus (motor cortex).

(2) The **precentral gyrus** gives rise to the following tracts:

(a) Corticobulbar tract

–innervates cranial nerve nuclei.

(b) Lateral corticospinal tract

–regulates volitional synergistic motor activity.

(c) Corticopontocerebellar tracts

–regulate the output of the neocerebellum.

c. Inferior olivary nucleus pathway

(1) The inferior olivary nucleus **receives direct input from the dentate nucleus** via the crossed descending fibers of the superior cerebellar peduncle.

(2) The inferior olivary nucleus **projects directly to the dentate nucleus** via the contralateral inferior cerebellar peduncle.

V. Cerebellar Dysfunction

–is characterized by the triad **hypotonia, disequilibrium, and dyssynergia.**

A. Hypotonia

–is a loss in the resistance normally offered by muscles to palpation or to passive manipulation.

—results in a floppy, loose-jointed, rag-doll appearance with pendular re-flexes; the patient appears inebriated.

B. Disequilibrium

—refers to loss of balance, characterized by gait and trunk dystaxia.

C. Dyssynergia

—is a loss of coordinated muscle activity and includes:

1. Dysarthria

—is slurred or scanning speech.

2. Dystaxia

—is a lack of coordination in the execution of voluntary movement (e.g., gait, trunk, leg, and arm dystaxia).

3. Dysmetria

—is the inability to arrest muscular movement at the desired point (past pointing).

4. Intention tremor

—occurs during a voluntary movement (a type of dysmetria).

5. Dysdiadochokinesia

—is the inability to perform rapid alternating movements (rapid suppination and pronation of the hands).

6. Nystagmus

—is a form of dystaxia consisting of to-and-fro eye movements (ocular dysmetria).

7. Decomposition of movement ("by-the-numbers" phenomenon)

—consists of breaking down a smooth muscle act into a number of jerky awkward component parts.

VI. Cerebellar Lesions

A. Anterior vermis syndrome

—involves the leg region of the anterior lobe.
—results from atrophy of the rostral vermis, most commonly caused by alcohol abuse.
—results in gait, trunk, and leg dystaxia.

B. Posterior vermis syndrome

—involves the flocculonodular lobe.
—is usually the result of brain tumors in children.
—is most frequently caused by ependymomas or medulloblastomas.
—results in truncal dystaxia.

C. Hemispheric syndrome

—usually involves one cerebellar hemisphere.
—is frequently the result of a brain tumor or an abscess.
—results in arm, leg, trunk, and gait dystaxia.
—results in cerebellar signs that are ipsilateral to the lesion.

D. Tumors of the cerebellum

    1. Astrocytomas

        –constitute 30% of all brain tumors in children.

        –are most frequently found in the cerebellar hemisphere.

        –after surgical removal, survival for many years is common.

    2. Ependymomas

        –constitute 20% of all brain tumors in children.

        –occur most frequently in the fourth ventricle.

        –usually obstruct cerebrospinal fluid (CSF) passage and cause hydrocephalus.

    3. Medulloblastomas

        –are malignant and constitute 20% of all brain tumors in children.

        –occur most frequently in the cerebellar vermis.

        –are thought to originate from the superficial granular layer of the cerebellar cortex.

        –usually obstruct CSF passage and cause hydrocephalus.

Review Test

Directions: Each of the numbered items or incomplete statements in this section is followed by answers or by completions of the statement. Select the **one** lettered answer or completion that is **best** in each case.

1. The inferior cerebellar peduncle contains all of the following afferent connections EXCEPT

(A) the cuneocerebellar tract.
(B) the ventral spinocerebellar tract.
(C) the dorsal spinocerebellar tract.
(D) the olivocerebellar tract.
(E) the trigeminocerebellar fibers.

2. All of the following statements concerning the superior cerebellar peduncle are correct EXCEPT

(A) it connects the cerebellum to the midbrain.
(B) it is primarily an efferent bundle of fibers.
(C) it represents the major output from the cerebellum.
(D) it contains dentatothalamic fibers.
(E) it contains the juxtarestiform body.

3. All of the following statements concerning the vestibulocerebellar pathway are correct EXCEPT

(A) it plays a role in the initiation, planning, and timing of voluntary motor activities.
(B) it projects via the MLF to the ocular motor nuclei.
(C) it receives input from the cristae ampullares.
(D) it receives input from the maculae of the utricle and saccule.
(E) it includes the flocculonodular lobe.

4. All of the following statements concerning the red nucleus are correct EXCEPT

(A) it influences the cerebellum via the inferior olivary nucleus.
(B) its primary effect is on truncal and proximal muscles.
(C) it receives bilateral input from the motor and premotor cortex.
(D) it receives contralateral input from the nucleus interpositus.
(E) it receives modest input from the contralateral dentate nucleus.

5. All of the following statements concerning the neocerebellar pathway are correct EXCEPT

(A) the neocerebellar pathway influences the motor cortex via the ventral anterior thalamic nucleus.
(B) the dentatothalamic tract decussates in the midbrain.
(C) the corticopontocerebellar tract decussates in the base of the pons.
(D) the neocerebellum expresses itself via the corticospinal tract.
(E) the dentate nucleus is reciprocally connected with the inferior olivary nucleus.

6. Signs of cerebellar dysfunction include all of the following EXCEPT

(A) hypotonia.
(B) slurred or scanning speech.
(C) resting static pill-rolling tremor.
(D) dysdiadochokinesia.
(E) decomposition of movement.

7. All of the following statements concerning cerebellar nuclei are correct EXCEPT

(A) the fastigial nucleus projects to the thalamus.
(B) the fastigial nucleus projects to the brainstem via the superior and inferior cerebellar peduncles.
(C) the fastigial nucleus and the emboliform nucleus are called the interposed nucleus.
(D) the dentate nucleus produces the bulk of the axons found in the superior cerebellar peduncle.
(E) Purkinje cells project to all of the cerebellar nuclei.

8. All of the following statements concerning the cerebellum are correct EXCEPT

(A) it contains four pairs of nuclei within its medullary body.
(B) it contains two pairs of cerebellar peduncles.
(C) it consists of a midline vermis and two lateral hemispheres.
(D) it is located infratentorially within the posterior fossa.
(E) it has a three-layered cortex.

9. All of the following statements concerning the cerebellum are correct EXCEPT

(A) it projects to the red nucleus.
(B) it projects to the vestibular nuclei.
(C) it projects to the lateral ventral nucleus of the thalamus.
(D) it receives input from the superior olivary nucleus.
(E) it receives the olivocerebellar tract via the inferior cerebellar peduncle.

10. All of the following statements concerning the cerebellum are correct EXCEPT

(A) it is derived from the alar plate.
(B) it develops from the rhombic lips.
(C) it is part of the metencephalon.
(D) it is part of the rhombencephalon.
(E) it is part of the brainstem.

11. All of the following statements concerning the dentate nucleus are correct EXCEPT

(A) it receives input from climbing and mossy fibers.
(B) it receives inhibitory input from Purkinje cells.
(C) it gives rise to the superior cerebellar peduncle.
(D) it gives rise to the fascia dentata.
(E) it projects to the ventral lateral nucleus of the thalamus.

12. The most common cause of anterior vermis syndrome is

(A) alcohol abuse.
(B) an abscess.
(C) a tumor.
(D) vascular occlusion.
(E) lead intoxication.

Answers and Explanations

1–B. The ventral spinocerebellar tract enters the cerebellum via the superior cerebellar peduncle.

2–E. The inferior cerebellar peduncle includes the restiform body and the juxtarestiform body. The juxtarestiform body contains vestibulocerebellar, cerebellovestibular, and cerebelloreticular fibers.

3–A. The vestibulocerebellum (archicerebellum) plays a role in the maintenance of posture and balance and in the coordination of head and eye movements.

4–B. The red nucleus gives rise to the crossed rubrospinal tract, which has its primary effect on distal muscle groups. The red nucleus is a way station in the paravermal spinocerebellar pathway, a system dedicated to distal motor control and ongoing execution of motor acts.

5–A. In the neocerebellar pathway, the dentate nucleus projects to the contralateral ventral lateral nucleus of the thalamus, which in turn projects to the motor cortex. The motor cortex gives rise to the crossed corticopontocerebellar tract, which then modifies further cerebellar output to the neocortex. The motor cortex also gives rise to the corticospinal and corticobulbar tracts. The neocerebellum thus expresses itself via the corticospinal (pyramidal) and corticobulbar (corticonuclear) tracts.

6–C. Cerebellar signs include hypotonia, disequilibrium, muscle incoordination (dyssynergia), and nystagmus. Intention tremor is a variation of dysmetria (inability to correctly meter distances) and is commonly seen in lesions of the cerebellar hemispheres or their central projections. Dysdiadochokinesia is the inability to perform rapid alternating movements. Decomposition of movement is a breakdown of smooth muscular movement into a number of component steps. A static resting pill-rolling tremor is seen in Parkinson's disease.

7–C. The emboliform and globose nuclei are called the interposed nucleus. The fastigial nucleus projects to the vestibular nuclei via the uncinate fasciculus (a component of the superior cerebellar peduncle) and via the juxtarestiform body (a component of the inferior cerebellar peduncle). The dentate nucleus, the largest of the cerebellar nuclei, gives rise to the bulk of the axons in the superior cerebellar peduncle.

8–B. The cerebellum is attached to the brainstem by three pairs of cerebellar peduncles: Superior cerebellar peduncles connect to the pons and midbrain; middle cerebellar peduncles connect to the pons; and inferior cerebellar peduncles attach to the medulla.

9–D. The superior olivary nucleus is a relay nucleus of the auditory system and does not project to the cerebellum. The inferior olivary nucleus of the medulla projects to the cerebellum via the inferior cerebellar peduncle.

10–E. The cerebellum develops from the rhombic lips of the alar plates. The metencephalon (afterbrain) consists of the pons and cerebellum; the rhombencephalon (hindbrain) includes the metencephalon and the myelencephalon (medulla oblongata). The brainstem (truncus cerebri) includes the midbrain, pons, and medulla oblongata; some authorities also include the diencephalon.

11–D. The dentate nucleus is innervated by climbing and mossy fibers and receives inhibitory input from the Purkinje cells of the cerebellar cortex. It gives rise to most of the fibers in the superior cerebellar peduncle (i.e., the dentatorubrothalamic tract). The dentate nucleus projects to the ventral lateral and ventral posterolateral nuclei of the thalamus; these thalamic nuclei project to the motor cortex. The fascia dentata (dentate gyrus) is a structure of the hippocampal formation.

12–A. Anterior vermis syndrome is a result of chronic alcohol abuse. Patients present with dystaxia of the lower limb and trunk. Posterior vermis syndrome involves the flocculonodular lobe; it is most frequently caused by an ependymoma or a medulloblastoma. Patients have truncal dystaxia. Hemispheric syndrome usually is the result of a tumor (astrocytoma) or abscess; patients have arm, leg, trunk, and gait dystaxia.

16

Thalamus

I. Introduction—The Thalamus

–is the largest division of the diencephalon.

–receives precortical sensory input from all sensory systems except the olfactory system.

–receives its largest input from the cerebral cortex.

–projects primarily to the cerebral cortex and, to a lesser degree, to the basal ganglia and hypothalamus.

–plays an important role in sensory and motor systems integration.

II. Boundaries of the Thalamus

–consist of the following **six boundaries**:

A. Anterior: interventricular foramen

B. Posterior: free pole of the pulvinar

C. Dorsal: free surface underlying the fornix and the lateral ventricle

D. Ventral: plane connecting the hypothalamic sulci

E. Medial: third ventricle

F. Lateral: posterior limb of the internal capsule

III. Main Thalamic Nuclei and Their Major Connections (Figures 16.1 and 16.2)

A. Anterior nucleus

–receives hypothalamic input from the mamillary nucleus via the mamillo-thalamic tract.

–receives hippocampal input via the fornix.

–projects to the cingulate gyrus.

–is part of the Papez circuit of emotion (the limbic system).

B. Mediodorsal nucleus (dorsomedial nucleus)

–is reciprocally connected to the prefrontal cortex.

–has abundant connections with the intralaminar nuclei.

–receives input from the amygdaloid nucleus and the temporal neocortex.

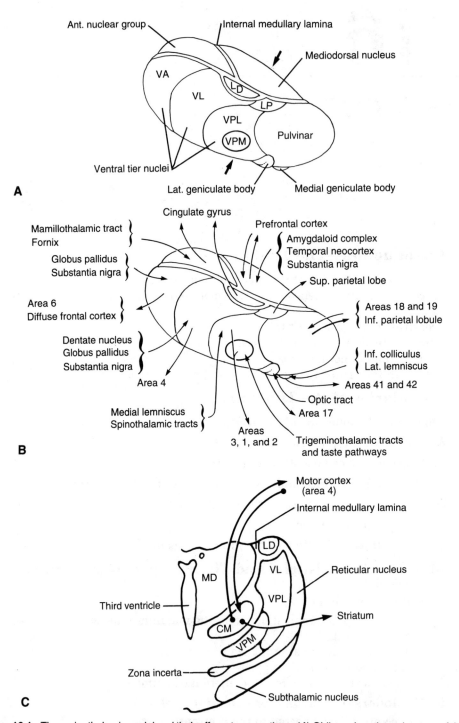

Figure 16.1. The major thalamic nuclei and their afferent connections. (*A*) Oblique dorsolateral aspect of the thalamus and major nuclei. (*B*) The major afferent and efferent connections of the thalamus. (*C*) The transverse section of the thalamus at the level of the *arrows* in (*A*), showing the major connections of the centromedian nucleus. *CM* = centromedian nucleus; *MD* = mediodorsal nucleus; *LD* = lateral dorsal nucleus; *LP* = lateral posterior nucleus; *VA* = ventral anterior nucleus; *VL* = ventral lateral nucleus; *VPL* = ventral posterior lateral nucleus; *VPM* = ventral posterior medial nucleus.

A

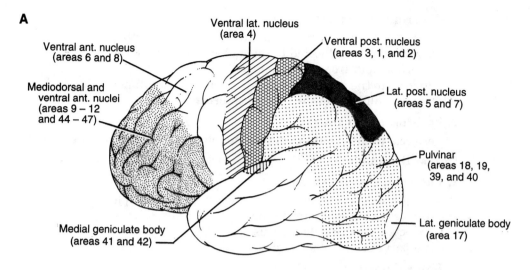

B

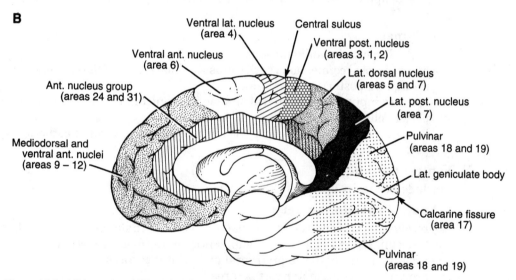

Figure 16.2. (*A*) Lateral and (*B*) medial views of the cerebral hemisphere showing the cortical projection areas of the major thalamic nuclei.

–is part of the limbic system.
–when destroyed, causes memory loss (Wernicke-Korsakoff syndrome).
–plays a role in the expression of affect, emotion, and behavior (limbic function).

C. Intralaminar nuclei

–receive input from the brainstem reticular formation, the ascending reticular system, and other thalamic nuclei.
–receive spinothalamic and trigeminothalamic input.
–projects diffusely to the entire neocortex.
–include the following nuclei:

1. Centromedian nucleus
   —is the largest of the intralaminar nuclei.
   —is reciprocally connected to the motor cortex (area 4).
   —receives input from the globus pallidus.
   —projects to the striatum (caudate nucleus and putamen).
   —projects diffusely to the entire neocortex.

2. Parafascicular nucleus
   —projects to the striatum and the supplementary motor cortex (area 6).

D. Dorsal tier nuclei

1. Lateral dorsal nucleus
   —is a posterior extension of the anterior nuclear complex.
   —receives mamillothalamic input.
   —projects to the cingulate gyrus.
   —is a part of the limbic system.

2. Lateral posterior nucleus
   —is located between the lateral dorsal nucleus and the pulvinar.
   —has reciprocal connections with the superior parietal cortex (areas 5 and 7).

3. Pulvinar
   —is the largest thalamic nucleus.
   —has reciprocal connections with the association cortex of the occipital, parietal, and posterior temporal lobes.
   —receives input from the lateral and medial geniculate bodies and the superior colliculus.
   —is concerned with the integration of visual, auditory, and somesthetic input.

E. Ventral tier nuclei
   —include primarily specific relay nuclei:

1. Ventral anterior nucleus
   —receives input from the globus pallidus (via the thalamic and lenticular fasciculi, H_1 and H_2) and the substantia nigra (motor function).
   —projects diffusely to the prefrontal and orbital cortices.
   —projects to the premotor cortex (area 6).

2. Ventral lateral nucleus
   —receives input from the globus pallidus (via the thalamic and lenticular fasciculi, H_1 and H_2), substantia nigra, and the cerebellum (dentate nucleus).
   —projects to the motor cortex (area 4) and to the supplementary motor area (area 6).
   —influences somatic motor mechanisms via the striatal motor system and the cerebellum.

3. Ventral posterior nucleus
   —is the nucleus of termination of general somatic afferent (GSA; pain and temperature) and special visceral afferent (SVA; taste) pathways.

  −contains **three subnuclei**:

  a. Ventral posterolateral (VPL) nucleus
    −receives the spinothalamic tracts and the medial lemniscus.
    −projects to the somesthetic (sensory) cortex (areas 3, 1, and 2).

  b. Ventral posteromedial (VPM) nucleus
    −receives the trigeminothalamic tracts.
    −receives the taste pathway via the solitary nucleus and the parabrachial nucleus.
    −projects to the somesthetic cortex (areas 3, 1, and 2).

  c. Ventral posteroinferior (VPI) nucleus
    −receives vestibulothalamic fibers from the vestibular nuclei.
    −projects to the vestibular area of the somesthetic cortex.

F. Lateral geniculate body
  −is a visual relay nucleus.
  −receives retinal input via the optic tract.
  −projects to the primary visual cortex (area 17, the lingual gyrus and the cuneus) via the optic radiation.

G. Medial geniculate body
  −is an auditory relay nucleus.
  −receives auditory input via the brachium of the inferior colliculus.
  −projects to the primary auditory cortex (areas 41 and 42) via the auditory radiation.

IV. Blood Supply of the Thalamus

−irrigates the thalamus via three arteries:

A. Posterior communicating artery

B. Posterior cerebral artery

C. Anterior choroidal artery (lateral geniculate body)

V. Internal Capsule (Figure 16.3; see Figures 1.9–1.11)

−is a layer of white matter (myelinated axons) that separates the caudate nucleus and thalamus medially from the lentiform nucleus laterally.
−consists of three divisions:

A. Anterior limb
  −is located between the caudate nucleus and the lentiform nucleus (the globus pallidus and the putamen).

B. Genu
  −contains corticobulbar fibers.

C. Posterior limb
  −is located between the thalamus and the lentiform nucleus.
  −contains the sensory radiations (pain, temperature, and touch).
  −contains the corticospinal fibers.
  −contains the visual and auditory radiations.

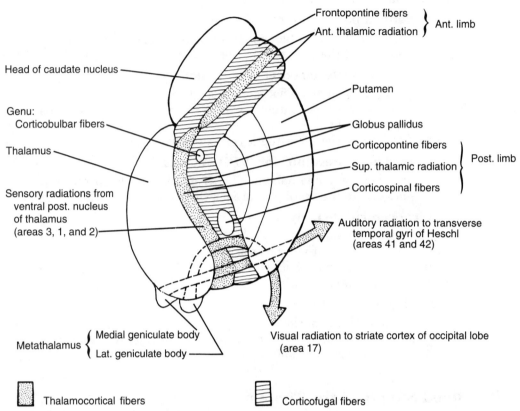

Frontopontine fibers

Ant. thalamic radiation

Ant. limb

Head of caudate nucleus

Putamen

Genu:
Corticobulbar fibers

Globus pallidus

Corticopontine fibers

Thalamus

Sup. thalamic radiation

Post. limb

Corticospinal fibers

Sensory radiations from
ventral post. nucleus
of thalamus
(areas 3, 1, and 2)

Auditory radiation to transverse
temporal gyri of Heschl
(areas 41 and 42)

Metathalamus { Medial geniculate body
Lat. geniculate body

Visual radiation to striate cortex of occipital lobe
(area 17)

Thalamocortical fibers

Corticofugal fibers

Figure 16.3. Horizontal section of the right internal capsule showing the fiber components of the anterior limb, the genu, and the posterior limb. The corticobulbar fibers are found in the genu; the corticospinal fibers are found in the posterior third of the posterior limb. The auditory and visual radiations are found in the sublenticular portion of the posterior limb. (Modified with permission from Carpenter MB and Sutin J: *Human Neuroanatomy,* 8th ed. Baltimore, Williams & Wilkins 1983, p 537.)

VI. Blood Supply of the Internal Capsule (see Figure 3.5)

   —the **anterior limb** is irrigated by the medial striate branches of the anterior cerebral artery and by the lateral striate branches (lenticulostriate) of the middle cerebral artery.

   —the **genu** is perfused either by direct branches from the internal carotid artery or by pallidal branches of the anterior choroidal artery.

   —the **posterior limb** is supplied by branches of the anterior choroidal artery and lenticulostriate branches of the middle cerebral arteries.

Review Test

Directions: Each of the numbered items or incomplete statements in this section is followed by answers or by completions of the statement. Select the **one** lettered answer or completion that is **best** in each case.

1. The thalamus receives precortical sensory input from all of the following modalities EXCEPT

(A) general somatic sense.
(B) gustation.
(C) vision.
(D) audition.
(E) olfaction.

2. Which of the following thalamic nuclei has a motor function?

(A) Lateral dorsal nucleus
(B) Mediodorsal nucleus
(C) Ventral lateral nucleus
(D) Ventral posterior nucleus
(E) Lateral posterior nucleus

3. All of the following statements concerning the mediodorsal nucleus are correct EXCEPT

(A) it receives input from the amygdaloid nucleus.
(B) it receives input from the intralaminar nuclei.
(C) it is part of the limbic system.
(D) it is part of the extrapyramidal motor system.
(E) it has reciprocal connections with the prefrontal cortex.

4. All of the following statements concerning the lateral geniculate body are correct EXCEPT

(A) it projects to the lingual gyrus.
(B) it projects to the cuneus.
(C) it receives input from the retina.
(D) it receives input from the lateral lemniscus.
(E) it receives its blood supply from the anterior choroidal artery.

5. Spinothalamic fibers project to which one of the following thalamic nuclei?

(A) Ventral posteromedial (VPM) nucleus
(B) Pulvinar
(C) Ventral anterior nucleus
(D) Ventral posterolateral (VPL) nucleus
(E) Anterior nucleus

6. Cerebellar fibers project to which one of the following thalamic nuclei?

(A) VPM nucleus
(B) Lateral dorsal nucleus
(C) Lateral posterior nucleus
(D) Ventral lateral nucleus
(E) Anterior nucleus

7. The globus pallidus projects to which one set of thalamic nuclei?

(A) Centromedian, ventral anterior, and ventral lateral nuclei
(B) Ventral anterior, ventral lateral, and anterior nuclei
(C) Ventral lateral, lateral dorsal, and lateral posterior nuclei
(D) Mediodorsal, VPL, and VPM nuclei
(E) Centromedian, lateral dorsal, and lateral ventral nuclei

8. All of the following statements concerning the pulvinar are correct EXCEPT

(A) it is the largest nucleus of the thalamus.
(B) it receives input from the visual association cortex.
(C) it receives input from the superior colliculus.
(D) it has reciprocal connections with the parietal association cortex.
(E) a lesion results in a contralateral hemianopia.

Directions: The group of items in this section consists of lettered options followed by a set of numbered items. For each item, select the **one** lettered option that is most closely associated with it. Each lettered option may be selected once, more than once, or not at all.

Questions 9–13

Match each nucleus with the pathway from which it receives input.

(A) Anterior nucleus
(B) Ventral lateral nucleus
(C) Medial geniculate (nucleus) body
(D) Ventral posteromedial nucleus
(E) Ventral posterior inferior nucleus

9. Brachium of the inferior colliculus

10. Thalamic fasciculus (H_1)

11. Mamillothalamic tract

12. Dentatothalamic tract

13. Gustatory (taste) pathway

Answers and Explanations

1–E. The thalamus receives precortical input from all sensory systems except the olfactory system. The olfactory pathway reaches the primary olfactory cortex (prepiriform and periamygdaloid cortex) without a relay in the thalamus.

2–C. The ventral lateral nucleus receives motor input from the extrapyramidal (striatal) motor system (globus pallidus and substantia nigra) and from the cerebellum (dentate nucleus).

3–D. The mediodorsal nucleus plays an important role in the expression of affect, emotion, and behavior. It is a limbic structure. The mediodorsal nucleus is not a part of the extrapyramidal motor system.

4–D. The lateral geniculate body receives input from the retina and projects to the visual cortex (lingual gyrus and cuneus). It is irrigated by the anterior choroidal artery and the posterior cerebral artery (thalamogeniculate arteries). The lateral lemniscus is an auditory pathway.

5–D. Spinothalamic fibers project to the VPL nucleus, which receives the medial lemniscus.

6–D. Cerebellar fibers (dentatocerebellar) project to the ventral lateral and VPL nuclei, which project to the motor cortex (area 4).

7–A. The globus pallidus, a nucleus of the extrapyramidal (striatal) motor system, projects to three thalamic nuclei: the centromedian, the ventral anterior, and the ventral lateral nuclei of the thalamus.

8–E. The pulvinar, the largest nucleus of the thalamus, is a dorsal tier nucleus and has reciprocal connections with the visual association cortex (areas 18 and 19). The pulvinar is reciprocally connected with the parietal association cortex (areas 39 and 40). It also receives input from the superior colliculus and the pretectal area. Destruction of the pulvinar does not result in a visual field deficit (hemianopia).

9–C. The medial geniculate body receives auditory input via the brachium of the inferior colliculus.

10–B. The ventral lateral nucleus receives input from the globus pallidus via the thalamic fasciculus (H_1).

11–A. The anterior nucleus receives input from the mamillary nuclei via the mamillothalamic tract. This is a major link in the Papez circuit.

12–B. The ventral lateral nucleus receives cerebellar input from the dentate nucleus via the dentatothalamic tract.

13–D. The VPM nucleus receives SVA (taste) fibers from the central tegmental tract.

17

Visual System

I. Introduction—The Visual System

—is served by the **optic nerve, cranial nerve II,** which is a special somatic afferent (**SSA**) nerve.

II. The Retina

—is the innermost layer of the eye.
—is derived from the optic vesicle of the diencephalon.
—contains efferent fibers that give rise to the optic nerve, which is actually a fiber tract of the diencephalon.
—is sensitive to wavelengths from 400 nm to 700 nm.

A. Structures of the ocular fundus

1. Optic disk (optic papilla)

—is located nasal to the fovea centralis.
—contains unmyelinated axons from the ganglion cell layer of the retina.
—is the blind spot (contains no rods or cones).
—contains a central disk margin, a peripheral disk margin, and retinal vessels.

2. Macula lutea

—is a yellow-pigmented area that surrounds the fovea centralis.

3. Fovea centralis

—is located within the macula lutea, temporal to the optic disk.
—contains only cones and is the site of highest visual acuity.
—is avascular and receives nutrients by diffusion via the choriocapillaris.
—subserves color or day (photopic) vision.

4. Retinal blood supply

—is provided by the **choriocapillaris** of the choroid layer and the **central retinal artery,** a branch of the ophthalmic artery.
—occlusion of the central retinal artery results in blindness.

B. Cells of the retina

—constitute a chain of three neurons that project visual impulses via the optic nerve and lateral geniculate body to the visual cortex.

1. Rods and cones

—are first-order receptor cells that respond directly to light stimulation.

a. Rods (100 million)

—contain **rhodopsin** (visual purple) and are sensitive to low intensity light.

—subserve night (scotopic) vision.

b. Cones (7 million)

—contain the photopigment **iodopsin**.

—operate only at high illumination levels.

—are concentrated in the fovea centralis.

—are responsible for day vision, color vision, and high visual acuity.

2. Bipolar neurons

—are second-order neurons that relay stimuli from the rods and cones to the ganglion cells.

3. Ganglion cells

—are third-order neurons with axons that form the optic nerve.

—project directly to the hypothalamus, superior colliculus, pretectal nucleus, and lateral geniculate body.

C. Meridional divisions of the retina

1. The visual field illustrated in Figure 17.1 is the environment seen by one eye (**monocular field**) or by both eyes (**binocular field**).

2. The vertical meridian divides the retina into **hemiretinae,** and the horizontal meridian divides the hemiretinae into **upper and lower quadrants**.

a. Temporal hemiretina

—receives image input from the nasal visual field.

b. Nasal hemiretina

—receives image input from the temporal visual field.

c. Upper retinal quadrants

—receive image input from the lower visual fields.

d. Lower retinal quadrants

—receive image input from the upper visual fields.

D. Concentric divisions of the retina

1. Macular area

—is a small area surrounding and including the fovea centralis that serves central vision (high visual acuity).

—projects to the posterior part of the visual cortex.

2. Paramacular area

—is a large area surrounding the macular area that contains predominantly rods.

—projects to the visual cortex posterior to the macular representation.

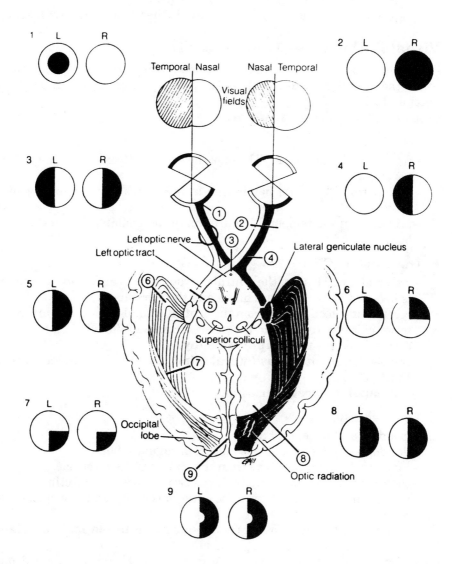

Figure 17.1. Visual pathway from the retina to the visual cortex, showing the common visual field defects at sites 1–9. Note the monocular visual fields; the temporal visual field projects to the nasal retina, and the nasal visual field projects to the temporal retina. Note also that temporal fibers remain ipsilateral, and nasal fibers decussate. (*1*) Central scotoma, due to optic or retrobulbar neuritis. (*2*) Total blindness of the right eye, due to complete lesion of a right optic nerve. (*3*) Bitemporal hemianopia, due to the pressure exerted on the optic chiasm by a pituitary tumor. (*4*) Right nasal hemianopia, due to a perichiasmal lesion such as a calcified internal carotid artery. (*5*) Right homonymous hemianopia, due to a lesion of the left optic tract. (*6*) Right homonymous superior quadrantanopia, due to partial involvement of the optic radiation by a lesion in the left temporal lobe (Meyer's loop). (*7*) Right homonymous inferior quadrantanopia, due to partial involvement of the optic radiation by a lesion in the left parietal lobe. (*8*) Right homonymous hemianopia, due to complete involvement of the left optic radiation. A similar defect may also result from a destructive lesion at 9. (*9*) Right homonymous hemianopia with macular sparing, due to posterior cerebral artery occlusion. (Reprinted with permission from Simon RP, Aminoff MJ, and Greenberg DA: *Clinical Neurology.* Norwalk, CT, Appleton & Lange 1989, p 112.)

3. Monocular area

–represents the peripheral monocular field.
–projects to the visual cortex posterior to the paramacular representation.

III. Visual Pathway (see Figures 1.2 and 17.1)

–transmits visual impulses from the retina to the lateral geniculate body and from the lateral geniculate body to the primary visual cortex (area 17) of the occipital lobe.
–consists of the following structures:

A. Ganglion cells

–constitute the ganglion cell layer of the retina with axons that form the optic nerve (CN II).
–project from the nasal hemiretina to the contralateral lateral geniculate body.
–project from the temporal hemiretina to the ipsilateral lateral geniculate body.

B. Optic nerve (CN II)

–is a myelinated tract of the central nervous system and is **not a true nerve**.
–is invested by the pia–arachnoid and the dura mater.
–receives its blood supply from the central retinal artery, pial arteries, posterior ciliary arteries, and the arterial circle of Willis.
–compression results in **optic atrophy**.
–transection results in **ipsilateral blindness** and in **no direct pupillary light reflex**.
–is **incapable of regeneration**.

C. Optic chiasm

–is a part of the diencephalon.
–lies dorsal to the hypophysis and diaphragma sellae.
–contains decussating fibers from the two nasal hemiretinae.
–contains noncrossing fibers from the two temporal hemiretinae.
–receives its blood supply from the anterior cerebral and internal carotid arteries.
–midsagittal transection or pressure results in **bitemporal hemianopia** (frequently from a pituitary tumor).
–bilateral lateral compression results in **binasal hemianopia** (calcified internal carotid arteries).

D. Optic tract

–contains fibers from the ipsilateral temporal hemiretina and the contralateral nasal hemiretina.
–contains **pupillary reflex fibers**.
–projects to the lateral geniculate body and, via the brachium of the superior colliculus, to the pretectal nuclei and to the superior colliculus.
–receives its blood supply from the posterior communicating artery and the anterior choroidal artery.
–transection results in a **contralateral homonymous hemianopia** and in **transsynaptic degeneration of the ipsilateral geniculate body**.

E. Lateral geniculate body

–is a thalamic relay nucleus that subserves vision.
–receives fibers from the ipsilateral temporal hemiretina and the contralateral nasal hemiretina.
–projects, via the geniculocalcarine tract, to the primary visual cortex (area 17).
–is irrigated by branches of the posterior cerebral artery and the anterior choroidal artery.
–destruction results in a **contralateral homonymous hemianopia**.

F. Geniculocalcarine tract (visual radiation) [Figure 17.2]

–extends from the lateral geniculate body to the banks of the calcarine sulcus, the visual cortex (area 17).
–is irrigated by branches of the middle cerebral artery, anterior choroidal artery, and calcarine artery (a branch of the posterior cerebral artery).
–transection results in a **contralateral homonymous hemianopia**.
–has two divisions (see Figure 17.2):

1. Upper division

–projects to the upper bank of the calcarine sulcus, the **cuneus**.
–contains input from the superior retinal quadrants, representing inferior visual field quadrants.
–transection results in a **contralateral lower homonymous quadrantanopia**.

2. Lower division

–loops from the lateral geniculate body anteriorly (Meyer's loop), then posteriorly to terminate in the lower bank of the calcarine sulcus, the **lingual gyrus**.

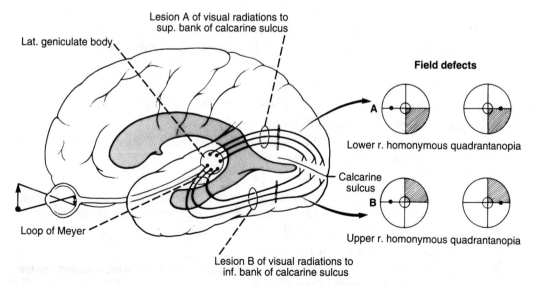

Figure 17.2. Relationships of the left upper and left lower divisions of the geniculocalcarine tract to the lateral ventricle and the calcarine sulcus. Transection of the upper division (*A*) results in a right lower homonymous quadrantanopia; transection of the lower division (*B*) results in a right upper homonymous quadrantanopia.

–contains input from the inferior retinal quadrants, representing superior visual field quadrants.

–transection of Meyer's loop results in a **contralateral upper homonymous quadrantanopia**.

G. Visual (striate) cortex (area 17)

–is located in the banks of the calcarine sulcus.

–receives retinal input via the ipsilateral lateral geniculate body.

–receives its blood supply from the calcarine artery, a branch of the posterior cerebral artery; anastomosis with the middle cerebral artery may be substantial (with macular sparing).

–lesions result in a **contralateral homonymous hemianopia with macular sparing**.

–has **retinotopic organization**:

1. Posterior third of the visual cortex

–receives macular input (central vision).

2. Intermediate area of the visual cortex

–receives paramacular input (peripheral input).

3. Anterior area of the visual cortex

–receives monocular input.

IV. Pupillary Light Reflexes and Pathway (Figure 17.3)

A. Pupillary light reflexes

–result when light shone into one eye causes both pupils to constrict.

1. Direct pupillary light reflex

–is the response in the stimulated eye.

2. Consensual pupillary light reflex

–is the response in the unstimulated eye.

B. Pupillary light reflex pathway

–comprises an afferent limb, **CN II,** and an efferent limb, **CN III**.

–consists of the following structures:

1. Ganglion cells of the retina

–project bilaterally to the pretectal nuclei.

2. Pretectal nucleus of the midbrain

–projects crossed (in the posterior commissure) and uncrossed fibers to the Edinger-Westphal nucleus.

3. Edinger-Westphal nucleus of the midbrain

–gives rise to preganglionic parasympathetic fibers, which exit the midbrain with the oculomotor nerve and synapse with postganglionic parasympathetic neurons of the ciliary ganglion.

4. Ciliary ganglion of the orbit

–gives rise to postganglionic parasympathetic fibers, which innervate the sphincter muscle of the iris.

V. Pupillary Dilation Pathway

–is mediated by the sympathetic division of the autonomic nervous system.

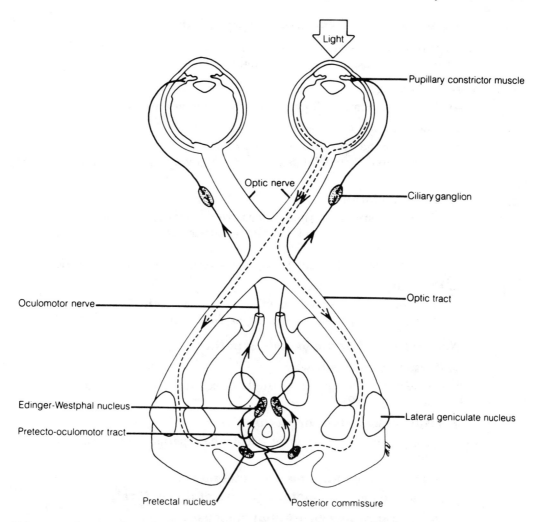

Figure 17.3. Diagram of the pupillary light pathway. Light shone into one eye causes both pupils to constrict. The response in the stimulated eye is called the direct pupillary light reflex; the reponse in the opposite eye is called the consensual pupillary light reflex. (Reprinted with permission from Walsh FB and Hoyt WF: *Clinical Neuro-ophthalmology,* vol 1, 3rd ed. Baltimore, Williams & Wilkins, 1969, p 473.)

—interruption at any level results in **Horner's syndrome**.

—consists of the following structures:

A. Hypothalamus

—hypothalamic neurons project directly to the ciliospinal center (T1–T2) of the intermediolateral cell column.

B. Ciliospinal center of Budge (T1–T2)

—projects preganglionic sympathetic fibers via the sympathetic trunk to the superior cervical ganglion.

C. Superior cervical ganglion

—projects postganglionic sympathetic fibers via the perivascular plexus of the carotid system to the dilator muscle of the iris. Postganglionic sympathetic fibers pass through the cavernous sinus and enter the orbit via the superior orbital fissure.

VI. Near Reflex and Accommodation Reaction

–is essential for visual fixation and acuity at close range.
–is initiated by conscious visual fixation or by a blurred retinal image.

A. Reflex changes

–with accommodative effort, three reflex changes are evoked:

1. Convergence

–occurs as the eyes focus on a near point.
–is mediated by medial recti innervation via the oculomotor nerve (CN III).

2. Accommodation

–is the adjustment of the eye for various distances.
–occurs as contraction of the ciliary muscle results in a thickening of the lens and an increase in refractive power.
–is mediated by the caudal Edinger-Westphal nucleus via CN III.

3. Pupillary constriction

–results in an increase in depth of field and depth of focus.
–is mediated by the rostral Edinger-Westphal nucleus via CN III.

B. Near reflex and accommodation pathway

1. Cortical visual pathway

–projects from the primary visual cortex (area 17) to the visual association cortex (area 19).

2. Visual association cortex (area 19)

–projects via the corticotectal tract to the superior colliculus and pretectal nucleus.

3. Superior colliculus and pretectal nucleus

–project to the **oculomotor complex of the midbrain**:

a. Rostral Edinger-Westphal nucleus

–mediates pupillary constriction via the ciliary ganglion.

b. Caudal Edinger-Westphal nucleus

–mediates contraction of the ciliary muscle, resulting in an increase in refractive power.

c. Medial rectus subnucleus of CN III

–mediates convergence.

VII. Centers for Ocular Motility

A. Frontal eye field

–is located in the caudal part of the middle frontal gyrus (area 8).
–is a center for voluntary eye movements.
–stimulation (an irritative lesion) results in **contralateral deviation of the eyes** (i.e., away from the lesion).
–destruction results in **transient ipsilateral conjugate deviation of the eyes** (i.e., toward the lesion).

B. Occipital eye fields

  –are located in areas 18 and 19 of the occipital lobe.

  –are cortical centers for involuntary pursuit and tracking movements.

  –stimulation results in **contralateral conjugate deviation of the eyes**.

C. Subcortical center for lateral conjugate gaze

  –is located in the abducent nucleus of the pons.

  –receives input from the contralateral frontal eye field.

  –projects to the ipsilateral lateral rectus muscle.

  –projects, via the medial longitudinal fasciculus (MLF), to the contralateral medial rectus subnucleus of the oculomotor complex.

D. Subcortical center for vertical conjugate gaze

  –is located in the midbrain at the level of the posterior commissure.

  –is associated with **Parinaud's syndrome** (see Chapter 14).

VIII. Clinical Correlations

A. MLF syndrome

  –is a condition in which there is damage (demyelination) to the MLF between the abducent and the oculomotor nuclei.

  –results in **medial rectus palsy** on attempted lateral conjugate gaze and **monocular horizontal nystagmus** in the abducting eye (convergence is normal).

B. Anisocoria (unequal pupils)

  –is a condition in which the pupils are not equal.

  –is present in 10% of the population.

  –is seen in **Horner's syndrome** and in **palsies of CN III**.

C. Argyll Robertson pupil (pupillary light–near dissociation)

  –is the absence of a miotic reaction to light, both direct and consensual, with preservation of a miotic reaction to near stimulus (accommodation-convergence).

  –may be present in **syphilis and diabetes**.

D. Afferent pupil (Marcus Gunn pupil)

  1. This condition results from a **lesion in the afferent limb of the pupillary light reflex** (e.g., retrobulbar neuritis of the optic nerve seen in multiple sclerosis).

  2. Diagnosis can be made by the **swinging flashlight test**.

   a. Light shone into the normal eye results in brisk **pupillary constriction** in both the normal eye and in the affected eye (consensual reaction).

   b. Light is then immediately shone into the affected eye with the afferent lesion, which results in **dilation of the afferent pupil**. The consensual stimulation of the constrictor pupillae muscle is much greater than the direct stimulation through a defective optic nerve.

E. Transtentorial herniation (uncal herniation)

  –occurs as the result of **increased supratentorial pressure**, commonly due to a brain tumor or a hematoma (subdural or epidural).

1. The pressure cone forces the parahippocampal uncus through the tentorial incisure.

2. The impacted uncus forces the contralateral crus cerebri against the tentorial edge and brings pressure to bear on ipsilateral CN III and the posterior cerebral artery, resulting in the following neurologic deficits:

    a. Ipsilateral hemiparesis due to pressure on the corticospinal tract located in the crus cerebri

    b. A fixed and dilated pupil, ptosis, and a "down and out" eye, due to pressure on the ipsilateral oculomotor nerve

    c. Contralateral homonymous hemianopia, due to compression of the ipsilateral posterior cerebral artery, which irrigates the visual cortex

F. Papilledema (choked disk)

    −is a noninflammatory congestion of the optic disk caused by increased intracranial pressure.

    −is most commonly caused by **brain tumors, subdural hematoma, and hydrocephalus**.

    −usually does not alter visual acuity or result in visual field deficits.

    −is frequently asymmetric and will be greater on the side of the supratentorial lesion.

Review Test

Directions: Each of the numbered items or incomplete statements in this section is followed by answers or by completions of the statement. Select the **one** lettered answer or completion that is **best** in each case.

1. All of the following statements concerning the optic chiasm are correct EXCEPT

(A) it is irrigated by the anterior cerebral and internal carotid arteries.
(B) it lies dorsal to the pituitary gland.
(C) midsagittal section results in binasal hemianopia.
(D) it contains uncrossed fibers from the temporal hemiretinae.
(E) it contains pupillary fibers en route to the pretectum.

2. All of the following statements concerning the lateral geniculate body are correct EXCEPT

(A) it is a thalamic nucleus.
(B) it receives input from the contralateral visual field.
(C) it is irrigated by the posterior cerebral artery and the anterior choroidal artery.
(D) destruction results in bitemporal hemianopia.
(E) it projects to the lingual gyrus and the cuneus.

3. All of the following statements concerning the visual cortex are correct EXCEPT

(A) it corresponds to area 17.
(B) it is located in the banks of the calcarine sulcus.
(C) destruction of the upper bank of the calcarine sulcus results in a lower ipsilateral homonymous quadrantanopia.
(D) cortical lesions are characterized by macular sparing.
(E) it is irrigated by the posterior cerebral artery.

4. All of the following statements concerning the pupillary light pathway are correct EXCEPT

(A) transection of the optic tract eliminates the direct pupillary light response.
(B) transection of the optic nerve would not eliminate the consensual pupillary light reflex.
(C) destruction of the lateral geniculate body would not interrupt the pupillary light pathway.
(D) the efferent limb of the pupillary light reflex is the oculomotor nerve (CN III).
(E) axons of retinal ganglion cells mediating the pupillary light reflex terminate in the pretectal nucleus.

5. All of the following statements concerning the retina are correct EXCEPT

(A) it is derived from the optic vesicle of the diencephalon.
(B) it is sensitive to wavelengths from 400 nm to 700 nm.
(C) retinal ganglion cells project directly to the visual cortex.
(D) retinal ganglion cells project directly to the hypothalamus.
(E) retinal ganglion cells project directly to the midbrain.

6. All of the following statements concerning the optic disk are correct EXCEPT

(A) it is found nasal to the fovea centralis.
(B) it is the blind spot.
(C) it contains the retinal vessels.
(D) it contains myelinated axons from the ganglion cell layer.
(E) it contains neither rods nor cones.

7. All of the following statements concerning the fovea centralis are correct EXCEPT

(A) it plays a role in photopic vision.
(B) it lies within the macula lutea.
(C) it contains only cones.
(D) it is the optic papilla.
(E) it is the site of highest visual acuity.

8. All of the following statements concerning the ganglion cells of the retina are correct EXCEPT they

(A) give rise to the optic nerve.
(B) receive direct input from the rods and cones.
(C) are derived from the diencephalon.
(D) project to the lateral geniculate body.
(E) project directly to the hypothalamus.

9. All of the following statements concerning the optic nerve are correct EXCEPT

(A) it is a myelinated tract of the CNS.
(B) it is a true peripheral nerve.
(C) it is invested by leptomeninges.
(D) it is incapable of regeneration.
(E) its cells of origin are found in the ganglion cell layer of the retina.

10. All of the following statements concerning the subcortical center for lateral gaze are correct EXCEPT

(A) it receives input from the contralateral frontal lobe.
(B) it projects to the contralateral MLF.
(C) it is found in the pons.
(D) it is found in the midbrain.
(E) it is found within a cranial nerve nucleus.

11. Interruption of the MLF at pontine levels

(A) results in miosis and ptosis.
(B) results in paralysis of upward gaze on command.
(C) results in paralysis of lateral gaze on command.
(D) abolishes convergence.
(E) abolishes accommodation.

Directions: Each group of items in this section consists of lettered options followed by a set of numbered items. For each item, select the **one** lettered option that is most closely associated with it. Each lettered option may be selected once, more than once, or not at all.

Questions 12–19

Match each defect below with the condition it causes.

(A) Bitemporal hemianopia
(B) Binasal hemianopia
(C) Left upper homonymous quadrantanopia
(D) Right lower homonymous quadrantanopia
(E) Left homonymous hemianopia

12. Transection of the right optic tract

13. Transection of the right side of Meyer's loop

14. Midsagittal section of the optic chiasm

15. Tumor of the right lateral geniculate body

16. Pituitary tumor

17. Tumor of the left cuneus

18. Trauma to the right lingual gyrus

19. Bilateral lateral constriction of the optic chiasm

Answers and Explanations

1–C. Midsagittal section of the optic chiasm transects fibers from the nasal hemiretinae and results in a bitemporal hemianopia. This visual field defect is frequently the result of a pituitary tumor (e.g., a chromophobic adenoma).

2–D. Complete destruction of the optic tract, the lateral geniculate body, or the geniculocalcarine tract all result in the same visual field defect, a contralateral homonymous hemianopia.

3–C. Destruction of the upper bank of the calcarine sulcus interrupts the fibers of the lateral geniculate body that represent the upper ipsilateral retinal quadrants. The field defect is called a lower contralateral homonymous quadrantanopia.

4–A. Transection of the optic tract would not eliminate the direct pupillary response. Pupillary fibers in the optic tract project to the pretectal nuclei, which discharge to the ipsilateral and contralateral Edinger-Westphal nuclei.

5–C. Retinal ganglion cells project to the lateral geniculate body, which projects to the primary visual cortex. Retinal ganglion cells project directly to the suprachiasmatic nucleus of the hypothalamus and to the pretectal nuclei and superior colliculus of the midbrain. The retina is derived from the optic vesicle of the diencephalon.

6–D. The optic disk, the optic papilla, is found nasal (medial) to the fovea centralis. It contains no rods or cones and thus represents a blind spot in the retina. The retinal vessels emerge from the optic disk. Myelineated axons usually are not found in the retina; when they are present, they may produce a central scotoma. Myelination of the optic nerve extends from the external part of the lamina cribrosa to the lateral geniculate body.

7–D. The fovea centralis lies within the macula lutea and represents the locus of highest visual acuity. The fovea contains only cones, thus subserving color or day (photopic) vision. The fovea centralis lies temporal (lateral) to the optic disk. The optic disk is the optic papilla.

8–B. The ganglion cells of the retina give rise to the optic nerve and project to the lateral geniculate body, the hypothalamus, the pretectal nucleus, and the superior colliculus. Input from the rods and cones is conducted to the ganglion cells via the bipolar cells. The retina is derived from the optic vesicle of the diencephalon. The hypothalamic projection is to the suprachiasmatic nucleus, a circadian pacemaker.

9–B. The optic nerve is a myelinated tract of the CNS that is invested by the leptomeninges and the dura mater. Its cells of origin are found in the ganglion cell layer of the retina. It is incapable of regeneration.

10–D. The subcortical center for lateral gaze is found in the abducent nucleus of the pons, receives input from the contralateral frontal eye field (area 8), and projects to the contralateral MLF. Destruction of the abducent nucleus results in an ipsilateral lateral rectus paralysis and a contralateral medial rectus palsy on attempted lateral gaze. The subcortical center for vertical conjugate gaze is located in the midbrain at the level of the posterior commissure.

11–C. Interruption of the pontine MLF results in a medial rectus palsy on attempted conjugate lateral gaze. Convergence remains intact. This syndrome, called internuclear ophthalmoplegia or MLF syndrome, is commonly seen in multiple sclerosis.

12–E. Transection of the right optic tract results in a left homonymous hemianopia.

13–C. Transection of Meyer's loop on the right side results in a left upper quadrantanopia, "pie in the sky." Meyer's loop is the inferior geniculocalcarine pathway that conveys information from the inferior retinal quadrants to the inferior bank of the calcarine sulcus, the lingual gyrus.

14–A. A midsagittal section of the optic chiasm interrupts the decussating fibers from the nasal hemiretinae and results in a bitemporal hemianopia.

15–E. A lesion of the right lateral geniculate body produces a left homonymous hemianopia. A lesion of the optic tract, the lateral geniculate body, or the visual pathway all produce the same field deficit, a contralateral homonymous hemianopia.

16–A. A pituitary tumor most commonly produces a bitemporal hemianopia. The pituitary (hypophysis) gland lies ventral to the optic chiasm.

17–D. Destruction of the left cuneus produces a right lower homonymous quadrantanopia. Upper retinal quadrants project to the upper banks of the calcarine sulcus.

18–C. Destruction of the right lingual gyrus produces a left upper homonymous quadrantanopia. Lower retinal quadrants project to the lower banks of the calcarine sulcus.

19–B. Bilateral lateral constriction of the optic chiasm damages the nondecussating fibers from the temporal hemiretinae and produces a binasal hemianopia.

18
Autonomic Nervous System

I. Overview—The Autonomic Nervous System (ANS)

—is a general visceral efferent (**GVE**) motor system that controls and regulates smooth muscle, cardiac muscle, and glands.

—consists of two types of projection neurons: **preganglionic neurons** and **postganglionic neurons** (sympathetic ganglia have interneurons).

—autonomic output is influenced by the hypothalamus.

—has three divisions: the **sympathetic,** the **parasympathetic,** and the **enteric.**

II. Divisions of the Autonomic Nervous System

A. Sympathetic division (Figure 18.1; Table 18.1)

—is also called the **thoracolumbar,** or **adrenergic, system**.

—stimulates activities that are mobilized during emergency stress situations, the "fight, fright, and flight" responses, which include increased heart rate and force of contraction and increased blood pressure.

1. Preganglionic neurons (see Figures 6.2 and 6.3)

—are located in the intermediolateral cell column (T1–L3).

—project via ventral roots and white communicating rami to the sympathetic trunk or via splanchnic nerves to prevertebral ganglia. They synapse at both locations with postganglionic neurons.

2. Postganglionic neurons (see Figures 6.2 and 6.3)

—are located in the sympathetic trunk (paravertebral ganglia) and in prevertebral (collateral) ganglia.

—in the sympathetic trunk, they project via gray communicating rami to spinal nerves and innervate blood vessels, arrector pili muscles, and sweat glands.

—in prevertebral ganglia, they project to abdominal and pelvic viscera.

3. Interneurons

—are called **small intensely fluorescent (SIF) cells**.

—are located in sympathetic ganglia.

—are dopaminergic and inhibitory.

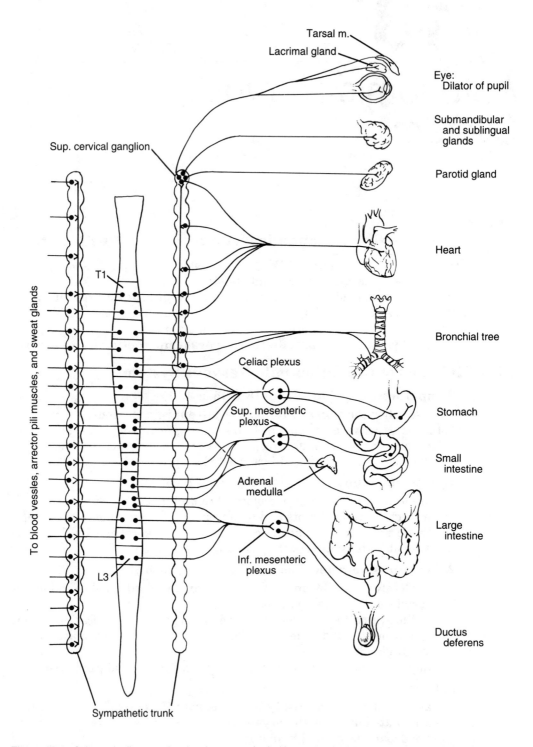

Figure 18.1. Schematic diagram showing the sympathetic (thoracolumbar) innervation of the ANS. Note that the entire sympathetic innervation of the head is via the superior cervical ganglion. Gray communicating rami are found at all spinal cord levels; white communicating rami are found only in spinal segments T1–L3.

Table 18.1. Sympathetic and Parasympathetic Activity on Organ Systems

Structure	Sympathetic Function	Parasympathetic Function
Eye		
Radial muscle of iris	Dilates pupil (mydriasis)	
Circular muscle of iris		Constricts pupil (miosis)
Ciliary muscle of ciliary body		Contracts for near vision
Lacrimal gland		Stimulates secretion
Salivary glands	Viscous secretion	Watery secretion
Sweat glands		
Thermoregulatory	Increases	
Apocrine (stress)	Increases	
Heart		
Sinoatrial node	Accelerates	Decelerates (vagal arrest)
Atrioventricular node	Increases conduction velocity	Decreases conduction velocity
Contractility	Increases	Decreases (atria)
Vascular smooth muscle		
Skin, splanchnic vessels	Contracts	
Skeletal muscle vessels	Relaxes	
Bronchiolar smooth muscle	Relaxes	Contracts
Gastrointestinal tract		
Smooth muscle		
Walls	Relaxes	Contracts
Sphincters	Contracts	Relaxes
Secretion and motility	Decreases	Increases
Genitourinary tract		
Smooth muscle		
Bladder wall	Little or no effect	Contracts
Sphincter	Contracts	Relaxes
Penis, seminal vesicles	Ejaculation	Erection
Adrenal medulla	Secretes epinephrine and norepinephrine	
Metabolic functions		
Liver	Gluconeogenesis and glycogenolysis	
Fat cells	Lipolysis	
Kidney	Renin release	

4. Neurotransmitters

a. Acetylcholine

—is the neurotransmitter of **preganglionic neurons**.

b. Norepinephrine

—is the neurotransmitter of **postganglionic neurons,** with the exception of sweat glands and some blood vessels that receive cholinergic sympathetic innervation.

c. Dopamine

—is the neurotransmitter of the **SIF cells**.

B. Parasympathetic division (Figure 18.2; see Table 18.1)

–is called the **craniosacral, or cholinergic, system**.

–stimulates activities that conserve energy and restore body resources, including reduction of heart rate and increases in digestion and absorption of food.

–**uses acetylcholine** as the neurotransmitter for both preganglionic and postganglionic synapses.

1. Cranial division

–is associated with four cranial nerves:

a. Oculomotor nerve (CN III) [see Figure 17.3]

(1) Edinger-Westphal nucleus (midbrain)

–projects preganglionic fibers to the ciliary ganglion.

(2) Ciliary ganglion

–projects postganglionic fibers to the sphincter muscle of the iris (miosis) and to the ciliary muscle (accommodation).

b. Facial nerve (CN VII) [see Figure 13.3]

(1) Superior salivatory nucleus

–projects preganglionic fibers to the pterygopalatine and submandibular ganglia.

(2) Pterygopalatine ganglion

–projects postganglionic fibers to the lacrimal gland and to the mucosa of the nose and palate.

(3) Submandibular ganglion

–projects postganglionic fibers to the submandibular and sublingual glands.

c. Glossopharyngeal nerve (CN IX) [see Figure 9.5]

(1) Inferior salivatory nucleus

–projects preganglionic fibers to the otic ganglion.

(2) Otic ganglion

–projects postganglionic fibers to the parotid gland.

d. Vagal nerve (CN X) [see Figures 9.3 and 9.4]

(1) Dorsal motor nucleus

–projects preganglionic fibers to intramural (terminal) ganglia located within or adjacent to visceral organs.

(2) Intramural (terminal) ganglia

–innervate, via short postganglionic fibers, viscera of the thorax and abdomen as far as the left colic flexure.

(3) Nucleus ambiguus

–projects preganglionic fibers to the intramural ganglia of the heart (sinoatrial and atrioventricular nodes).

2. Sacral division

–originates from the sacral parasympathetic nucleus of sacral segments S2–S4.

–its postganglionic neurons lie on, near, or in the wall of the innervated viscus (intramural ganglia).

–innervates, via pelvic nerves, the lower abdomen and pelvic viscera, including the colon distal to the left colic flexure, urinary bladder (detrusor muscle), and genital viscera.

–is involved with **micturition, defecation, and sexual function**.

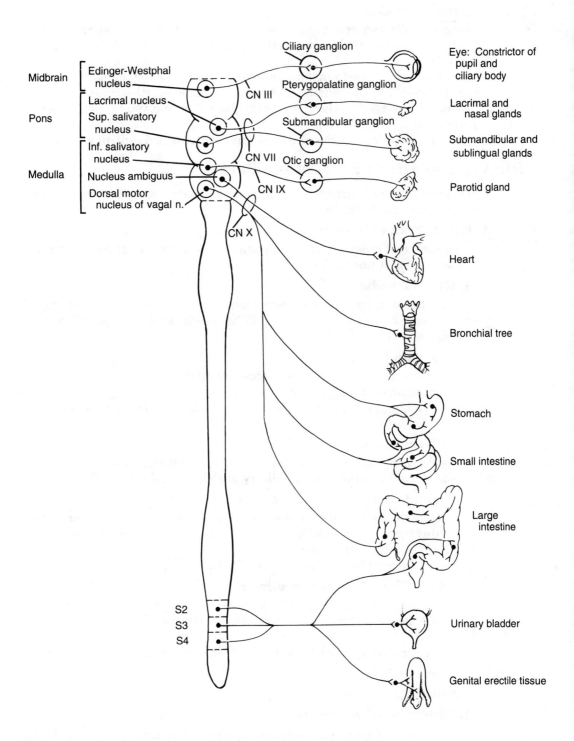

Figure 18.2. Schematic diagram showing the parasympathetic (craniosacral) innervation of the ANS. Sacral outflow includes segments S2–S4. Cranial outflow is mediated via four cranial nerves: CN III, CN VII, CN IX, and CN X. Note that the preganglionic parasympathetic innervation of the heart is from the nucleus ambiguus via the vagal nerve.

C. Enteric division

—consists of intramural (enteric) ganglia and plexuses of the gastrointestinal tract, including the submucosal (Meissner's) plexus and the myenteric (Auerbach's) plexus.

—is influenced by postganglionic adrenergic sympathetic input.

—is influenced by preganglionic cholinergic parasympathetic input.

—functions independently when deprived of central nervous system innervation.

—plays a major role in the control of **gastrointestinal motility**.

III. Visceral Afferent Fibers and Pain

—all sympathetic and parasympathetic nerves contain both general visceral afferent (**GVA**) and **GVE** fibers.

A. GVA fibers and innervated structures

—most visceral reflexes and organic sensations are mediated by parasympathetic afferent fibers.

1. GVA cell bodies

—are found in dorsal root ganglia, inferior ganglia of the glossopharyngeal nerve (CN IX), the vagal nerve (CN X), and the geniculate ganglion of the facial nerve (CN VII).

2. GVA pain fibers

—are found in the white communicating rami.

—accompany sympathetic nerves exclusively.

—have their cell bodies in the dorsal root ganglia of the thoracolumbar region (T1–L3).

3. GVA reflex fibers

—accompany both sympathetic and parasympathetic nerves.

—terminate centrally in the solitary nucleus (i.e., the gag reflex).

4. Carotid sinus

—is a slight dilation of the common carotid artery at the bifurcation; it contains baroreceptors, which, when stimulated, cause bradycardia and a decrease in blood pressure.

—is innervated by GVA fibers from CN IX.

5. Carotid body (glomus caroticum)

—is a small structure located just above the bifurcation of the common carotid artery; it contains chemoreceptors that respond to CO_2, O_2, and pH levels.

—is innervated by GVA fibers from CN IX and CN X.

B. Visceral pain

—results from the following conditions:

1. Distension of any viscus

2. Spasms or strong contractions, especially when accompanied by ischemia

3. Mechanical stimulation, especially when the organ is hyperemic

4. Myocardial ischemia with the release of kinins

C. Referred visceral pain

–is the false reference or localization of a painful visceral stimulus to a somatic dermatome of the same spinal cord segment.

–can be explained by the **convergence-projection mechanism:**

1. For example, in angina pectoris, painful impulses from the myocardium are projected to sensory dorsal horn relay neurons of thoracic segments T1–T4. These same relay neurons also receive cutaneous input from their corresponding dermatomes.

2. Painful impulses are projected to the somesthetic cortex via the spinothalamic and thalamocortical tracts. These impulses are misperceived as coming from nociceptors of the left chest (T2–T4) and radiating down the left arm (T1 and T2).

IV. Autonomic Innervation of Selected Organs

A. Eye

1. Sympathetic input

a. **Hypothalamic neurons** project directly to the intermediolateral cell column at T1 and T2, the ciliospinal center of Budge.

b. The **intermediolateral cell column** (T1–T2) projects preganglionic fibers via the sympathetic trunk to the superior cervical ganglion.

c. The **superior cervical ganglion** projects postganglionic fibers via the internal carotid artery to the cavernous sinus.

d. Pupillodilator fibers reach the dilator pupillae muscle of the iris via the superior orbital fissure and via the nasociliary and long ciliary nerves (CN V).

e. Fibers to the tarsal muscles of Müller reach the eyelids via the **ophthalmic artery** (optic canal).

f. Interruption of sympathetic input to the eye at any level results in **Horner's syndrome** (ptosis, enophthalmos, miosis, flushing, and heminanhydrosis).

2. Parasympathetic input (see Figure 17.3)

a. The **Edinger-Westphal nucleus** projects preganglionic fibers via the oculomotor nerve (CN III) to the ciliary ganglion.

b. The **ciliary ganglion** projects postganglionic fibers via the short ciliary nerves to the sphincter pupillae and ciliary muscles (accommodation).

c. **Postganglionic fibers** mediate the efferent limb of the pupillary light reflex.

d. Interruption of the parasympathetic input results in **internal ophthalmoplegia** (fixed [unresponsive] and dilated pupil).

B. Blood vessels

–receive their predominant innervation from the noradrenergic supply via the sympathetic division.

1. Arteries and arterioles

–are well innervated.

—those located in skeletal muscles contain cholinergic (muscarinic) receptors in their walls; these are innervated by postganglionic sympathetic fibers and cause vasodilation.

2. Large veins and venules

—are moderately innervated.

3. Capillaries

—seem to have no innervation.

C. Heart

1. Sympathetic input

a. The **intermediolateral cell column** (T1–T5) projects preganglionic fibers to the upper thoracic ganglia and to the three cervical ganglia of the sympathetic trunk.

b. The **rostral sympathetic trunk** projects postganglionic fibers via cardiac nerves to the ventricular and atrial walls and the pacemaker tissue.

c. Stimulation of cardiac nerves results in an increase in heart rate and in the force of cardiac contractility (β_1-adrenergic receptors).

2. Parasympathetic input

a. The **nucleus ambiguus** projects preganglionic fibers via the vagal nerve to the intramural ganglia of the atria and the sinoatrial node.

b. Postganglionic fibers from the intramural ganglia innervate the heart.

c. Vagal stimulation lowers the strength and rate of cardiac contraction.

V. Clinical Correlations

A. Megacolon (Hirschsprung's disease)

—is also called **congenital aganglionic megacolon.**

—is characterized by extreme dilation and hypertrophy of the colon with fecal retention and by the absence of ganglion cells in the myenteric plexus.

—results from the **failure of neural crest cells to migrate into the colon.**

B. Familial dysautonomia (Riley-Day syndrome)

—affects Jewish children, predominantly.

—is an **autosomal recessive trait** characterized by abnormal sweating, blood pressure instability (orthostatic hypotension), difficulty in feeding due to inadequate muscle tone in the gastrointestinal tract, and progressive sensory loss.

—results in a **loss of neurons in autonomic and sensory ganglia.**

C. Raynaud's disease

—is a painful disorder of the terminal arteries of the extremities.

—is characterized by idiopathic paroxysmal bilateral cyanosis of the digits, due to arterial and arteriolar contraction caused by cold or emotion.

—may be treated by **preganglionic sympathectomy.**

D. Peptic ulcer

—results from **excessive production of hydrochloric acid** because of increased parasympathetic (tone) stimulation.

Review Test

Directions: Each of the numbered items or incomplete statements in this section is followed by answers or by completions of the statement. Select the **one** lettered answer or completion that is **best** in each case.

1. Which of the following statements concerning preganglionic sympathetic fibers is false?

(A) They arise from the intermediolateral cell column.
(B) They project without synapse to the adrenal medulla.
(C) Their terminals elaborate acetylcholine.
(D) They are found in splanchnic nerves.
(E) They synapse in the myenteric plexus.

2. Which of the following ganglia does not contain postganglionic parasympathetic neurons?

(A) Otic
(B) Celiac
(C) Pterygopalatine
(D) Submandibular
(E) Ciliary

3. The viscera are insensitive to all of the following stimuli EXCEPT

(A) distension.
(B) cold.
(C) heat.
(D) cutting.
(E) touch.

4. Parasympathetic stimulation results in all of the following responses EXCEPT

(A) contraction of the ductus deferens.
(B) secretion of the salivary glands.
(C) increased peristalsis.
(D) bronchial constriction.
(E) penile erection.

5. All of the following statements concerning gray communicating rami are correct EXCEPT they

(A) contain preganglionic sympathetic fibers.
(B) are found at all spinal cord levels.
(C) contain GVE fibers.
(D) contain postganglionic sympathetic fibers.
(E) are gray because they contain no myelinated fibers.

6. Postganglionic sympathetic cholinergic fibers innervate the

(A) sweat glands.
(B) lacrimal gland.
(C) ductus deferens.
(D) trigone of the urinary bladder.
(E) detrusor muscle.

7. Sympathectomy of the superior cervical ganglion results in all of the following signs EXCEPT

(A) vasodilation of the cutaneous vessels of the face.
(B) miosis.
(C) sweating of the face.
(D) exophthalmos.
(E) ptosis.

8. Destruction of the ciliary ganglion results in which one of the following deficits?

(A) Severe ptosis
(B) Loss of corneal reflex
(C) Loss of lacrimation
(D) Loss of direct pupillary reflex
(E) Miosis

9. All of the following statements concerning the sacral division of the ANS are correct EXCEPT

(A) it innervates the transverse colon.
(B) it innervates the descending colon.
(C) it innervates the detrusor muscle of the urinary bladder.
(D) it includes sacral segments S2, S3, and S4.
(E) its postganglionic parasympathetic neurons are found in, on, or near the walls of the organs that they innervate.

10. All of the following statements concerning the innervation of blood vessels are correct EXCEPT

(A) blood vessels receive a predominant sympathetic input.
(B) blood vessels contain cholinergic (muscarinic) receptors.
(C) arterioles are well innervated.
(D) capillaries seem to have no innervation.
(E) the predominant innervation is cholinergic.

11. Sympathetic stimulation results in all of the following responses EXCEPT

(A) dilation of the pupil.
(B) contraction of the bladder.
(C) dilation of the bronchial lumina.
(D) increased perspiration.
(E) ejaculation.

12. All of the following statements concerning the vagal nerve are correct EXCEPT

(A) it supplies the transverse colon.
(B) it supplies the esophagus.
(C) it contains fibers from the carotid sinus.
(D) it contains GVE fibers from the nucleus ambiguus.
(E) it contains fibers from the carotid body.

13. All of the following statements concerning preganglionic parasympathetic fibers are correct EXCEPT they

(A) are found in the pelvic nerves.
(B) arise from the Edinger-Westphal nucleus.
(C) arise from the nuclei of cranial nerves III, VII, IX, and X.
(D) traverse the white communicating rami.
(E) project to the otic ganglion.

14. Horner's syndrome may result from all of the following lesions EXCEPT

(A) carcinoma of the lung apex.
(B) tumorous involvement of the cervical lymph nodes.
(C) hemisection of the cervical spinal cord.
(D) thrombosis of the posterior inferior cerebellar artery.
(E) destruction of the ciliary ganglion.

Directions: Each group of items in this section consists of lettered options followed by a set of numbered items. For each item, select the **one** lettered option that is most closely associated with it. Each lettered option may be selected once, more than once, or not at all.

Questions 15–19

Match each of the characteristics below with the condition it best describes.

(A) Hirschsprung's disease
(B) Horner's syndrome
(C) Peptic ulcer disease
(D) Riley-Day syndrome
(E) Raynaud's disease

15. Results from increased parasympathetic stimulation

16. Is a painful vasospastic disorder affecting the digits

17. Is an autosomal recessive trait characterized by abnormal sweating and blood pressure instability

18. Results from congenital absence of ganglion cells in the myenteric plexus

19. Consists of anisocoria and lack of sweating

Answers and Explanations

1–E. The myenteric plexus receives postganglionic sympathetic input from the prevertebral (collateral) ganglia. The adrenal medulla receives preganglionic sympathetic cholinergic fibers via the lesser splanchnic nerve.

2–B. The celiac ganglion is a sympathetic prevertebral (collateral) ganglion that contains postganglionic neurons.

3–A. Visceral pain results from distension, strong contractions, mechanical stimulation of hyperemic organs, and ischemia with release of kinins.

4–A. Contraction of the smooth muscles of the ductus deferens and seminal vesicle (ejaculation) results from sympathetic stimulation.

5–A. Gray communicating rami are associated with all spinal nerves; they contain only nonmyelinated postganglionic sympathetic fibers. All autonomic visceromotor fibers are GVE fibers.

6–A. Postganglionic sympathetic cholinergic fibers innervate the eccrine (merocrine) sweat glands and some blood vessels; blood vessels, however, are predominantly innervated by postganglionic sympathetic adrenergic fibers. Apocrine sweat glands of the axilla are innervated by adrenergic fibers; these glands secrete in response to mental stress.

7–D. Sympathectomy of the superior cervical ganglion interrupts sympathetic innervation to the head, resulting in Horner's syndrome: mild ptosis (lid droop), miosis, facial hemianhydrosis, vasodilation, and an apparent enophthalmos due to ptosis.

8–D. Destruction of the ciliary ganglion interrupts postganglionic parasympathetic fibers, which innervate the sphincter muscle of the iris and the ciliary muscle; this results in loss of the direct pupillary reflex, mydriasis and paralysis of accommodation. In addition, postganglionic sympathetic vasomotor fibers are interrupted, resulting in a hyperemic globe. Postganglionic sympathetic pupillodilator fibers reach the iris via the nasociliary and long ciliary nerve. Severe ptosis results from an oculomotor paralysis involving the fibers that innervate the levator palpebrae muscle. Mild ptosis results from a lesion of the oculosympathetic fibers, which innervate the smooth tarsal muscle (Horner's syndrome).

9–A. The sacral division (S2–S4) of the ANS innervates the lower abdominal and pelvic viscera, including the colon distal to the left colic flexure, the urinary bladder (detrusor muscle), and the genital viscera. Postganglionic parasympathetic neurons are found in or on the viscera that they innervate.

10–E. Blood vessels receive a predominant noradrenergic innervation and a predominant sympathetic input and contain cholinergic (muscarinic) receptors. Arterioles are well innervated. Capillaries seem to have no innervation. Cerebral blood vessels respond more to circulating metabolites (CO_2 and O_2) than to innervation by the ANS.

11–B. Sympathetic stimulation results in dilation of the pupils (mydriasis), dilation of the lumina of the bronchi, increased perspiration (sudation), and constriction of the ductus deferens (resulting in ejaculation). Contraction of the detrusor muscle is a parasympathetic function.

12–C. The vagal nerve (CN X) contains preganglionic fibers from the nucleus ambiguus that terminate in the cardiac ganglia. It innervates the esophagus, thoracic viscera, and abdominal viscera, excluding the descending colon, sigmoid colon, and rectum, which are innervated by the pelvic nerve (S2–S4). The carotid sinus (baroreceptor) is innervated by the glossopharyngeal nerve (CN IX; sinus nerve). The carotid body (chemoreceptor) is innervated by the glossopharyngeal and vagal nerves.

13–D. Preganglionic parasympathetic fibers arise from the Edinger-Westphal nucleus of CN III, superior salivatory nucleus of CN VII, inferior salivatory nucleus of CN IX, and dorsal motor nucleus and nucleus ambiguus of CN X. Preganglionic parasympathetic fibers from sacral segments (S2–S4) traverse the pelvic nerves; they do not traverse the white communicating rami. The otic ganglion receives preganglionic parasympathetic input from the inferior salivatory nucleus of CN IX.

14–E. Horner's syndrome is caused by all lesions that interrupt sympathetic input to the eye. A lesion of the ciliary ganglion results in denervation of the sphincter pupillae muscle of the iris and the ciliary muscle. Postganglionic sympathetic fibers that innervate the dilator pupillae muscle and the smooth tarsal muscle do not traverse the ciliary ganglion.

15–C. Peptic ulcer disease results from increased parasympathetic tone.

16–E. Raynaud's disease is a benign symmetric disease characterized by painful vasospasms affecting the digits.

17–D. Riley-Day syndrome, familial dysautonomia, is an autosomal recessive trait characterized by abnormal sweating and blood pressure instability.

18–A. Congenital aganglionic megacolon, or Hirschsprung's disease, results from failure of the neural crest cells to migrate into the wall of the distal colon (sigmoid colon and rectum) and form the myenteric plexus. It is characterized by extreme dilation and hypertrophy of the colon, with fecal retention.

19–B. Anisocoria (unequal pupils) and hemianhydrosis (lack of sweating on half of the face) result from Horner's syndrome (ptosis, miosis, and hemianhydrosis).

19

Hypothalamus

I. Overview—The Hypothalamus

—is a division of the diencephalon.
—lies within the floor and ventral part of the walls of the third ventricle.
—functions primarily in the **maintenance of homeostasis**.
—subserves three systems: the **autonomic nervous system (ANS)**, the **endocrine system**, and the **limbic system**.

II. Surface Anatomy—The Hypothalamus (see Figures 1.2 and 1.5)

—is visible only from the ventral aspect of the brain.
—lies between the optic chiasm and the interpeduncular fossa (posterior perforated substance).
—lies below the hypothalamic sulcus.
—includes the following **ventral surface structures:**

A. Infundibulum

—is the stalk of the hypophysis.
—contains the hypophyseal portal vessels.
—contains the supraopticohypophyseal and tuberohypophyseal tracts.

B. Tuber cinereum

—is the prominence between the infundibulum and the mamillary bodies.
—includes the **median eminence,** which contains the **arcuate nucleus** (infundibular nucleus).

C. Mamillary bodies

—contain the **mamillary nuclei.**

D. Optic chiasm

—is the floor of the optic recess of the third ventricle.

E. Arterial circle of Willis

—surrounds the ventral surface of the hypothalamus and provides its blood supply.

III. Hypothalamic Regions and Nuclei

—the hypothalamus is divided into a lateral area and a medial area. These areas are separated by the fornix and the mamillothalamic tract.

A. Lateral hypothalamic area

—is traversed by the **medial forebrain bundle**.
—includes two major nuclei:

1. Lateral preoptic nucleus

—is the anterior telencephalic portion.

2. Lateral hypothalamic nucleus

—when stimulated, induces eating.
—lesions cause anorexia and starvation.

B. Medial hypothalamic area (Figure 19.1)

—is divided into four regions, from anterior to posterior:

1. Preoptic region

—is the anterior telencephalic portion.
—contains the **medial preoptic nucleus,** which regulates the release of gonadotropic hormones from the adenohypophysis. The medial preoptic nucleus contains the sexually dimorphic nucleus, whose development is dependent on testosterone levels.

2. Supraoptic region

—lies dorsal to the optic chiasm.

a. Suprachiasmatic nucleus

—receives direct input from the retina.
—plays a role in the **control of circadian rhythms**.

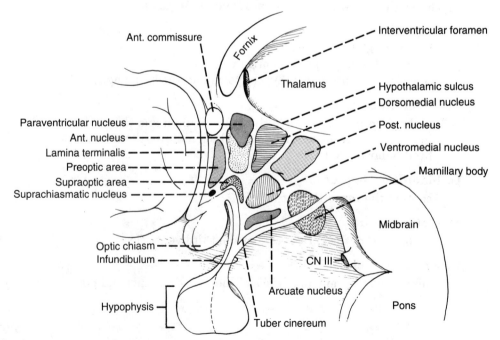

Figure 19.1. The medial hypothalamic nuclei and structures surrounding the midline ventricle.

b. Anterior nucleus

–plays a role in **temperature regulation**.
–stimulates the parasympathetic nervous system.
–destruction results in **hyperthermia**.

c. Paraventricular nucleus

–neurosecretory cells synthesize and release antidiuretic hormone (**ADH**), **oxytocin,** and corticotropin-releasing hormone (**CRH**).
–regulates water balance (conservation of water).
–gives rise to the supraopticohypophyseal tract, which projects to the neurohypophysis.
–destruction results in **diabetes insipidus**.

d. Supraoptic nucleus

–synthesizes **ADH** and **oxytocin**.
–projects to the neurohypophysis via the supraopticohypophyseal tract.

3. Tuberal region

–lies dorsal to the tuber cinereum.

a. Dorsomedial nucleus

–when stimulated in animals, results in savage behavior.

b. Ventromedial nucleus

–is considered a **satiety center**.
–when stimulated, inhibits the urge to eat.
–bilateral destruction results in hyperphagia, obesity, and savage behavior.

c. Arcuate (infundibular) nucleus

–is located in the tuber cinereum.
–contains neurons that produce **hypothalamic-releasing factors** and gives rise to the tuberhypophyseal tract, which terminates in the hypophyseal portal system of the infundibulum.
–effects, via hypothalamic-releasing factors, the release-nonrelease of adenohypophyseal hormones into the systemic circulation.

4. Mamillary region

–lies dorsal to the mamillary bodies.

a. Mamillary nuclei

–receive input from the **hippocampal formation** (specifically the subiculum) via the **fornix**.
–receive input from the dorsal and ventral tegmental nuclei and the raphe nuclei, via the mamillary peduncle.
–project to the anterior nucleus of the thalamus via the mamillothalamic tract.
–contain hemorrhagic lesions in Wernicke's encephalopathy.

b. Posterior nucleus

–plays a role in **thermal regulation** (i.e., conservation and increased production of heat).
–lesions result in **poikilothermia,** the inability to thermoregulate.

IV. Major Hypothalamic Connections (Figures 19.2 and 19.3)

A. Afferent connections to the hypothalamus

—**derive** from the following structures:

1. Septal area and nuclei and orbitofrontal cortex

—via the medial forebrain bundle

2. Hippocampal formation

—primarily from the subiculum via the fornix

3. Amygdaloid complex

—via the stria terminalis and ventral amygdalofugal pathway

4. Primary olfactory cortex

—via the medial forebrain bundle

5. Mediodorsal nucleus of the thalamus

—via the inferior thalamic peduncle

6. Brainstem nuclei

a. Tegmental nuclei (dorsal and ventral)

—project via the mamillary peduncle

b. Raphe nuclei (dorsal and superior central)

—project serotonergic fibers via the medial forebrain bundle and the mamillary peduncle (see Figure 22.4).

c. Locus ceruleus

—projects noradrenergic fibers via the medial forebrain bundle (see Figure 22.4).

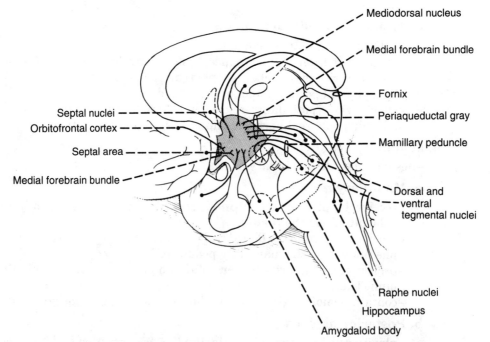

Figure 19.2. Major afferent (input) connections of the hypothalamus. The fornix projects from the hippocampal formation to the mamillary bodies. The medial forebrain bundle conducts afferent and efferent fibers.

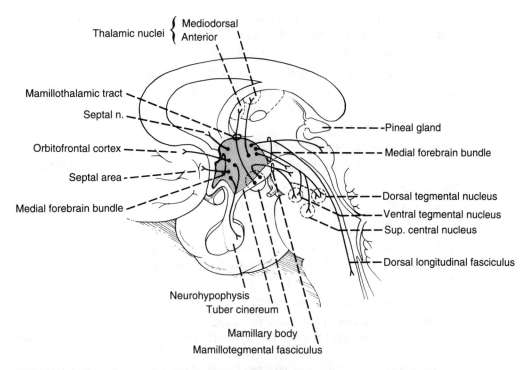

Figure 19.3. Major efferent (output) connections of the hypothalamus. The medial forebrain bundle conducts afferent and efferent fibers. The hypothalamus projects directly to the autonomic visceral nuclei of the brainstem and spinal cord.

B. Efferent connections from the hypothalamus

 —**project** to the following structures:

1. Septal area and nuclei

 —via the medial forebrain bundle

2. Anterior nucleus of the thalamus

 —via the mamillothalamic tract

3. Mediodorsal nucleus of the thalamus

 —via the inferior thalamic peduncle

4. Amygdaloid complex

 —via the stria terminalis and the ventral amygdalopetal pathway

5. Brainstem nuclei and spinal cord

 —via the dorsal longitudinal fasciculus and the medial forebrain bundle

6. Adenohypophysis

 —via the tuberohypophyseal tract and hypophyseal portal system

7. Neurohypophysis

 —via the supraopticohypophyseal tract

V. Major Fiber Systems

A. Fornix (see Figures 1.4, 1.5, 19.1, 20.3, and 20.4)

 —has five parts: the **alveus, fimbria, crus, body,** and **column**.

−projects from the hippocampal formation to the mamillary nucleus, anterior nucleus of the thalamus, and septal area.

−is the largest projection to the hypothalamus.

B. Medial forebrain bundle (see Figures 19.2 and 19.3)

−traverses the entire lateral hypothalamic area.

−interconnects the septal area and nuclei, the hypothalamus, and the midbrain tegmentum.

C. Mamillothalamic tract (see Figure 20.4)

−projects from the mamillary nuclei to the anterior nucleus of the thalamus.

D. Mamillary peduncle (see Figure 19.2)

−conducts fibers from the dorsal and ventral tegmental nuclei and the raphe nuclei to the mamillary body.

E. Mamillotegmental tract (see Figure 19.3)

−conducts fibers from the mamillary nuclei to the dorsal and ventral tegmental nuclei.

F. Stria terminalis (see Figure 20.3)

−is the most prominent pathway from the amygdaloid complex.

−interconnects the septal area, the hypothalamus, and the amygdaloid complex.

−lies in the sulcus terminalis between the caudate nucleus and the thalamus.

G. Ventral amygdalofugal pathway (see Figure 20.3)

−interconnects the amygdaloid complex and the hypothalamus.

H. Supraopticohypophyseal tract (Figure 19.4)

−conducts fibers from the supraoptic and paraventricular nuclei to the **neurohypophysis** (the release site for ADH and oxytocin).

I. Tuberohypophyseal (tuberoinfundibular) tract (see Figure 19.4)

−conducts fibers from the arcuate nucleus to the hypophyseal portal system of the infundibulum.

J. Dorsal longitudinal fasciculus (see Figure 19.3)

−extends from the hypothalamus to the caudal medulla.

−projects to the parasympathetic nuclei of the brainstem.

K. Hypothalamospinal tract

−contains direct descending autonomic fibers that influence preganglionic sympathetic neurons of the intermediolateral cell column and preganglionic neurons of the sacral parasympathetic nucleus.

−interruption above T1 results in Horner's syndrome.

VI. Functional Considerations

A. Autonomic function

−the ANS is regulated by hypothalamic nuclei.

1. Anterior hypothalamus

−has an excitatory effect on the parasympathetic nervous system.

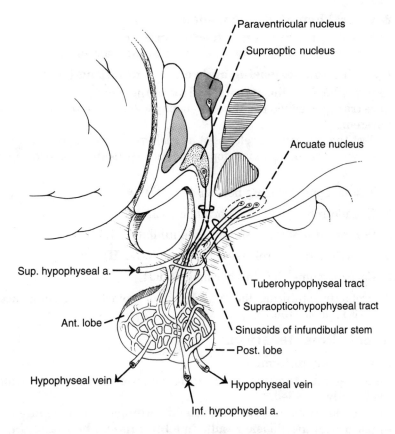

Figure 19.4. The hypophyseal portal system. The paraventricular and supraoptic nuclei produce antidiuretic hormone (ADH) and oxytocin and transport the substances via the supraopticohypophyseal tract to the capillary bed of the neurohypophysis. The arcuate nucleus of the infundibulum transports releasing hormones via the tuberohypophyseal tract to the sinusoids of the infundibular stem, which drain into the secondary capillary plexus in the adenohypophysis.

2. Posterior hypothalamus

–has an excitatory effect on the sympathetic nervous system.

B. Temperature regulation

1. Anterior hypothalamus

–helps **regulate and maintain body temperature**.
–destruction causes **hyperthermia**.

2. Posterior hypothalamus

–helps **produce and conserve heat**.
–destruction causes the **inability to thermoregulate**.

C. Water balance regulation

–ADH controls water excretion by the kidneys.

D. Food intake regulation

–two hypothalamic nuclei play roles in the control of appetite:

1. Ventromedial nucleus

–is discussed on p 243, tuberal region.

2. Lateral hypothalamic nucleus

–is called the **hunger or feeding center**.

–destruction causes **starvation and emaciation**.

E. Hypothalamic-releasing and release-inhibiting factors

–are produced in the arcuate nucleus of the median eminence.

–are transported via the tuberohypophyseal tract to the hypophyseal portal system.

–effect the release-nonrelease of adenohypophyseal hormones.

–are, with the exception of dopamine, **peptides** (hypophysiotropins), which include:

1. Thyrotropin-releasing hormone (**TRH**)

2. Gonadotropin-releasing hormone (**GnRH**)

3. Somatostatin (growth hormone-inhibiting hormone)

4. Growth hormone-releasing hormone (**GHRH**)

5. Corticotropin-releasing hormone (**CRH**)

6. Prolactin-inhibiting factor (**PIF**) and prolactin-releasing factor (**PRF**) [PIF is dopamine.]

VII. Clinical Considerations

A. Craniopharyngioma

–is a congenital tumor thought to originate from remnants of Rathke's pouch.

–is usually calcified.

–is the most common **supratentorial tumor** found in children.

–pressure on the chiasm results in a **bitemporal hemianopia**.

–pressure on the hypothalamus causes **hypothalamic syndrome** with adiposity, diabetes insipidus, disturbance of temperature regulation, and somnolence.

B. Pituitary adenoma

–constitutes 15% of cases of clinically symptomatic **intracranial tumors**.

–is rarely seen in children.

–when endocrine-active, produces endocrine abnormalities (e.g., amenorrhea and galactorrhea from a prolactin-secreting adenoma, the most common type).

–pressure on the chiasm results in a **bitemporal hemianopia** (most cases show asymmetry of field defects).

–pressure on the hypothalamus may cause **hypothalamic syndrome**.

Review Test

Directions: Each of the numbered items or incomplete statements in this section is followed by answers or by completions of the statement. Select the **one** lettered answer or completion that is **best** in each case.

1. All of the following structures are surface landmarks of the hypothalamus EXCEPT the

(A) infundibulum.
(B) tuber cinereum.
(C) optic chiasm.
(D) tuberculum cinereum.
(E) mamillary bodies.

2. The fornix consists of all of the following parts EXCEPT the

(A) alveus.
(B) calcar avis.
(C) fimbria.
(D) crus.
(E) column.

3. Which of the following statements concerning the paraventricular nucleus is incorrect?

(A) It contains neurosecretory neurons that produce ADH.
(B) It projects to the posterior pituitary gland.
(C) Its magnocellular neurons elaborate oxytocin.
(D) It gives rise to the supraopticohypophyseal tract.
(E) It plays a role in regulating the release of gonadotropin.

4. All of the following statements concerning hypothalamic releasing-nonreleasing hormones are correct EXCEPT

(A) they are predominantly neuropeptides.
(B) they are transported to the neurohypophysis.
(C) they include somatostatin.
(D) they include dopamine.
(E) they are produced in the arcuate nucleus.

5. Which of the following statements concerning the medial forebrain bundle is incorrect?

(A) It is a major thoroughfare of the hypothalamus.
(B) It traverses the entire lateral hypothalamus.
(C) It interconnects the mamillary body with the anterior nucleus of the thalamus.
(D) It receives input from the septal area.
(E) It receives input from the midbrain tegmentum.

6. The sexually dimorphic nucleus is located in

(A) the anterior nucleus.
(B) the arcuate nucleus.
(C) the medial preoptic nucleus.
(D) the posterior nucleus.
(E) the ventromedial nucleus.

7. All of the following statements concerning the hypothalamus are correct EXCEPT

(A) it is a division of the diencephalon.
(B) it is perfused by the posterior communicating artery.
(C) it is visible only from the ventral aspect of the brain.
(D) it lies within the walls of the fourth ventricle.
(E) it includes the mamillary body.

8. The supraoptic region contains all of the following nuclei EXCEPT

(A) a nucleus that plays a role in temperature regulation.
(B) a nucleus that receives substantial input from the hippocampal formation.
(C) a nucleus that manufactures ADH.
(D) a nucleus that manufactures oxytocin.
(E) a nucleus that receives direct input from the retina.

249

9. All of the following statements concerning the mamillary nucleus are correct EXCEPT

(A) it projects to the ventral anterior nucleus of the thalamus.
(B) it receives input from the hippocampal formation.
(C) it receives input from the dorsal and ventral tegmental nuclei.
(D) it receives input from the subiculum via the fornix.
(E) it contains hemorrhagic lesions in Wernicke's encephalopathy.

10. All of the following statements concerning craniopharyngiomas are correct EXCEPT they

(A) frequently cause a bitemporal hemianopia.
(B) usually can be seen on x-ray.
(C) are rarely seen in children.
(D) are thought to originate from Rathke's pouch.
(E) may cause adiposity and diabetes insipidus.

Directions: Each group of items in this section consists of lettered options followed by a set of numbered items. For each item, select the **one** lettered option that is most closely associated with it. Each lettered option may be selected once, more than once, or not at all.

Questions 11–17

Match the description below with the structure it best describes.

(A) Fornix
(B) Medial forebrain bundle
(C) Stria terminalis
(D) Mamillary peduncle
(E) Dorsal longitudinal fasciculus

11. Extends from the posterior hypothalamic nucleus to the caudal medulla

12. Interconnects the hypothalamus and the amygdaloid complex

13. Is the largest projection to the hypothalamus

14. Connects the septal area to the midbrain tegmentum

15. Conducts fibers from the hippocampal formation to the mamillary nucleus

16. Lies between the caudate nucleus and the thalamus

17. Separates the medial hypothalamus from the lateral hypothalamus

Questions 18–22

Match each defect below with the condition it best describes.

(A) Diabetes insipidus
(B) Hyperthermia
(C) Hyperphagia and savage behavior
(D) Inability to thermoregulate
(E) Anorexia

18. Bilateral lesion of the ventromedial hypothalamic nucleus

19. Bilateral lesion of the posterior hypothalamic nuclei

20. Lesions involving the supraoptic and paraventricular nuclei

21. Destruction of the anterior hypothalamic nuclei

22. Stimulation of the ventromedial nuclei

Answers and Explanations

1–D. The tuberculum cinereum is a surface eminence of the medulla, overlying the spinal trigeminal tract and nucleus. The tuber cinereum is a hypothalamic prominence found on the ventral surface between the optic chiasm and the mamillary bodies.

2–B. The calcar avis (hippocampus minor), an eminence of the medial wall of the occipital horn of the lateral ventricle, overlies the calcarine fissure.

3–E. The medial preoptic nucleus plays a role in regulating the release of gonadotropic hormones from the anterior pituitary gland.

4–B. Hypothalamic releasing-nonreleasing hormones are transported via the tuberinfundibular (tuberohypophyseal) tract to the sinusoids of the hypophyseal portal system, which are located in the infundibular stalk.

5–C. The medial mamillary nucleus projects via the mamillothalamic tract to the anterior nucleus of the thalamus. The medial forebrain bundle interconnects the septal area, the lateral hypothalamus, and the midbrain tegmentum.

6–C. The sexually dimorphic nucleus is located in the medial preoptic nucleus of the preoptic region.

7–D. The hypothalamus, a division of the diencephalon, is visible only from the ventral surface of the brain. It is perfused by all vessels of the arterial circle of Willis, including the posterior communicating artery. The hypothalamus lies below the thalamus and within the walls of the third ventricle. The thalamus is the longest and most conspicuous part of the diencephalon.

8–B. The hippocampal formation projects massive input to the mamillary nucleus, a nucleus of the mamillary region. The supraoptic region contains the anterior, suprachiasmatic, paraventricular, and supraoptic nuclei. The anterior nucleus plays a role in temperature regulation. The paraventricular and supraoptic nuclei elaborate ADH and oxytocin. The suprachiasmatic nucleus receives direct input from the retina.

9–A. The mamillary nucleus projects via the mamillothalamic tract to the anterior nucleus of the thalamus.

10–C. A craniopharyngioma is a congenital tumor thought to originate from remnants of Rathke's pouch and is the most common supratentorial tumor in children. These tumors are usually calcified and can be seen on plain film. Pressure on the chiasm produces a bitemporal hemianopia. Pressure on the hypothalamus causes hypothalamic syndrome (e.g., adiposity and diabetes insipidus).

11–E. The dorsal longitudinal fasciculus extends from the posterior hypothalamic nucleus to the caudal medulla and projects to autonomic centers of the brainstem. It contains both ascending and descending fibers.

12–C. The amygdaloid complex is interconnected with the hypothalamus via the stria terminalis and the ventral amygdalofugal pathway.

13–A. The fornix contains 2.7 million fibers and is the largest projection to the hypothalamus.

14–B. The medial forebrain bundle interconnects the septal area, the hypothalamus, and the midbrain tegmentum.

15–A. The fornix projects from the subiculum of the hippocampal formation to the mamillary nucleus of the hypothalamus. The fornix projects to the anterior nucleus of the thalamus, septal nuclei, lateral preoptic region, and the nucleus of the diagonal band of Broca.

16–C. The stria terminalis lies in the sulcus terminalis with the vena terminalis, separates the head of the caudate nucleus from the thalamus, and interconnects the amygdaloid nuclear complex with the hypothalamus.

17–A. The column of the fornix lies between the medial and lateral hypothalamus.

18–C. A bilateral lesion of the ventromedial hypothalamic nucleus results in hyperphagia and savage behavior.

19–D. A bilateral lesion of the posterior hypothalamic nucleus results in the inability to thermoregulate (poikilothermia). Bilateral destruction of only the posterior aspect of the lateral hypothalamic nucleus results in anorexia and emaciation.

20–A. Lesions involving the supraoptic and paraventricular nuclei or the supraopticohypophyseal tract result in diabetes insipidus with polydipsia and polyuria.

21–B. Destruction of the anterior hypothalamic nuclei results in hyperthermia.

22–E. Stimulation of the ventromedial nuclei inhibits the urge to eat, resulting in emaciation (cachexia). Destruction of these nuclei results in hyperphagia and savage behavior.

20

Olfactory, Gustatory, and Limbic Systems

I. Olfactory System

–mediates the special visceral afferent (SVA) modality of **smell** via the olfactory nerve (**CN I**).

–is the only sensory system that has no precortical relay in the thalamus.

–projects to the thalamus and hypothalamus and the hippocampal formation.

A. Olfactory pathway (Figure 20.1)

1. Olfactory receptor cells

–number 25 million on each side.

–are replaced throughout life (they may regenerate).

–are found in the nasal mucosa.

–are **first-order neurons** in the olfactory pathway.

–are unmyelinated bipolar neurons whose central processes are CN I.

–have axons that enter the olfactory bulb and synapse in the olfactory glomeruli with mitral cells.

2. Olfactory bulb (see Figure 1.2)

–lies on the cribriform plate of the ethmoid bone and receives the olfactory nerve.

–contains **mitral cells** (second-order neurons) that project via the olfactory tract and the lateral olfactory stria to the primary olfactory cortex and the amygdaloid nucleus.

3. Olfactory tract (see Figure 1.2)

–contains the **anterior olfactory nucleus**.

–gives rise to the **medial and lateral olfactory striae**.

–projects to the contralateral olfactory tract via the anterior commissure.

4. Lateral olfactory stria (see Figure 1.2)

–projects to the primary olfactory cortex.

5. Primary olfactory cortex (see Figure 1.2)

–overlies the **uncus** of the parahippocampal gyrus.

–receives input from the lateral olfactory stria.

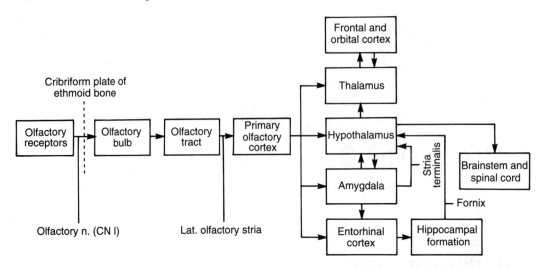

Figure 20.1. The pathways of the olfactory system. The olfactory nerve enters the olfactory bulb via the cribriform plate. Mitral cells of the olfactory bulb project via the lateral olfactory stria to the primary olfactory cortex (prepiriform and periamygdaloid cortices). The primary olfactory cortex projects to the hypothalamus, thalamus, amygdaloid nucleus, and to the entorhinal area. The olfactory system is the only sensory system that projects directly to the cortex of the telencephalon without a precortical relay in the thalamus.

—consists of **prepiriform** and **periamygdaloid cortices**.

—projects to the mediodorsal nucleus of the thalamus, via the amygdaloid nucleus to the hypothalamus, and via the entorhinal cortex (area 28) to the hippocampal formation.

6. Mediodorsal nucleus of the thalamus

—projects to the **orbitofrontal cortex,** where the conscious perception of smell takes place.

B. Clinical considerations

1. Anosmia, the loss of smell, may occur as a result of a lesion of the olfactory nerve.

2. Olfactory nerves may be damaged by **fractures of the cribriform plate,** by **meningitis, meningiomas, gliomas,** or by **abscesses of the frontal lobes**.

3. Olfactory hallucinations (uncunate fits) may be a consequence of lesions of the parahippocampal uncus.

4. Foster Kennedy syndrome

—results from a **meningioma of the olfactory groove** that compresses the olfactory tract and the optic nerve.

—results in ipsilateral anosmia, optic atrophy, and contralateral papilledema.

II. Gustatory System

—mediates the SVA modality of **taste**.

—mediates gustation, which, like smell, is a chemical sense.

A. Gustatory pathway (Figure 20.2)

1. Taste receptor cells

—are modified epithelial cells, not neurons.

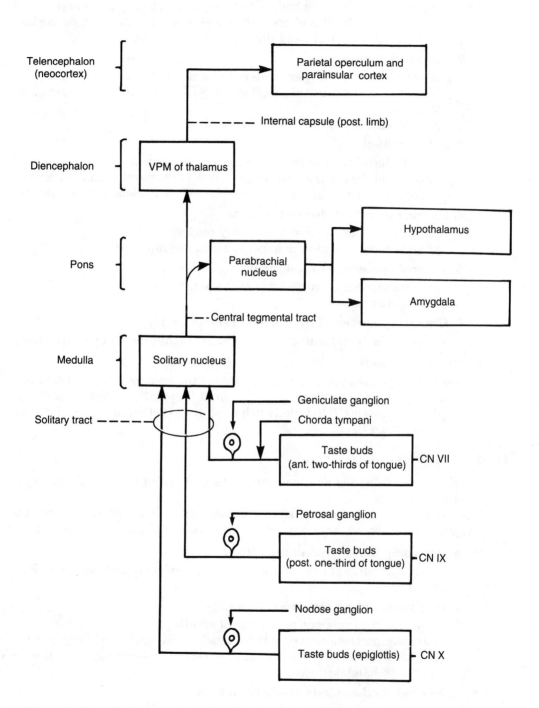

Figure 20.2. The gustatory pathway. Cranial nerves VII, IX, and X transmit taste (SVA) information from the anterior two-thirds of the tongue, the posterior one-third of the tongue, and the epiglottis to the solitary tract and nucleus; from the solitary nucleus via the central tegmental tract to the medial parabrachial nucleus; and to the ventral posteromedial (VPM) nucleus of the thalamus, hypothalamus, and amygdaloid complex. The gustatory cortex is located in the parietal operculum and in the parainsular cortex.

—are continuously being regenerated.

—are located in the taste buds of the tongue, epiglottis, and palate.

—are innervated by SVA fibers of the facial nerve (CN VII), the glossopharyngeal nerve (CN IX), and the vagal nerve (CN X).

2. First-order neurons

—are **pseudounipolar ganglion cells** located in the geniculate ganglion of CN VII, in the petrosal ganglion of CN IX, and in the nodose ganglion of CN X.

—project centrally to the solitary nucleus.

3. Solitary nucleus

—receives taste input from the tongue and epiglottis.

—projects via the **central tegmental tract** to the parabrachial nucleus of the pons and to the ventral posteromedial (VPM) nucleus of the thalamus.

4. Parabrachial nucleus of the pons

—receives taste input from the solitary nucleus.

—projects taste input to the hypothalamus and amygdala.

5. Ventral posteromedial nucleus

—projects to the gustatory cortex of the parietal operculum (area 43) and parainsular cortex.

6. Gustatory cortex of the insular area (area 43)

—projects via the entorhinal cortex (area 28) to the hippocampal formation.

B. Clinical consideration

—**ageusia** (gustatory anesthesia), the lack of the sense of taste, is most commonly caused by heavy smoking. It is most frequently associated with peripheral lesions of CN VII (Bell's palsy and disease of the middle ear [chorda tympani]) and CN IX.

III. Limbic System

—is considered to be the anatomic substrate underlying behavioral and emotional expression.

—plays a role in feeling, feeding, fighting, fleeing, and undertaking mating activity.

—expresses itself through the hypothalamus via the autonomic nervous system.

A. Major components and connections

—include structures of the telencephalon, diencephalon, and midbrain (Figure 20.3).

1. Orbitofrontal cortex (see Figure 1.2)

—mediates the conscious perception of **smell**.

—has reciprocal connections with the mediodorsal nucleus of the thalamus.

—is interconnected via the medial forebrain bundle with the septal area and hypothalamic nuclei.

2. Mediodorsal nucleus of the thalamus

—has reciprocal connections with the orbitofrontal and prefrontal cortices and the hypothalamus.

—receives input from the amygdaloid nucleus.

—plays a role in **affective behavior and memory**.

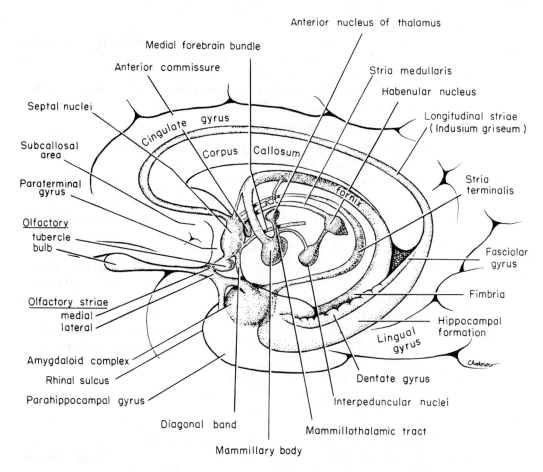

Figure 20.3. Major subcortical structures of the limbic system. The fornix projects from the hippocampal formation to the septal nuclei (precommissural fornix) and to the mamillary body (postcommissural fornix). The major pathway from the amygdaloid nucleus is the stria terminalis, which terminates in the septal nuclei and in the hypothalamus. The stria medullaris of the thalamus connects the septal nuclei to the habenular nucleus. (Reprinted with permission from Carpenter MB and Sutin J: *Human Neuroanatomy*. Baltimore, Williams & Wilkins, 1983, p 618.)

3. Anterior nucleus of the thalamus

– receives input from the mamillary nucleus via the mamillothalamic tract and fornix.

– projects to the cingulate gyrus.

– is a major link in the limbic **circuit of Papez**.

4. Septal area (see Figures 1.4 and 23.1*B*)

– is a telencephalic structure.

– consists of a cortical septal area, which includes the paraterminal gyrus and the subcallosal area.

– consists of a subcortical septal area (the septal nuclei), which lies between the septum pellucidum and the anterior commissure.

– has reciprocal connections with the hippocampal formation via the fornix.

– has reciprocal connections with the hypothalamus via the medial forebrain bundle.

– projects via the **stria medullaris** (thalami) to the **habenular nucleus**.

5. Limbic lobe (see Figure 23.1*B*)

–includes the **subcallosal area,** the **par0aterminal gyrus,** the **cingulate gyrus and isthmus,** and the **parahippocampal gyrus,** which includes the **uncus** (see Figure 1.4).

–contains, buried in the parahippocampal gyrus, the **hippocampal formation** and the **amygdaloid nuclear complex.**

6. Hippocampal formation

–functions in learning, memory, and recognition of novelty.

–receives major input via the entorhinal cortex.

–projects major output via the fornix.

a. Major structures of the hippocampal formation

–project output via the fornix to the septal area and the mamillary nuclei.

–receive input via the fornix from the septal area.

–receive input via the entorhinal cortex (area 28) as the alvear pathway to the hippocampus and the perforant pathway to the dentate gyrus.

(1) Dentate gyrus (see Figure 1.4)

–has a three-layered archicortex.

–contains **granule cells** that receive hippocampal input and project it to the pyramidal cells of the hippocampus and subiculum.

(2) Hippocampus (cornu ammonis)

–has a three-layered archicortex.

–contains **pyramidal cells** that project via the fornix to the septal area and the hypothalamus.

(3) Subiculum

–receives input via the hippocampal pyramidal cells.

–projects via the fornix to the mamillary nuclei and the anterior nucleus of the thalamus.

b. Major afferent connections to the hippocampal formation

(1) Cerebral association cortices (areas 19, 22, and 7)

(2) Septal area

(3) Anterior nucleus of the thalamus

–via the cingulate gyrus, cingulum, and entorhinal cortex (Figure 20.4)

c. Major efferent connections from the hippocampal formation

(1) Mamillary nucleus of the hypothalamus

(2) Septal area

(3) Anterior nucleus of the thalamus

7. Amygdaloid complex (amygdala)

–is a **basal ganglion** underlying the parahippocampal uncus.

–when stimulated, produces activities associated with feeding and nutrition.

–when stimulated, may cause rage and aggressive behavior.

–lesions result in placidity and hypersexual behavior.

a. Major afferent connections to the amygdaloid complex (see Figure 20.4)

–**from** the following structures:

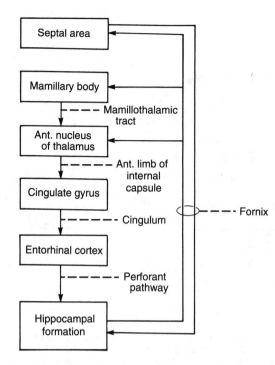

Figure 20.4. Major connections of the amygdaloid nucleus. The amygdaloid nucleus receives input from three major sources: the olfactory system, the sensory association and limbic cortices, and the hypothalamus. The major output from the amygdaloid nucleus is via two channels: The stria terminalis projects to the hypothalamus and the septal area, and the ventral amygdalofugal pathway (VAFP) projects to the hypothalamus, brainstem, and spinal cord. A smaller efferent bundle, the diagonal band of Broca, projects to the septal area. Afferent fibers from the hypothalamus and brainstem enter the amygdaloid nucleus via the ventral amygdalopetal pathway (VAPP).

(1) **Olfactory bulb and olfactory cortex**
(2) **Cerebral cortex** (includes the limbic and temporal cortices)
(3) **Hypothalamus**
(4) **Parabrachial nucleus of the pons** (taste input)

b. **Major efferent connections from the amygdaloid complex** (see Figure 20.4)

–**to** the following structures:
(1) **Cerebral cortex** (entire frontal cortex)
(2) **Hypothalamus**
(3) **Brainstem and spinal cord**

8. **Hypothalamus**

–is a major part of the limbic system that projects to the brainstem and spinal cord (see Chapter 19).

9. **Limbic midbrain nuclei**

a. **Ventral tegmental area** (see Figure 22.2)

–projects ascending dopaminergic fibers to all limbic structures.

b. **Raphe nuclei of the midbrain** (see Figure 22.4)

–project ascending serotonergic fibers to all limbic structures.

c. **Locus ceruleus** (see Figure 22.3)

–projects ascending noradrenergic fibers to all limbic structures.

B. **Major limbic fiber systems** (see Figures 20.3, 20.4, and 20.5)

1. **Fornix** (see Figures 1.4, 1.5, and 20.3)

–projects from the hippocampal formation to the hypothalamus (mamil-

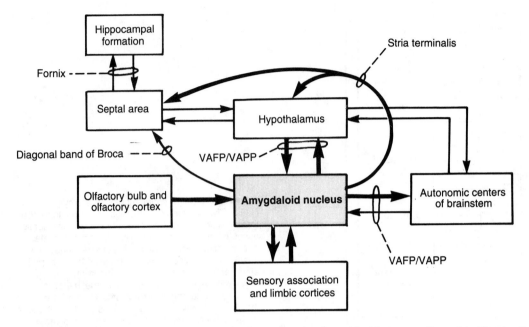

Figure 20.5. Limbic connections. Major afferent and efferent connections of the hippocampal formation. The circuit of Papez is: hippocampal formation → mamillary nucleus → anterior thalamic nucleus → cingulate gyrus → hippocampal formation. The hippocampal formation consists of three components: the hippocampus per se (cornu ammonis), the subiculum, and the dentate gyrus. The hippocampus projects to the septal area; the subiculum projects to the mamillary nuclei; and the dentate gyrus does not project beyond the hippocampal formation.

lary nucleus), the anterior nucleus of the thalamus, and the septal area.

–projects from the septal area to the hippocampal formation.

2. Stria terminalis

–lies between the thalamus and the caudate nucleus.

–projects from the amygdala to the hypothalamus and the septal area.

3. Ventral amygdalofugal pathway

–projects from the amygdala to the hypothalamus, thalamus, brainstem, and spinal cord.

4. Stria medullaris (thalami)

–projects from the septal area to the habenular nucleus.

5. Diagonal band of Broca

–forms the medial border of the anterior perforated substance.

–interconnects the amygdaloid nucleus and the septal area.

6. Tractus retroflexus (habenulointerpeduncular tract)

–projects from the habenular nucleus (epithalamus) to the interpeduncular nucleus (midbrain).

C. Papez circuit (see Figure 20.5)

–is a circular pathway that interconnects the major limbic structures.

–contains the following stations:

1. Hippocampal formation

–projects via the **fornix** to the mamillary nucleus.

2. Mamillary body

–projects via the **mamillothalamic tract** to the anterior nucleus of the thalamus.

3. Anterior nucleus of the thalamus

–projects to the **cingulate gyrus**.
–receives the mamillothalamic tract.

4. Cingulate gyrus

–projects via the entorhinal cortex to the hippocampal formation.

D. Functional and clinical considerations

1. Hippocampus

–has a low threshold for seizure activity.
–is involved in learning and memory.
–bilateral ablation results in the **inability to form long-term memories.**

2. Cingulate gyrus

–lesions result in **akinesia, mutism, apathy, and indifference to pain**.

3. Amygdaloid nucleus

–modulates hypothalamic and endocrine activities.
–has the highest concentration of opiate receptors in the brain.
–has a high concentration of estradiol receptors.
–bilateral lesions result in **placidity, with loss of fear, rage, and aggression**.

4. Anterior temporal lobe

–contains the amygdala and the hippocampus.
–bilateral ablation results in **Klüver-Bucy syndrome** (psychic blindness [visual agnosia], hyperphagia, docility, and hypersexuality).

5. Mamillary bodies and the mediodorsal nucleus of the thalamus

–are damaged by chronic alcoholism and thiamine (vitamin B_1) deficiency, which results in **Korsakoff's syndrome** (amnestic-confabulatory syndrome). This syndrome is considered to be a late chronic stage of Wernicke's encephalopathy.
–clinical signs include memory disturbances (amnesia), confabulation, and temporospatial disorientation.

Review Test

Directions: Each of the numbered items or incomplete statements in this section is followed by answers or by completions of the statement. Select the **one** lettered answer or completion that is **best** in each case.

1. The hippocampal formation includes all of the following structures EXCEPT the

(A) dentate gyrus.
(B) cornu ammonis.
(C) subiculum.
(D) amygdala
(E) alveus.

2. All of the following statements concerning the hippocampal formation are correct EXCEPT

(A) it is a three-layered paleocortex.
(B) it receives mossy fiber input from the dentate gyrus.
(C) the output cell is the pyramidal neuron.
(D) major input is via the entorhinal cortex.
(E) major output is via the fornix.

3. Which of the following signs and symptoms is not related to Klüver-Bucy syndrome?

(A) Hyperphagia
(B) Psychic blindness
(C) Docility
(D) Hypersexuality
(E) Amnestic confabulation

4. All of the following statements concerning the primary olfactory cortex are correct EXCEPT

(A) it receives olfactory input from the lateral olfactory stria.
(B) it projects to the thalamus.
(C) it projects to the amygdala.
(D) it includes the entorhinal cortex.
(E) it includes the prepiriform and periamygdaloid cortices.

5. All of the following statements concerning the olfactory tract are correct EXCEPT

(A) it is a telencephalic structure.
(B) it contains a nucleus.
(C) it projects fibers to the anterior commissure.
(D) it projects via the lateral olfactory stria to the primary olfactory cortex.
(E) it conducts fibers to the thalamus.

6. All of the following statements concerning taste receptor cells are correct EXCEPT they

(A) are found in the palate.
(B) mediate a SVA modality.
(C) are innervated by the vagal nerve.
(D) are innervated by fibers that traverse the chorda tympani.
(E) project to the solitary tract of the medulla.

7. The taste pathway includes all of the following way stations EXCEPT

(A) the geniculate ganglion.
(B) the semilunar ganglion.
(C) the solitary nucleus.
(D) cortical area 43.
(E) the central tegmental tract.

8. All of the following statements concerning the circuit of Papez are correct EXCEPT

(A) the hippocampal formation projects via the fornix to the mamillary body.
(B) the mamillothalamic tract interconnects the mamillary body and the anterior nucleus of the thalamus.
(C) the anterior nucleus of the thalamus projects to the cingulate gyrus.
(D) the mamillary nucleus projects via the fornix to the hippocampal formation.
(E) the cingulate gyrus projects via the entorhinal cortex to the hippocampal formation.

Directions: Each group of items in this section consists of lettered options followed by a set of numbered items. For each item, select the **one** lettered option that is most closely associated with it. Each lettered option may be selected once, more than once, or not at all.

Questions 9–13

Match the characteristic with the structure it best describes.

(A) Stria terminalis
(B) Stria medullaris
(C) Medial forebrain bundle
(D) Tractus retroflexus
(E) Diagonal band of Broca

9. Consists of septohabenular fibers

10. Forms the medial border of the anterior perforated substance

11. Lies between the thalamus and the caudate nucleus

12. Projects from the epithalamus to the midbrain tegmentum

13. Is a major efferent pathway from the amygdala

Questions 14–17

Match each characteristic with the structure it most appropriately describes.

(A) Amygdala
(B) Hippocampal formation
(C) Both A and B
(D) Neither A nor B

14. Is located in the temporal lobe

15. Is destroyed in Klüver-Bucy syndrome

16. Projects via the stria terminalis

17. Receives direct olfactory input

Answers and Explanations

1–D. The hippocampal formation consists of the dentate gyrus, the hippocampus (cornu ammonis), and the subiculum. The alveus, a fiber layer of the hippocampus, is the origin of the fornix.

2–A. The olfactory (piriform) cortex is paleocortex; the hippocampal cortex is archicortex. Archicortex and paleocortex are both three-layered cortex and are classified as allocortex (heterogenetic cortex). The cingulate gyrus is mesocortex or juxtallocortex, a transitional cortex between the neocortex and allocortex.

3–E. Psychic blindness (visual agnosia), docility, hyperphagia, and hypersexuality are all signs and symptoms of Klüver-Bucy syndrome. Amnestic confabulation is the classic manifestation of Korsakoff's syndrome, a late stage of Wernicke's encephalopathy.

4–D. The primary olfactory cortex (prepiriform and periamygdaloid cortices) projects to the thalamus (dorsomedial nucleus) and to the amygdaloid complex. The lateral olfactory stria projects to the primary olfactory cortex. The entorhinal cortex (also known as the second olfactory cortex; area 28) receives input from the primary olfactory cortex.

5–E. The olfactory tract, a telencephalic structure, contains a relay nucleus, the anterior olfactory nucleus, which projects fibers via the anterior commissure to the opposite olfactory bulb. The olfactory tract projects via the lateral olfactory stria to the primary olfactory cortex.

6–E. Taste receptor cells are found in the tongue, epiglottis, palate, and esophagus. They are SVA receptors and are innervated by the facial nerve (CN VII), the glossopharyngeal nerve (CN IX), and the vagal nerve (CN X). The chorda tympani contains taste fibers from the anterior two-thirds of the tongue with cell bodies located in the geniculate ganglion of CN VII of the petrous part of the temporal bone. Taste receptor cells are modified epithelial cells; unlike olfactory receptor cells, which are first-order neurons, they do not project to the central nervous system.

7–B. The peripheral taste pathway includes the geniculate ganglion of CN VII, the petrosal ganglion of CN IX, the nodose ganglion of CN X, the solitary tract and nucleus, the central tegmental tract, the ventral posteromedial nucleus of the thalamus, and the gustatory cortex, which is located in the parietal operculum (area 43) and in the parainsular cortex. The semilunar ganglion, the terminal ganglion of CN V, is not a structure of gustation.

8–D. The mamillary body projects via the mamillothalamic tract to the anterior nucleus of the thalamus and via the mamillotegmental tract to the tegmental nuclei of the midbrain.

9–B. The stria medullaris (thalami) contains septohabenular fibers (i.e., fibers that project from the septal nuclei to the habenular nuclei). The stria medullaris (singular) should not be confused with the striae medullares (plural). The striae medullares (rhombencephali) arise from the arcuate nuclei of the medulla and are seen on the floor of the rhomboid fossa.

10–E. The diagonal band of Broca is the medial border of the anterior perforated substance. This fiber bundle contains amygdaloseptal and septoamygdalar fibers. The nucleus of the diagonal band projects via the fornix to the hippocampal formation.

11–A. The stria terminalis and the vena terminalis lie in the sulcus terminalis between the thalamus and the caudate nucleus.

12–D. The tractus retroflexus contains habenulointerpeduncular fibers that project from the habenular nuclei of the epithalamus to the interpeduncular nucleus of the midbrain tegmentum.

13–A. The stria terminalis is a major efferent pathway from the amygdala. It projects to the septal area and to the bed nucleus of the stria terminalis.

14–C. Both the hippocampal formation and the amygdala are found in the parahippocampal gyrus of the temporal (limbic) lobe.

15–C. The hippocampal formation and the amygdala are both involved in Klüver-Bucy syndrome.

16–A. The amygdala projects via the stria terminalis and via the ventral amygdalofugal pathway. The stria terminalis is the most prominent projection from the amygdaloid complex.

17–A. The amygdala receives both direct and indirect olfactory input.

21

Basal Ganglia and the Striatal Motor System

I. Basal Ganglia (Figure 21.1)

—consist of subcortical nuclei (gray matter) located within the cerebral hemispheres.

A. Components

1. **Caudate nucleus**
2. **Putamen**
3. **Globus pallidus**
4. **Amygdala (amygdaloid nuclear complex)** [See Chapter 20, amygdaloid complex system.]
5. **Claustrum**

    —is located between the putamen and the insular cortex and between the external capsule and the extreme capsule.

B. Groupings of the basal ganglia

1. **Striatum (neostriatum)**

    —consists of the **caudate nucleus** and the **putamen,** which are similar in structure and connections and have a common embryological origin.
2. **Lentiform nucleus**

    —consists of the **putamen** and the **globus pallidus**.
3. **Corpus striatum**

    —consists of the **lentiform nucleus** and the **caudate nucleus**.

II. Striatal Motor System (see Figure 21.1)

—is also called the **extrapyramidal motor system**.

—plays a role in the initiation and execution of somatic motor activity, especially willed movement.

—is involved in automatic stereotyped motor activity of a postural and reflex nature.

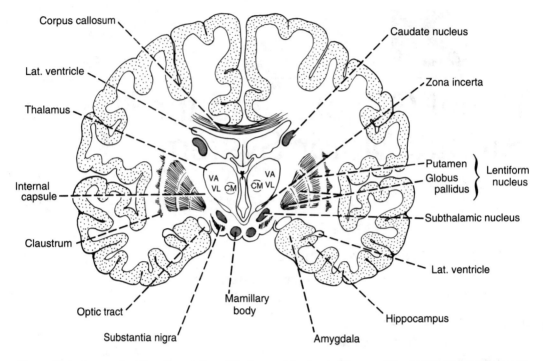

Figure 21.1. A coronal section through the midthalamus at the level of the mamillary bodies. The basal ganglia are all prominent at this level and include the striatum (caudate nucleus and putamen) and the lentiform nucleus (globus pallidus and putamen). The subthalamic nucleus and substantia nigra are important components of the striatal motor system.

—exerts its influences on motor activities via the thalamus, motor cortex, and corticobulbar and corticospinal systems.

A. Components of the striatal system

—consist of the following nuclei:

1. Striatum (caudatoputamen or neostriatum)

a. Caudate nucleus (caudatum)

b. Putamen

2. Globus pallidus (pallidum or paleostriatum)

a. Medial (internal) segment

—is adjacent to the internal capsule.

b. Lateral (external) segment

—is adjacent to the putamen.

3. Subthalamic nucleus

—lies between the internal capsule and the thalamus and between the internal capsule and the lenticular fasciculus.

4. Thalamus

a. Ventral anterior nucleus

b. Ventral lateral nucleus

c. Centromedian nucleus

5. Substantia nigra

a. Pars compacta

–contains dopaminergic neurons, which contain the pigment melanin.

b. Pars reticularis

–contains GABA-ergic neurons.

6. Pedunculopontine nucleus

–lies in the lateral tegmentum of the caudal midbrain.

B. Major connections of the striatal system (Figure 21.2)

1. Striatum (caudate nucleus and putamen)

–receives its largest input from the **neocortex,** from virtually all neocortical areas.

–receives input from the **thalamus** (centromedian nucleus) and from the **substantia nigra**.

–projects fibers to two major nuclei: the **globus pallidus** and the **substantia nigra**.

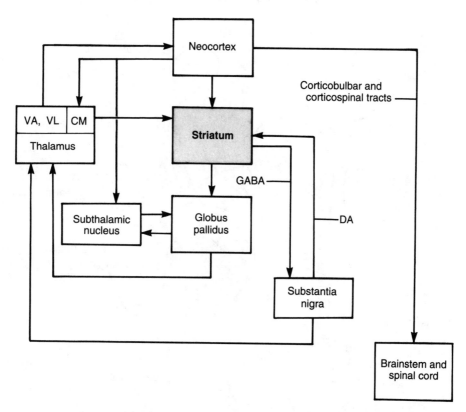

Figure 21.2. Major afferent and efferent connections of the striatal system. The striatum (caudate nucleus and putamen) receives major input from three sources: the thalamus, the neocortex, and the substantia nigra. The striatum projects to the globus pallidus and the substantia nigra. The globus pallidus is the effector nucleus of the striatal system; it projects to the thalamus and to the subthalamic nucleus. The substantia nigra also projects to the thalamus. The striatal motor system expresses itself via the corticobulbar and corticospinal tracts. *CM* = centromedian nucleus; *DA* = dopamine; *GABA* = γ-aminobutyric acid; *VA* = ventral anterior nucleus; *VL* = ventral lateral nucleus.

2. Globus pallidus (Figure 21.3)

–receives input from two major nuclei: the **striatum** and the **subthalamic nucleus**.

–projects fibers to three major nuclei: the **subthalamic nucleus;** the **thalamus** (ventral anterior, ventral lateral, and centromedian nuclei); and the **pedunculopontine nucleus**.

3. Subthalamic nucleus

–receives input from the **globus pallidus** and from the **motor cortex**.

–projects fibers to the globus pallidus.

4. Thalamus (see Figure 16.1)

a. Input to the thalamus

(1) Globus pallidus

–projects to the **ventral anterior, ventral lateral,** and **centromedian nuclei**.

(2) Substantia nigra

–projects from the pars reticularis to the **ventral anterior and ventral lateral nuclei**.

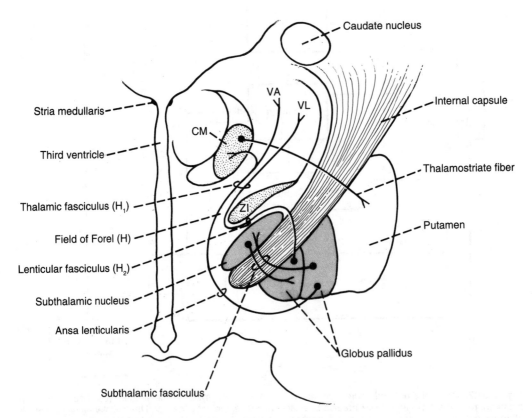

Figure 21.3. Major efferent projections from the globus pallidus, including the fields of Forel (H_1 and H_2). The globus pallidus is the principal effector nucleus of the striatal motor system, projecting to the thalamus (*VA, VL, CM*) and to the subthalamic nucleus. The zona incerta, *ZI,* lies between the thalamic and lenticular fasciculi.

b. Projections from the thalamus
    (1) Motor cortex (area 4)
        –from the **ventral lateral** and **centromedian nuclei**
    (2) Premotor cortex (area 6)
        –from the **ventral anterior** and **ventral lateral nuclei**
    (3) Supplementary motor cortex (area 6)
        –from the **ventral lateral** and **ventral anterior nuclei**
    (4) Striatum
        –from the **centromedian nucleus**

5. Substantia nigra
  –receives major input from the **striatum**.
  –projects fibers to the **striatum** and the **thalamus** (which projects to the ventral anterior and ventral lateral nuclei).

6. Pedunculopontine nucleus
  –receives input from the **globus pallidus**.
  –projects fibers to the **globus pallidus** and to the **substantia nigra**.

C. Major neurotransmitters of the neurons of the striatal system (Figure 21.4)

1. Glutamate-containing neurons (see Figure 22.10)
  –project from the cerebral cortex to the striatum.
  –project from the subthalamic nucleus to the globus pallidus.
  –excite **striatal GABA-ergic** and **cholinergic neurons**.

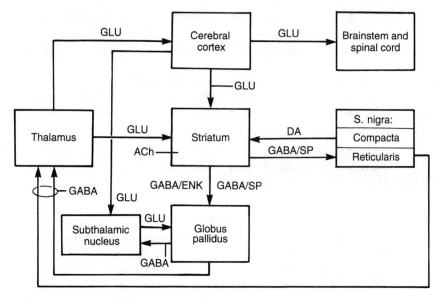

Figure 21.4 Major neurotransmitters of the striatal motor system. Within the striatum, globus pallidus, and pars reticularis of the substantia nigra, GABA is the predominant neurotransmitter. GABA may coexist in the same neuron with enkephalin or substance P. Dopamine-containing neurons are found in the pars compacta of the substantia nigra. Acetylcholine is found in local circuit neurons of the striatum. The subthalamic nucleus projects excitatory glutaminergic fibers to the globus pallidus. *ACh* = acetylcholine; *DA* = dopamine; *ENK* = enkephalin; *GABA* = γ-aminobutyric acid; *GLU* = glutamate and/or aspartate; *SP* = substance P.

2. γ-Aminobutyric acid (GABA)-containing neurons (see Figure 22.9)

–are the predominant neurons of the striatal system.

–are found in the striatum, globus pallidus, and substantia nigra (pars reticularis).

–give rise to the following **GABA-ergic projections:** striatopallidal, striatonigral, pallidothalamic, and nigrothalamic projections.

–degenerate in Huntington's disease.

3. Dopamine-containing neurons (see Figure 22.2)

–are found in the pars compacta of the substantia nigra.

–give rise to the dopaminergic nigrostriatal projection.

–are thought to regulate the production of striatal peptides and peptide mRNA.

–degenerate in Parkinson's disease.

4. Acetylcholine-containing neurons (see Figure 22.1)

–are local circuit neurons found in the striatum.

5. Neuropeptide-containing neurons (see Figures 22.6–22.8)

–include **enkephalin, dynorphin, substance P, somatostatin, neurotensin, neuropeptide Y, and cholectystokinin**.

–are also found in the basal ganglia.

–coexist with the major neurotransmitters (e.g., GABA and/or enkephalin and GABA and/or substance P).

D. Clinical considerations

1. Parkinson's disease

–is a common condition that is associated with degeneration and depigmentation of neurons in the substantia nigra.

–results in the **depletion of dopamine** in the caudate nucleus and putamen.

–includes clinical manifestations of **hypokinesia and bradykinesia** (difficulty in initiating and performing volitional movements); **rigidity** (cog-wheel rigidity); and **resting tremor** (pill-rolling tremor).

2. MPTP-induced parkinsonism

–is caused by MPTP (1-methyl-4-phenyl-1,2,3,6-tetrahydropyridine), a **meperidine analog** found in illicit recreational drugs.

–results in the destruction of dopaminergic neurons, which are located in the substantia nigra.

3. Huntington's disease (chorea)

–is an inherited **autosomal dominant movement disorder** associated with severe degeneration of the cholinergic and GABA-ergic neurons, which are located in the caudate nucleus and putamen.

–is usually accompanied by **gyral atrophy** in the frontal and temporal lobes.

–can be traced to a single gene defect on chromosome 4.

–results in clinical manifestations of **choreiform movements** and **progressive dementia**.

–results in **hydrocephalus ex vacuo,** due to the loss of neurons located in the head of the caudate nucleus.

4. Ballism and hemiballism

    —is an extrapyramidal motor disorder most often resulting from a vascular lesion (infarct) of the subthalamic nucleus.

    —is characterized by **violent flinging** (ballistic) **movements of one or both extremities;** symptoms appear on the contralateral side.

    —may be treated with dopamine-blocking drugs or with GABA-mimetic agents.

    —may be treated surgically by **ventrolateral thalamotomy.**

5. Hepatolenticular degeneration (Wilson's disease)

    —is an autosomal recessive disorder due to a **defect in the metabolism of copper** (ceruloplasmin).

    —has its gene locus on chromosome 13.

    —results in clinical manifestations of **tremor, rigidity,** and **choreiform or athetotic movements.**

    —results in a **corneal Kayser-Fleischer ring,** which is pathognomonic.

    —lesions are found in the liver (cirrhosis) and in the lentiform nuclei.

Review Test

Directions: Each of the numbered items or incomplete statements in this section is followed by answers or by completions of the statement. Select the **one** lettered answer or completion that is **best** in each case.

1. All of the following statements concerning Huntington's disease are correct EXCEPT

(A) it is inherited as an autosomal dominant trait.
(B) it is associated with severe degeneration of the subthalamic nucleus.
(C) it is associated with hydrocephalus.
(D) patients have dementia.
(E) patients have choreiform movements.

2. Wilson's disease is characterized by all of the following EXCEPT

(A) it is a disorder due to a defect in the metabolism of copper.
(B) it is inherited as an autosomal dominant trait.
(C) tremor, rigidity, athetotic or choreiform movements are present.
(D) a corneal Kayser-Fleischer ring is pathognomonic.
(E) lesions are found in the liver and lentiform nucleus.

3. The basal ganglia include all of the following structures EXCEPT the

(A) globus pallidus.
(B) caudate nucleus.
(C) putamen.
(D) lentiform nucleus.
(E) subthalamic nucleus.

4. Which of the following constellations is not correct?

(A) Lentiform nucleus = putamen and globus pallidus
(B) Neostriatum = striatum = caudate nucleus and putamen
(C) Paleostriatum = pallidum = globus pallidus
(D) Archistriatum = amygdaloid nucleus
(E) Corpus striatum = caudate nucleus, putamen, and claustrum

5. All of the following statements concerning neurotransmitters are correct EXCEPT

(A) the neocortex projects glutamatergic fibers to the striatum.
(B) the striatum projects GABA-ergic fibers to the globus pallidus and substantia nigra.
(C) dopaminergic neurons are found in the putamen.
(D) the substantia nigra projects dopaminergic fibers to the striatum.
(E) the globus pallidus projects GABA-ergic fibers to the thalamus.

6. All of the following statements concerning glutamatergic neurons are correct EXCEPT

(A) they are found in the globus pallidus.
(B) they excite GABA-ergic neurons of the putamen.
(C) they project from the subthalamic nucleus to the globus pallidus.
(D) they project from the cortex to the subthalamic nucleus.
(E) they project from the cortex to the thalamus.

7. All of the following statements concerning dopaminergic neurons are correct EXCEPT

(A) they are found in the pars compacta of the substantia nigra.
(B) they are found in the subthalamic nucleus.
(C) they project to the caudate nucleus.
(D) they project to the putamen.
(E) they are thought to regulate the production of striatal peptides and peptide mRNA.

8. Which thalamic nucleus projects to the striatum?

(A) Centromedian nucleus
(B) Mediodorsal nucleus
(C) Ventral lateral nucleus
(D) Ventral anterior nucleus
(E) Ventral posterolateral nucleus

9. All of the following statements concerning the substantia nigra are correct EXCEPT

(A) it receives input from the caudate nucleus.
(B) it receives input from the putamen.
(C) it receives dopaminergic input from the striatum.
(D) it projects to the thalamus.
(E) it is found in the midbrain.

10. The striatum receives major input from all of the following nuclei EXCEPT the

(A) substantia nigra.
(B) centromedian nucleus.
(C) motor cortex.
(D) sensory cortex.
(E) subthalamic nucleus.

11. All of the following statements concerning the globus pallidus are correct EXCEPT

(A) it receives input from the motor cortex.
(B) it receives input from the putamen.
(C) it receives input from the subthalamic nucleus.
(D) it projects to the ventral anterior nucleus.
(E) it projects to the ventral lateral nucleus.

12. All of the following statements concerning the subthalamic nucleus are correct EXCEPT

(A) it lies between the internal capsule and the lenticular fasciculus.
(B) it receives input from the globus pallidus.
(C) it projects to the putamen.
(D) it projects to the globus pallidus.
(E) its destruction results in violent flinging movements of the extremities.

13. The globus pallidus projects to the thalamus via the

(A) fasciculus retroflexus.
(B) stria medullaris
(C) ansa lenticularis.
(D) ansa peduncularis.
(E) stria terminalis.

14. All of the following statements concerning striatal connections are correct EXCEPT

(A) the major projections of the globus pallidus are to the thalamus and the subthalamic nucleus.
(B) the major projection of the subthalamic nucleus is to the caudate nucleus.
(C) the dopaminergic neurons of the striatal system are found in the substantia nigra (pars compacta).
(D) the striatum receives its largest input from the neocortex.
(E) the centromedian nucleus receives input from the motor cortex and projects to the putamen.

15. All of the following structures are part of the striatal system EXCEPT the

(A) lentiform nucleus.
(B) subthalamic nucleus.
(C) substantia nigra.
(D) red nucleus.
(E) globus pallidus.

Answers and Explanations

1–B. Huntington's chorea, inherited as an autosomal dominant trait, is associated with severe degeneration of the striatum and cell loss in the cerebral cortex. Striatal cell loss results in widening of the frontal horn of the lateral ventricle; this is called hydrocephalis ex vacuo. A DNA marker linked to Hungtington's chorea is located on chromosome 4.

2–B. Wilson's disease (hepatolenticular degeneration) is a familial metabolic disease transmitted as an autosomal recessive trait. Low serum ceruloplasmin, or low serum copper, and increased urinary copper excretion usually corroborate the diagnosis. In the early course of the disease, liver biopsy shows a high copper content. The corneal Kayser-Fleischer ring is pathognomonic of this disease. A gene locus has been found on chromosome 13.

3–E. The basal ganglia include the caudate nucleus, putamen, and globus pallidus. The putamen and globus pallidus together are called the lentiform (lenticular) nucleus. The subthalamic nucleus, a diencephalic nucleus, is not a basal ganglion but is a component of the striatal system. The amygdaloid nucleus (archistriatum) and the claustrum are, from an embryological standpoint, basal ganglia since they are derived from the telencephalic corpus striatum.

4–E. The corpus striatum includes the caudate nucleus, the putamen, and the globus pallidus. The enigmatic claustrum is found between the external capsule and the extreme capsule.

5–C. Dopamine-containing neurons (cell bodies) are found in the pars compacta of the substantia nigra in the ventral tegmental area of the midbrain. The predominant cell type in the putamen is the medium-sized GABA-ergic spiny neuron.

6–A. Glutamatergic neurons have not been identified in the globus pallidus; they have been located in the subthalamic nucleus and thalamus.

7–B. Dopaminergic neurons of the substantia nigra project via the nigrostriatal pathway to the striatum (caudate nucleus and putamen). Dopamine released in the striatum is thought to regulate the production of neuropeptides and peptide mRNA within the resident striatal neurons. The subthalamic nucleus receives GABA-ergic input from the lateral (external) segment of the globus pallidus. The subthalamic nucleus projects excitatory glutamatergic input to both segments of the globus pallidus.

8–A. The striatum (caudate nucleus and putamen) receives thalamic input from the centromedian nucleus, the largest of the intralaminar nuclei.

9–C. The substantia nigra receives GABA-ergic input from the caudate nucleus and putamen. It projects dopaminergic fibers to the caudate nucleus and putamen. It projects GABA-ergic fibers to the ventral lateral and ventral anterior thalamic nuclei.

10–E. The striatum (caudate nucleus and putamen) receives major input from three sources: the neocortex, including the motor and sensory cortices; the thalamus (centromedian nucleus); and the substantia nigra (pars compacta). The subthalamic nucleus has important reciprocal connections with the globus pallidus; it does not project to the striatum.

11–A. The globus pallidus, the major effector nucleus of the striatal system, projects to the ventral anterior, ventral lateral, and centromedian thalamic nuclei. It receives input from the striatum (the caudate nucleus and putamen). The globus pallidus also has reciprocal connections with the subthalamic nucleus. The motor cortex does not project to the globus pallidus.

12–C. The subthalamic nucleus is reciprocally connected to the globus pallidus via the subthalamic fasciculus. It lies between the posterior limb of the internal capsule and the lenticular fasciculus. Lesions of the subthalamic nucleus result in contralateral wild, flinging (ballistic), involuntary movements of the limbs (hemiballism).

13–C. The globus pallidus projects to the thalamus via the lenticular and thalamic fasciculi and via the ansa lenticularis. The ansa peduncularis (part of the inferior thalamic peduncle) interconnects the amygdaloid nucleus and the hypothalamus. It also interconnects the orbitofrontal cortex and the thalamus (mediodorsal nucleus). The fasciculus retroflexus (habenulointerpeduncular tract) interconnects the habenular nucleus and the interpeduncular nucleus. The stria medullaris (thalami) interconnects the septal area (nuclei) and the habenular nuclei. The stria terminalis projects from the amygdaloid complex to the septal area and the hypothalamus.

14–B. The subthalamic nucleus does not project to the striatum. It projects glutaminergic fibers to the globus pallidus and receives GABA-ergic fibers from the globus pallidus.

15–D. The red nucleus, a prominent nucleus of the midbrain, is not considered a part of the striatal system. The red nucleus receives major input from the cerebellar nuclei and the motor and premotor cortex and projects to the spinal cord and the inferior olivary nucleus of the medulla.

22

Neurotransmitters and Pathways

I. Introduction

A. Neurotransmitters (chemical messengers)

–are substances released on exitation from presynaptic neurons. They produce the effects of nerve stimulation in postsynaptic neurons or in receptor cells.

B. Neurochemical pathways

–can be classified according to the chemical composition of their neurotransmitters.

1. Monoaminergic pathways

–employ **monoamines** as their neurotransmitters; they contain one amine group. Monoamines include **dopamine, norepinephrine, epinephrine,** and **serotonin.**

a. Catecholaminergic pathways

–employ a monoamine that contains a catechol nucleus. Catecholamines include **dopamine, norepinephrine,** and **epinephrine.**
–include dopaminergic, noradrenergic (norepinephrinergic), and adrenergic (epinephrinergic) pathways.

b. Indolaminergic pathways

–employ a monoamine that contains an indole nucleus. **Serotonin** is an indolamine.
–include serotonergic pathways.

2. Cholinergic pathways

–employ **acetylcholine** as their neurotransmitter.

3. Peptidergic pathways

–employ **peptides** as their neurotransmitters.

4. GABA-ergic pathways

–employ γ-aminobutyric acid (**GABA**) as their neurotransmitter.

5. Glutamatergic pathways

–employ **glutamate** as their neurotransmitter.

6. Glycinergic pathways

—employ **glycine** as their neurotransmitter.

II. Acetylcholine (ACh)

A. Characteristics—ACh

—can be identified indirectly by the marker choline acetyltransferase.
—is the major transmitter of the peripheral nervous system (PNS), neuro-muscular junction, parasympathetic nervous system, preganglionic sympathetic fibers, and postganglionic sympathetic fibers to the sweat glands.
—is found in neurons of the somatic and visceral motor nuclei in the brainstem and spinal cord.

B. Major cholinergic pathways (Figure 22.1)

1. Septal nuclei

—project via the fornix to the hippocampal formation.

2. Basal nucleus of Meynert

—is located in the substantia innominata of the basal forebrain.
—is located between the globus pallidus and the anterior perforated substance.
—projects to the entire neocortex.
—degenerates in **Alzheimer's disease**.

3. Striatum (caudate nucleus and putamen)

—contains ACh in its local circuit neurons.
—cholinergic neurons degenerate in **Huntington's disease and Alzheimer's disease**.

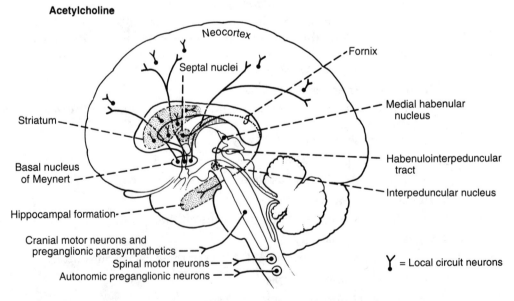

Figure 22.1. Distribution of acetylcholine- (ACh-) containing neurons and their axonal projections. The basal nucleus of Meynert projects to the entire cortex; this nucleus degenerates in Alzheimer's disease. Striatal ACh-local-circuit neurons degenerate in Huntington's chorea.

4. Neocortex

–contains ACh in its local circuit neurons.

III. Dopamine

A. Characteristics—dopamine

–is a **catecholamine**.
–can be identified by the marker tyrosine hydroxylase.
–plays a role in cognitive, motor, and neuroendocrine functions.
–is **depleted in Parkinson's disease**.
–transmission is **increased in schizophrenics** (dopamine hypothesis of schizophrenia).

B. Major dopaminergic pathways (Figure 22.2)

1. Nigrostriatal pathway

–the substantia nigra projects to the striatum.
–destruction of dopaminergic nigral neurons results in **parkinsonism**.

2. Mesolimbic pathway

–the ventral tegmental area projects to all cortical and subcortical structures of the limbic system.
–is linked to behavior and schizophrenia.

3. Tuberohypophyseal (tuberinfundibular) pathway

–the arcuate nucleus of the hypothalamus projects to the portal vessels of the infundibulum.

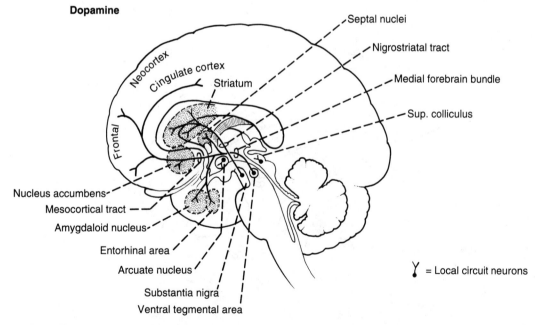

Figure 22.2. Distribution of dopamine-containing neurons and their projections. Two major ascending dopamine pathways arise in the midbrain: the nigrostriatal tract from the substantia nigra and the mesolimbic tract from the ventral tegmental area. In Parkinson's disease, loss of dopaminergic neurons occurs in the substantia nigra and in the ventral tegmental area.

—released dopamine inhibits the release of **prolactin** from the adenohypophysis.

IV. Norepinephrine (Noradrenalin)

A. Characteristics—norepinephrine

—is a **catecholamine**.
—can be localized by the marker dopamine β-hydroxylase.
—is the transmitter of the postganglionic sympathetic neurons.
—may play a role in the genesis and maintenance of **mood**. The catecholamine hypothesis of mood disorders states that reduced norepinephrine activity is related to **depression,** and that increased norepinephrine activity is related to **mania**.

B. Noradrenergic pathways (Figure 22.3)

1. Locus ceruleus

—contains the largest concentration of noradrenergic neurons in the CNS.
—is located in the pons and midbrain.
—projects to all parts of the central nervous system (CNS).
—receives multifarious input from the cortex, limbic system, reticular formation, raphe nuclei, cerebellum, and spinal cord.
—shows a significant loss of neurons in Alzheimer's disease and Parkinson's disease.
—is hypothesized to play a role in **anxiety and panic disorders**.

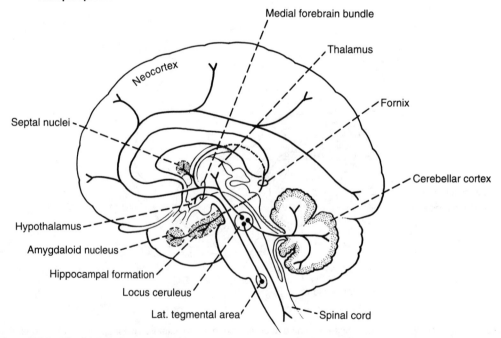

Figure 22.3. Distribution of norepinephrine-containing neurons and their projections. The locus ceruleus, located in the pons and midbrain, is the chief source of noradrenergic fibers. The locus ceruleus projects to all parts of the CNS.

2. Lateral tegmental area

– is located in the medulla and pons.
– projects via the central tegmental tract and the medial forebrain bundle to the hypothalamus and thalamus.

V. Serotonin (5-Hydroxytryptamine [5-HT]) [Figure 22.4]

A. Characteristics—5-HT

– is an **indoleamine**.
– can be identified by the marker tryptophan hydroxylase.
– plays an important role in influencing arousal, sensory perception, emotion, and higher cognitive functions.
– the **permissive serotonin hypothesis** states that reduced 5-HT activity permits reduced levels of catecholamines to cause depression and elevated levels to cause mania.
– **severe depression** and **insomnia** are associated with low 5-HT levels; **mania** is associated with high 5-HT activity.
– tricyclic antidepressants increase 5-HT availability by reduction of its re-uptake.

B. Major serotonergic pathways

– 5-HT neurons are found only in the **raphe nuclei** of the brainstem.
– raphe nuclei project diffusely to the entire CNS (see Figure 22.4).

Serotonin

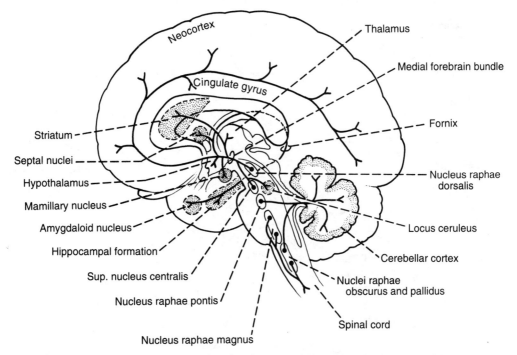

Figure 22.4. Distribution of serotonin-containing (5-HT) neurons and their projections. 5-HT neurons are found in nuclei of the raphe; they project widely to the forebrain, cerebellum, and spinal cord.

    1. Raphe nuclei of the medulla

      –project to the dorsal horns of the spinal cord.

    2. Raphe nuclei of the pons

      –project to the spinal cord and cerebellum.

    3. Raphe nuclei of the midbrain

      –project to widespread areas of the diencephalon and the telencephalon, including the striatum.

VI. Opioid Peptides

  A. Endorphins (Figure 22.5)

    –are derived from **pro-opiomelanocortin** (POMC), the precursor of adreno-corticotropin (ACTH).

    –include β-endorphin, the major endorphin found in the brain.

    –appear to play a major role in **endocrine function**.

    –endorphinergic neurons are found almost exclusively in the **hypothalamus** (arcuate and premamillary nuclei).

    –endorphinergic neurons project to the hypothalamus, amygdala, nucleus accumbens, septal area, thalamus, and locus ceruleus (midbrain and pons).

  B. Enkephalins (Figure 22.6)

    –are derived from **proenkephalin**.

    –are the most widely distributed and abundant opiate peptides.

    –are found in the highest concentrations in the **globus pallidus**.

    –are synthesized striatal neurons, which project to the globus pallidus.

    –are located mainly in local circuits of the limbic and striatal systems.

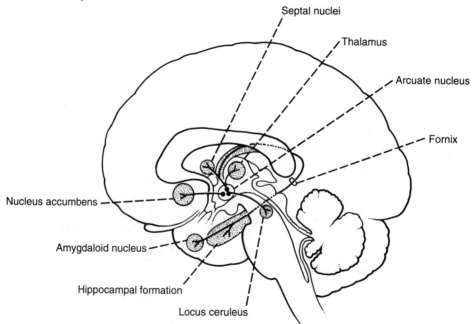

Figure 22.5. Distribution of endorphin-containing neurons and their projections. Endorphinergic neurons are found almost exclusively in the hypothalamus (arcuate nucleus).

Enkephalin

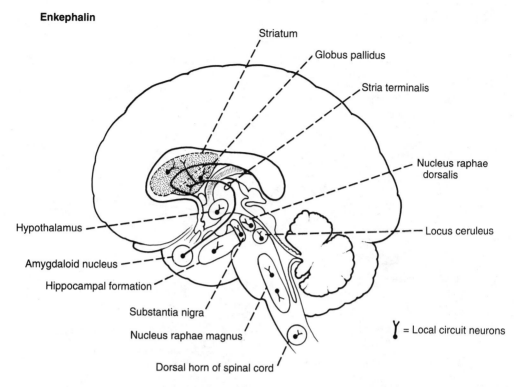

Figure 22.6. Distribution of enkephalin-containing neurons and their projections. They are found primarily in local circuits of the limbic and striatal systems. Enkephalinergic neurons of the brainstem and spinal cord play a role in pain-suppression mechanisms.

–play a role in **pain suppression** in the dorsal horn of the spinal cord.
–coexist with dopamine, norepinephrine, and acetylcholine.

C. Dynorphins

–are derived from **prodynorphin**.
–follow, in general, the distribution map for enkephalin.
–have high concentrations in the **hypothalamus** and **amygdala**.

VII. Nonopioid Neuropeptides

A. Substance P (Figure 22.7)

–is an excitatory neurotransmitter.
–is contained in dorsal root ganglion cells.
–plays a role in **pain transmission**.
–is synthesized in striatal neurons, which project to the globus pallidus and the substantia nigra.
–is found in highest concentration in the **substantia nigra** (striatonigral and pallidonigral tracts).

B. Somatostatin (Figure 22.8)

–is also called somatotropin-release–inhibiting factor.
–somatostatinergic neurons are found in the anterior hypothalamus and in the preoptic region, striatum, amygdala, cerebral cortex, and in dorsal root ganglion cells.

Substance P

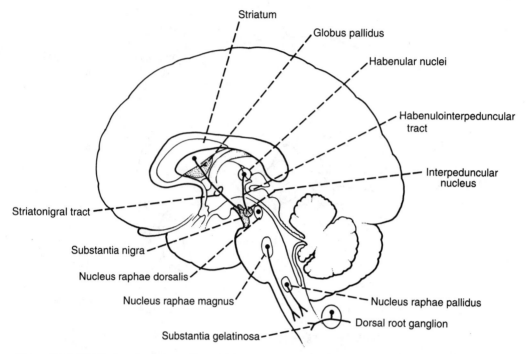

Figure 22.7. Distribution of substance P-containing neurons and their projections. Substance P is the neurotransmitter for nociceptive neurons of the dorsal root ganglia. Striatal substance P neurons project via the striatonigral tract to the substantia nigra.

–somatostatinergic neurons project their axons to the median eminence, where somatostatin enters the hypophyseal portal system and regulates the release of growth hormone (GH) and thyroid-stimulating hormone (THS).

–the concentration of somatostatin in the neocortex and hippocampus is significantly reduced in **Alzheimer's disease**.

VIII. Amino Acids

–are, from a quantitative standpoint, the major transmitters in the mammalian CNS.

A. Inhibitory amino acid transmitters

–are aliphatic amino acids that have **one acidic and one amine function**.

1. GABA (Figure 22.9)

–can be localized by the marker glutamic acid decarboxylase.

–is the major inhibitory neurotransmitter of the brain.

–coexists with substance P and with enkephalin.

–Purkinje, stellate, basket, and Golgi cells of the cerebellar cortex are GABA-ergic (see Figure 15.3).

–GABA-ergic striatal neurons project to the globus pallidus and the substantia nigra.

Somatostatin

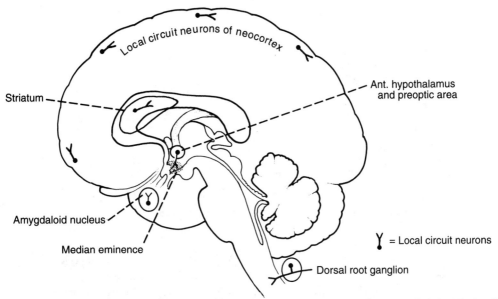

Figure 22.8. Distribution of somatostatin-containing neurons and their projections. Somatostatin is found primarily in the anterior hypothalamus and preoptic area. Somatostatinergic neurons project to the hypophyseal portal system and thus regulate the release of growth hormone.

—GABA-ergic pallidal neurons project to the thalamus.
—GABA-ergic nigral neurons project to the thalamus.

2. Glycine
—is the major inhibitory neurotransmitter of the spinal cord.
—is used by the Renshaw cells of the spinal cord.
—inhibitory action is blocked by strychnine.

B. Excitatory amino acid transmitters
—are aliphatic amino acids that have **two acidic functions and one alpha-amino group**.

1. Glutamate (Figure 22.10)
—is a major excitatory transmitter of the brain.
—neocortical glutamatergic neurons project to the striatum, the subthalamic nucleus, and the thalamus.
—the subthalamic nucleus projects glutamatergic fibers to the globus pallidus.
—is the neurotransmitter of the cerebellar granule cell.
—is used by the corticobulbar and corticospinal tracts.

2. Aspartate (see Figure 22.10)
—is a major excitatory transmitter of the brain.
—is the transmitter of the climbing fibers of the cerebellum.

GABA

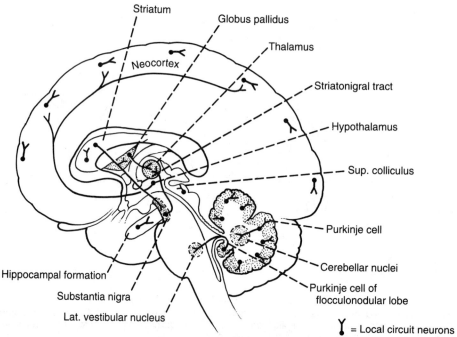

Figure 22.9. Distribution of GABA-containing neurons and their projections. GABA-ergic neurons are the major inhibitory cells of the CNS. GABA local circuit neurons are found in the neocortex, allocortex, and in the cerebellar cortex (Purkinje cells). Striatal GABA-ergic neurons project to the globus pallidus and the substantia nigra. Pallidal GABA-ergic neurons project to the thalamus and the subthalamic nucleus.

IX. Functional and Clinical Considerations

A. Endogenous pain control system

1. Ascending pathway

—spinoreticular pain impulses project to the periaqueductal gray of the midbrain.

2. Descending raphe–spinal pathway

—excitatory neurons of the periaqueductal gray project to the nucleus raphae magnus of the pons.

—excitatory neurons of the nucleus raphae magnus project serotonergic fibers to enkephalinergic inhibitory neurons of the substantia gelatinosa.

—enkephalinergic neurons of the substantia gelatinosa inhibit afferent pain fibers (substance P) and tract neurons that give rise to the spinoreticular and spinothalamic tracts.

3. Descending ceruleospinal pathway

—projects from the locus ceruleus to the spinal cord.

—is thought to directly inhibit tract neurons that give rise to the ascending pain pathways.

B. Parkinson's disease

—results from **degeneration of dopaminergic neurons** found in the pars compacta of the substantia nigra.

Glutamate and Aspartate

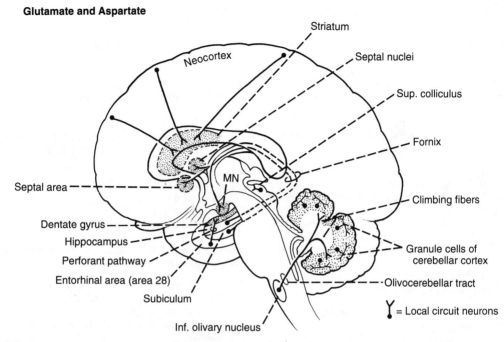

Figure 22.10. Distribution of glutamate- and aspartate-containing neurons and their projections. Glutamate is considered the major excitatory transmitter of the CNS. Cortical glutamatergic neurons project to the striatum; hippocampal and subicular glutamatergic neurons project via the fornix to the septal area and hypothalamus. Neurons of the inferior olivary nucleus project aspartatergic fibers to the cerebellum. The granule cells of the cerebellum are glutamatergic. *MN* = mamillary nucleus.

  —results in a **reduction of dopamine** in the striatum and in the substantia nigra.
  —results in the formation of **Lewy bodies,** intraneuronal inclusions in the substantia nigra.

C. Huntington's disease (Huntington's chorea)

  —results from a **loss of ACh- and GABA-containing neurons** in the striatum (caudatoputamen).
  —results in a **loss of GABA** in the striatum and substantia nigra.

D. Alzheimer's disease

  —results from the **degeneration of cortical neurons and cholinergic neurons** found in the basal nucleus of Meynert.
  —is associated with **60%–90% loss of choline acetyltransferase** in the cerebral cortex.
  —is characterized histologically by the presence of neurofibrillary tangles, senile plaques, granulovacuolar degeneration, and Hirano bodies.

E. Myasthenia gravis

  —is an autoimmune syndrome that occurs in the presence of antibodies to the nicotinic ACh receptor.
  —is caused by the action of antibodies that reduce the number of receptors in the neuromuscular junction, resulting in **muscle paresis**.

Review Test

Directions: Each of the numbered items or incomplete statements in this section is followed by answers or by completions of the statement. Select the **one** lettered answer or completion that is **best** in each case.

1. All of the following statements concerning acetylcholine (ACh) are correct EXCEPT

(A) it is the major transmitter of the peripheral nervous system.
(B) it is found in high concentrations in the striatum.
(C) it is found in high concentrations in the basal nucleus of Meynert.
(D) its levels are increased in Alzheimer's disease.
(E) it is the involved neurotransmitter in myasthenia gravis.

2. All of the following statements concerning dopamine are correct EXCEPT

(A) dopaminergic neurons are found chiefly in the midbrain.
(B) dopaminergic terminals are found chiefly in the striatum.
(C) dopaminergic fibers are found in the tuberohypophyseal pathway.
(D) dopamine contains an indole nucleus.
(E) dopamine is a catecholamine.

3. All of the following statements concerning the locus ceruleus are correct EXCEPT

(A) it is a mesencephalic structure.
(B) it contains noradrenergic neurons.
(C) it contains dopamine β-hydroxylase.
(D) its projections are limited to the cerebellar cortex.
(E) it is a pontine structure.

4. All of the following statements concerning serotonergic neurons are correct EXCEPT they

(A) are found in the raphe nuclei.
(B) are found in the cerebellum.
(C) innervate the basal ganglia.
(D) innervate the cerebellum.
(E) contain tryptophan hydroxylase.

5. All of the following statements concerning somatostatin are correct EXCEPT

(A) it is found in dorsal root ganglion cells.
(B) it is found in the hypothalamus.
(C) it is an endorphin.
(D) it is reduced in patients with Alzheimer's disease.
(E) it regulates the release of growth hormone (GH) and thyroid-stimulating hormone (TSH) from the hypophysis.

6. All of the following statements concerning substance P are correct EXCEPT it

(A) is found in the striatopallidal and striatonigral tracts.
(B) is contained in dorsal root ganglion cells.
(C) is produced in neurons of the raphe nuclei.
(D) plays a role in pain transmission.
(E) is a powerful inhibitory neurotransmitter.

Directions: The group of items in this section consists of lettered options followed by a set of numbered items. For each item, select the **one** lettered option that is most closely associated with it. Each lettered option may be selected once, more than once, or not at all.

Questions 7–15

Match each of the characteristics below with the neurotransmitter it best describes.

(A) Dopamine
(B) Serotonin
(C) β-Endorphin
(D) Glycine
(E) γ-Aminobutyric acid (GABA)

7. Is used by Purkinje cells

8. Is the major inhibitory neurotransmitter of the spinal cord

9. Contains an indole nucleus

10. Is associated with insomnia and depression

11. Is found almost exclusively in neurons of the hypothalamus

12. Is associated with glutamic acid decarboxylase

13. Shows reduced striatal levels in parkinsonism

14. Shows reduced striatal levels in chorea

15. Is produced primarily in the substantia nigra

Answers and Explanations

1–D. ACh is the major transmitter of the PNS. It is found in high concentrations in the striatum (caudate nucleus and putamen) and in the basal nucleus of Meynert. Striatal ACh-containing neurons are local circuit neurons. Cholinergic neurons from the basal nucleus project to the entire neocortex. Choline acetyltransferase (ChAT) levels are reduced in Alzheimer's disease. In myasthenia gravis, an autoimmune syndrome, there is a decrease in the number of ACh-receptor sites in the postsynaptic membrane.

2–D. Dopaminergic neurons are found chiefly in the midbrain (the pars compacta of the substantia nigra and the ventral tegmental area of Tsai). Dopamine is a monoamine and a catecholamine. The tuberohypophyseal tract contains dopaminergic axons from the arcuate nucleus of the hypothalamus. Dopamine inhibits the release of prolactin from the adenohypophysis. The indole nucleus is found in serotonin.

3–D. The locus ceruleus is located in the midbrain and rostral pons and contains noradrenergic neurons. The noradrenergic neurons contain the enzyme dopamine β-hydroxylase, which synthesizes noradrenaline from dopamine. The locus ceruleus projects to the entire brain, the cerebellum, and large parts of the brainstem and spinal cord; it contains the largest concentrations of noradrenergic neurons in the brain. There is a substantial loss of neurons in the locus ceruleus in Alzheimer's disease and Parkinson's disease.

4–B. Serotonergic (5-HT-containing) neurons are found in the raphe nuclei and contain tryptophan hydroxylase, which catalyzes the conversion of tryptophan to 5-hydroxytryptophan, the immediate precursor of 5-HT. The caudate nucleus and putamen (basal ganglia) and cerebellum are innervated by 5-HT cells of the raphe nuclei. Serotonergic neurons are found only in the raphe nuclei of the brainstem.

5–C. Somatostatin (somatotropin release-inhibiting hormone), a cyclic peptide, is found in dorsal root ganglia and in the anterior hypothalamus. Somatostatin is a growth hormone-inhibiting hormone that is released into the hypophyseal portal system. Somatostatin concentration in the neocortex and hippocampus is significantly reduced in patients with Alzheimer's disease.

6–E. Substance P is a powerful excitatory neurotransmitter that plays a role in pain transmission. The small nociceptive dorsal root ganglion cells use substance P. Raphe nuclei have been found to produce both serotonin (5-HT) and substance P. Substance P is also produced in striatal neurons (the caudate nucleus and the putamen), which project to the globus pallidus and the substantia nigra.

7–E. GABA is the inhibitory transmitter of the Purkinje cells of the cerebellum. The only output from the cerebellar cortex is via Purkinje cell axons.

8–D. Glycine is the major inhibitory neurotransmitter of the spinal cord.

9–B. Serotonin (5-HT) contains an indole nucleus and is therefore an indolamine.

10–B. Destruction of 5-HT neurons results in insomnia. Severe depression is associated with low 5-HT levels.

11–C. β-Endorphin is found almost exclusively in the neurons of the hypothalamus (arcuate and premamillary nuclei).

12–E. Glutamic acid decarboxylase is the marker for GABA; it converts L-glutamic acid to GABA.

13–A. Dopamine in the striatum is depleted in parkinsonism. This is due to the degeneration of nigral dopaminergic cells that project to the caudate nucleus and putamen.

14–E. GABA concentrations in the striatum are reduced in Huntington's chorea. This is the result of degeneration of GABA-ergic neurons in the striatum.

15–A. Dopamine is produced by the neurons in the pars compacta of the substantia nigra of the midbrain. The ventral tegmental area of the midbrain also contains dopaminergic neurons.

23

Cerebral Cortex

I. Overview—The Cerebral Cortex

—consists of the **neocortex** (90%) and the **allocortex** (10%).

A. Neocortex (isocortex; homogenetic cortex)
—is a six-layered cortex.

B. Allocortex (heterogenetic cortex)
—is three-layered and includes two types:

1. Archicortex
—includes the hippocampus and the dentate gyrus.

2. Paleocortex
—includes the olfactory cortex.

II. Six Layers of the Neocortex

—are expressed as Roman numerals I through VI:

A. Molecular layer (I)
—is the superficial layer located below the pia mater.

B. External granular layer (II)

C. External pyramidal layer (III)
—gives rise to association and commissural fibers.

D. Internal granular layer (IV)
—receives thalamocortical fibers from the thalamic nuclei of the ventral tier (e.g., ventral posterolateral [VPL] and ventral posteromedial [VPM] nuclei).
—in the striate cortex (area 17), receives input from the lateral geniculate body.
—myelinated fibers of this layer form the stripe of Gennari, which is visible to the naked eye.

E. Internal pyramidal layer (V)
—gives rise to corticobulbar, corticospinal, and corticostriatal fibers.

—contains the giant cells of Betz, which are found only in the motor cortex (area 4) of the precentral gyrus and the anterior paracentral lobule.

F. Multiform layer (VI)

—is the deepest layer of the cortex. It gives rise to projection, commissural, and association fibers.

III. Functional Areas—The Cerebral Cortex (Figure 23.1)

—is divided into 47 cytoarchitectural areas, the **Brodmann areas**.

A. Sensory areas

1. Primary somatosensory cortex (areas 3, 1, and 2)

—is located in the **postcentral gyrus** and in the posterior part of the **para-central lobule**.
—receives input from the ventral posterior nucleus.
—is somatotopically organized as the **sensory homunculus** (Figure 23.2A).
—stimulation results in numbness and tingling (paresthesiae).
—destruction results in a contralateral loss of tactile discrimination (**hyp-esthesia and astereognosis**).

2. Secondary somatosensory cortex

—lies ventral to the primary somatosensory area along the superior bank of the lateral sulcus.

3. Somatosensory association cortex

a. Superior parietal lobule (areas 5 and 7)

—receives input from areas 3, 1, and 2.
—area 7 receives visual input from area 19.
—destruction results in **contralateral loss of tactile discrimina-tion, stereognosis** (the ability to recognize form), and **statognosis** (the ability to recognize the position of body parts in space).
—destruction results in neglect of events occurring in the contralateral portion of the external world (more commonly seen with parietal damage on the right side).

b. Supramarginal gyrus (area 40)

—interrelates somatosensory, auditory, and visual input (multimodal sensory stimuli).
—destruction in the dominant hemisphere results in the following deficits:

(1) Ideomotor apraxia

—is the inability to perform complicated motor tasks (e.g., saluting or making a V-for-victory sign).

(2) Ideational apraxia

—is the inability to demonstrate the use of objects (e.g., tools placed in a patient's hands).

(3) Facial apraxia

—is the inability to perform facial movements on command (i.e., lick the lips).

(4) Conduction aphasia

—is associated with poor repetition of spoken language (results from interruption of the arcuate fasciculus; see p 295).

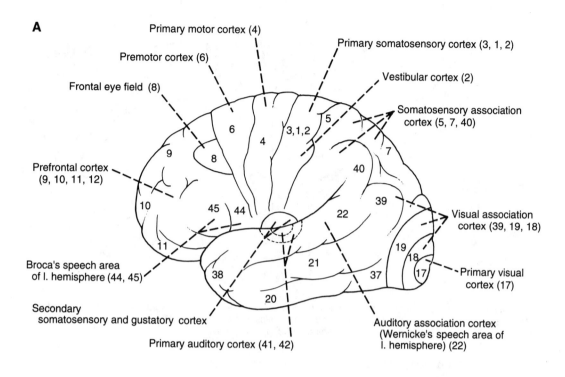

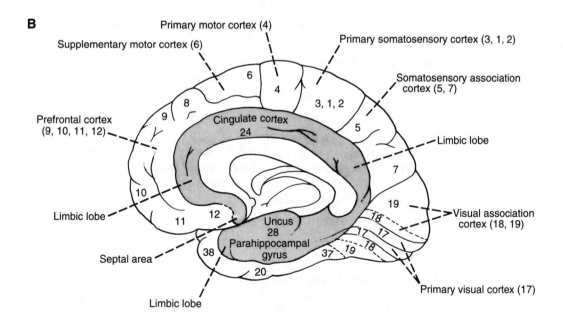

Figure 23.1. Some motor and sensory areas of the cerebral cortex. (*A*) Lateral convex surface of the hemisphere. (*B*) Medial surface of the hemisphere. The numbers refer to the Brodmann brain map, the Brodmann areas.

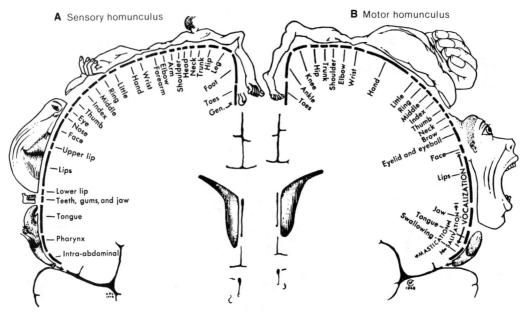

A Sensory homunculus   **B** Motor homunculus

Figure 23.2. The sensory and motor homunucli. (*A*) Sensory representation in the postcentral gyrus. (*B*) Motor representation in the precentral gyrus. (Reprinted with permission from Penfield, W and Rasmussen, T: *The Cerebral Cortex of Man*. New York, Hafner Publishing, 1968, pp 44 and 57.)

4. Primary visual cortex (area 17)

—is located in the occipital lobe in both banks of the calcarine sulcus.

—receives input from the lateral geniculate body.

—destruction results in **visual field deficits** (e.g., contralateral homonymous hemianopia) [see Figure 17.1].

5. Secondary and tertiary visual cortices

—include areas 18 and 19 of the occipital lobe.

—lesions may result in **visual hallucinations**.

6. Visual association cortex (angular gyrus [area 39])

—receives input from areas 18 and 19.

—destruction of the underlying visual radiation results in **contralateral homonymous hemianopia or lower quadrantanopia**.

—destruction in the dominant hemisphere results in **Gerstmann's syndrome** with the following deficits:

a. Right-left confusion

b. Finger agnosia (inability to recognize, name, or select own or another's fingers)

c. Agraphia (inability to express thoughts in writing with possible retention of the ability to copy written or printed words; often coexists with alexia)

d. Dyscalculia (difficulty with arithmetic)

7. Primary auditory cortex (areas 41 and 42)

—is located in the transverse gyri of Heschl.

—receives input from the medial geniculate body.

−unilateral destruction results in only **partial deafness** (due to bilateral cochlear representation).

8. Auditory association cortex (area 22)

−is located in the posterior part of the superior temporal gyrus.
−includes **Wernicke's speech area**.
−includes the **planum temporale** (part of Wernicke's speech area), which is larger in the dominant hemisphere.
−lesion in the dominant hemisphere results in **Wernicke's sensory aphasia.**
−lesion in the nondominant hemisphere results in **sensory dysprosodia** (inability to perceive pitch or rhythm of speech).

9. Gustatory cortex (area 43)

−is located in the parietal operculum and parainsular cortex.
−receives taste input from the VPM nucleus of the thalamus.

10. Vestibular cortex (area 2)

−is located in the postcentral gyrus.
−receives input from the ventral posteroinferior and the VPL nuclei of the thalamus.

B. Motor areas

1. Primary motor cortex (area 4)

−is located in the **precentral gyrus** and in the anterior part of the **paracentral lobule**.
−contributes to the corticospinal tract.
−is somatotopically organized as the **motor homunculus** (see Figure 23.2*B*).
−contains the giant cells of Betz in layer V.
−stimulation results in contralateral movements of voluntary muscles.
−ablation results in a **contralateral upper motor neuron lesion**.
−bilateral lesions of the paracentral lobule (e.g., parasagittal meningiomas) result in **urinary incontinence**.

2. Premotor cortex (area 6)

−is located anterior to the precentral gyrus.
−contributes to the corticospinal tract.
−plays a role in the **control of proximal and axial muscles;** it prepares the motor cortex for specific movements in advance of their execution.
−stimulation results in adversive movements of the head and trunk and flexion and extension of the extremities.
−lesions in the dominant hemisphere may cause **sympathetic apraxia** (motor apraxia in the left hand).

3. Supplementary motor cortex (area 6)

−is located on the medial surface of the hemisphere anterior to the paracentral lobule.
−contributes to the corticospinal tract.

—plays a role in **programming complex motor sequences** and in **co-ordinating bilateral movements;** it regulates the somatosensory input into the motor cortex.

—stimulation results in vocalization with associated facial movements and coordinated movements of the limbs.

—ablation in human subjects has resulted in transient **speech deficits or aphasias**.

—bilateral lesions result in **hypertonus of the flexor muscles** but no paralysis.

4. Frontal eye field (area 8)

—is located in the posterior part of the middle frontal gyrus.

—projects via the tectobulbar tract to the contralateral lateral gaze center of the pons (abducent nucleus).

—stimulation (irritative lesion) results in conjugate deviation of the eyes to the opposite side.

—destructive lesions result in **conjugate deviation of the eyes toward the side of the lesion**.

C. Areas of higher cortical function

1. Prefrontal cortex (areas 9–12)

a. Characteristics—prefrontal cortex

—extends from area 6 to the frontal pole (area 10).

—has reciprocal connections with the mediodorsal nucleus of the thalamus.

b. Frontal lobe syndrome (Phineas Gage syndrome)

—results from **lesions of the prefrontal cortex**.

—results in the following signs:

(1) Inappropriate social behavior

(2) Difficulty in adaptation and loss of initiative

(3) Sucking, groping, and grasping reflexes

(4) Gait apraxia, incontinence, abulia (loss of the ability to perform voluntary actions), or **akinetic mutism** (a coma-like state called coma vigil); these signs result from bilateral disease.

2. Broca's speech area (areas 44 and 45) [Figure 23.3]

a. Characteristics—Broca's speech area

—is located in the posterior part of the inferior frontal gyrus in the dominant hemisphere.

—is connected to Wernicke's speech area by the arcuate fasciculus.

b. Broca's aphasia

—results from lesions in Broca's speech area.

—is also called **motor, expressive, nonfluent, or anterior aphasia**.

—causes patients to speak slowly (nonfluent) and with effort; however, they have good comprehension of spoken and written language.

—is frequently accompanied by **contralateral weakness of the lower face and arm** and a **sympathetic apraxia** of the left hand (the inability to write with the nonparalyzed hand).

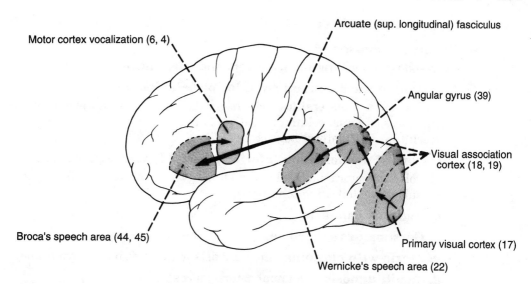

Figure 23.3. Cortical areas of the dominant hemisphere that play an important role in language production. The visual image of a word is projected from the visual cortex (17) to the visual association cortices (18 and 19) and then to the angular gyrus (39). Further processing occurs in Wernicke's speech area (22), where the auditory form of the word is recalled. Via the arcuate fasciculus, this information reaches Broca's speech area (44 and 45), where motor speech programs control the vocalization mechanisms of the precentral gyrus. Lesions of Broca's speech area, Wernicke's speech area, or the arcuate fasciculus result in dysphasias.

3. Wernicke's speech area (area 22) [see Figure 23.3]

a. Characteristics—Wernicke's speech area

- is located in the posterior part of the superior temporal gyrus in the dominant hemisphere.
- is connected to Broca's speech area by the arcuate fasciculus.

b. Wernicke's aphasia

- results from lesions in the dominant hemisphere.
- is also called **sensory, receptive, fluent, or posterior aphasia**.
- patients have poor comprehension of speech, speak faster than normal, and have difficulty in finding the right word to express themselves.
- patients appear unaware of the deficit.

4. Arcuate fasciculus

a. Characteristics—arcuate fasciculus

- underlies the supramarginal gyrus (area 40) and the frontoparietal operculum.
- connects the audiovisual association areas (areas 22, 39, and 40) with Broca's speech area (areas 44 and 45).

b. Conduction aphasia

- is a **fluent aphasia** associated with poor repetition of spoken language.
- speech comprehension and expression are relatively good.
- **paraphrasic errors** (using incorrect words) are common, and **object-naming is impaired** (nominal aphasia or amnestic aphasia).
- patients are aware of the deficit.

IV. Cerebral Dominance

A. Dominant hemisphere

—is responsible for **language, speech, and calculation**.

1. Lesions of the dominant superior parietal lobule

—result in contralateral loss of sensory discrimination (**astereognosis**) [i.e., loss of dorsal column modalities; area 5].

—result in contralateral neglect (area 7).

2. Lesions of the dominant inferior parietal lobule (Figure 23.4A)

—involve the supramarginal and angular gyri (areas 40 and 39).

—result in the following conditions:

a. Receptive aphasia

b. Gerstmann's syndrome

c. Alexia with agraphia (often coexists with Gerstmann's syndrome)

d. Tactile agnosia (bimanual astereognosis)

e. Ideomotor apraxia

f. Ideational apraxia

B. Nondominant hemisphere

—is primarily responsible for **three-dimensional** or **spatial perception** and **nonverbal ideation** (music and poetry).

1. Lesions of the nondominant superior parietal lobule (see Figure 23.4B)

—result in **contralateral loss of sensory discrimination** (i.e., loss of dorsal column modalities; area 5).

—result in **contralateral neglect** (area 7).

2. Lesions of the nondominant inferior parietal lobule

—involve the supramarginal and angular gyri.

—result in the following conditions:

a. Left-sided hemineglect

—results in a lack of awareness of the left half of space or the left half of the body.

—results in hemi-inattention or extinction; if, with the patient's eyes closed, both hands are touched simultaneously, the left hand stimulus often is not reported.

b. Topographic memory loss

—results in the inability to negotiate familiar surroundings.

c. Anosognosia (denial of deficit)

—results in indifference to the causal disease (e.g., hemiparesis or hemianopia).

d. Constructional apraxia

—results in the inability to draw simple designs (e.g., cross, star, or clock); the left side of the design is omitted.

—may also occur in lesions of the dominant hemisphere.

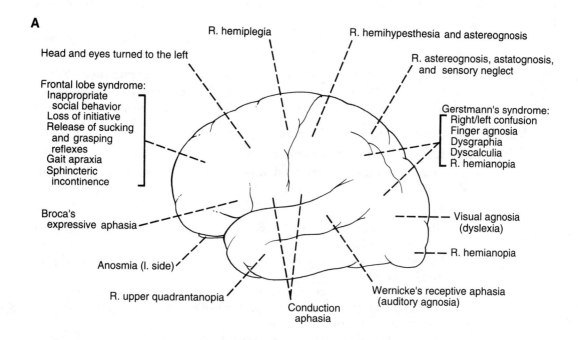

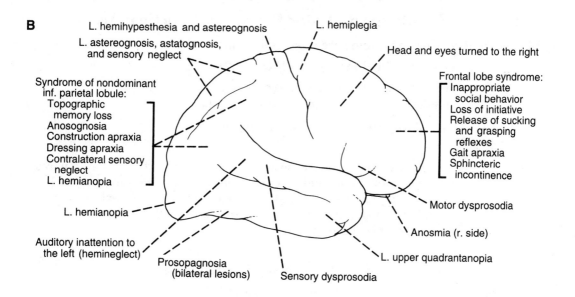

Figure 23.4. Focal destructive hemispheric lesions and resulting symptoms. (*A*) Lateral convex surface of the dominant left hemisphere. (*B*) Lateral convex surface of the nondominant right hemisphere.

e. Dressing apraxia

–results in the inability to dress properly.

3. Lesions of the nondominant inferior frontal gyrus (areas 44 and 45)

–correspond to Broca's speech area and result in **expressive dysprosodia** (the inability to articulate pitch and rhythm of speech).

4. Lesions of the nondominant superior temporal gyrus (area 22)

–correspond to Wernicke's speech area and result in **receptive dysprosodia** (the inability to perceive pitch and rhythm of speech).

V. Split-Brain Syndrome (Figure 23.5)

A. Description—split-brain syndrome

–represents a **disconnection syndrome** that results from transection (commissurotomy) of the corpus callosum.

B. Deficits

–inability of a blindfolded patient to match an object held in one hand with that held in the other hand

–inability, when blindfolded, to correctly name objects placed in the left hand (**anomia**)

–inability to match an object seen in the right half of the visual field with one seen in the left half (the test must be performed rapidly in order to eliminate bilateral visual scanning)

–**alexia** in the left visual fields (the verbal symbols seen in the right visual cortex have no access to the language centers of the left hemisphere)

VI. Blood Supply to the Major Functional Cortical Areas

–only **cortical branches** are discussed in this section.

A. Anterior cerebral artery (see Figure 3.2)

1. Territory—anterior cerebral artery

–supplies the medial aspect of the hemisphere.

2. Occlusion—affected areas and deficits

a. Paracentral lobule

–contralateral somatosensory loss in the lower extremity with paresthesia, numbness, and apallesthesia (loss of vibration sensation)

–contralateral weakness and hyperreflexia in the lower extremity with Babinski's sign (plantar reflex is the extensor)

–urinary incontinence

b. Corpus callosum: infarction

–dyspraxia and tactile agnosia of the left limbs

B. Middle cerebral artery (see Figure 3.3)

1. Territory—middle cerebral artery

–supplies the lateral convex surface of the hemisphere.

2. Occlusion—affected areas and deficits

a. Frontal lobe

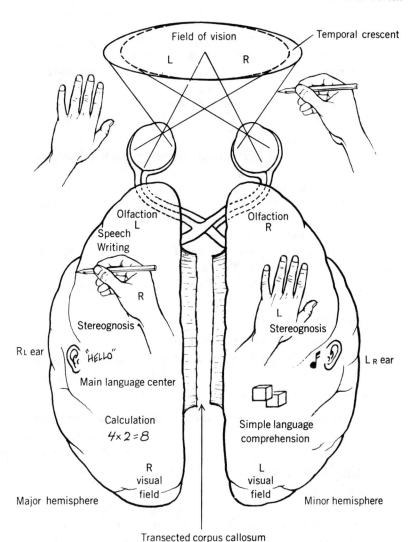

Figure 23.5. Functions of the split-brain after transection of the corpus callosum. Tactile and visual perception is projected to the contralateral hemisphere; olfaction is perceived on the same side; and audition is perceived predominantly in the opposite hemisphere. The left hemisphere is dominant for language; the right hemisphere is dominant for spatial construction and nonverbal ideation. (Reprinted with permission from Noback, CR and Demarest, RJ: *The Human Nervous System*. Malvern, Pa, Lea & Febiger, 1991, p 416.)

(1) Precentral gyrus
   −contralateral facial weakness and weakness in the upper extremity
(2) Frontal eye field
   −conjugate deviation of the eyes to the affected side
(3) Prefrontal cortex
   −affects judgment, insight, and mood (frontal lobe syndrome)
(4) Inferior frontal gyrus of the dominant side
   −Broca's expressive aphasia and contralateral weakness of the lower face and arm
   −sympathetic apraxia of the left hand

b. Temporal lobe

(1) Transverse temporal gyri of Heschl
–deafness with bilateral destruction

(2) Superior temporal gyrus of the dominant side
–Wernicke's receptive aphasia

(3) Superior and middle temporal gyri (superolateral parts)
–auditory illusions and hallucinations

c. Parietal lobe

(1) Postcentral gyrus and superior parietal lobule
–loss of sensory discrimination and stereognosis
–hemineglect (may occur with either left or right parietal lesions)

(2) Inferior parietal lobule of the dominant hemisphere
–ideomotor and ideational apraxia
–Gerstmann's syndrome

(3) Inferior parietal lobule of the nondominant hemisphere
–hemineglect syndrome
–topographic memory loss, anosognosia, constructional and dressing apraxia

C. Posterior cerebral artery (see Figure 3.4)

1. Territory—posterior cerebral artery

–supplies the occipital lobe, the inferior aspect of the temporal lobe (excluding the temporal pole), and the splenium of the corpus callosum.

2. Occlusion—affected areas and deficits

a. Occipital lobe: visual cortex (striate and extrastriate)

–if bilateral, cortical blindness (pupils are reactive to light)
–contralateral homonymous hemianopia with macular sparing

b. Temporal lobe (inferiomedial aspect): hippocampal formation and amygdala

–also perfused by the anterior choroidal artery
–if bilateral or in the dominant hemisphere, memory deficit (amnesia)
–incapacity to create and store new long-term memories; the patient retains and may recall old long-term memories.

c. Occipitotemporal region (ventromesial aspect)

–bilateral lesions may result in **prosopagnosia** (the inability to identify a familiar face) and **achromatopsia** (acquired color blindness).

D. Left posterior cerebral artery

1. Territory—left posterior cerebral artery

–supplies the splenium of the corpus collosum and the left visual cortex.

2. Occlusion

–results in **infarction** of the splenium of the corpus callosum and the left visual cortex; visual input from the right visual cortex cannot reach the parietal language centers of the dominant hemisphere.

–may cause **alexia without agraphia and aphasia;** because the left inferior parietal lobule and Wernicke's speech area are intact, the patient can write and is not dysphasic.

Review Test

Directions: Each of the numbered items or incomplete statements in this section is followed by answers or by completions of the statement. Select the **one** lettered answer or completion that is **best** in each case.

1. A lesion of the dominant inferior parietal lobule could result in all of the following deficits EXCEPT

(A) the inability to perform calculations.
(B) the inability to identify fingers.
(C) the inability to write from dictation.
(D) right-left disorientation.
(E) difficulty in dressing.

2. A lesion resulting in a nonfluent expressive aphasia would most likely be found in the

(A) temporal lobe.
(B) parietal lobe.
(C) frontal lobe.
(D) occipital lobe.
(E) limbic lobe.

3. Broca's aphasia is frequently associated with

(A) auditory hallucinations.
(B) finger agnosia.
(C) construction apraxia.
(D) an upper motor neuron (UMN) lesion.
(E) visual field deficits.

4. All of the following statements concerning the parietal lobe are correct EXCEPT

(A) it contains the primary somatosensory area.
(B) it contains the angular gyrus.
(C) it contains the supramarginal gyrus.
(D) it contains the visual radiation.
(E) it contains Wernicke's speech area.

5. All of the following statements concerning split-brain syndrome are correct EXCEPT

(A) the patient is alexic in the left visual fields.
(B) the patient, when blindfolded, cannot correctly name an object placed in the left hand.
(C) the patient, when blindfolded, cannot correctly name an object placed in the right hand.
(D) the patient, when blindfolded, cannot match an object held in one hand with that held in the other hand.
(E) the patient, if tested rapidly, cannot match an object seen in the right half of the visual field with one seen in the left half.

6. All of the following statements concerning the neocortex are correct EXCEPT

(A) it represents 90% of the cerebral mantle.
(B) it is a six-layered cortex.
(C) it gives rise to the pyramidal tract.
(D) it includes the olfactory cortex.
(E) it contains the giant cells of Betz.

7. All of the following statements concerning the allocortex are correct EXCEPT

(A) it represents 10% of the cortical mantle.
(B) it is a three-layered cortex.
(C) it includes paleocortex.
(D) it includes archicortex.
(E) it includes visual cortex.

8. Lesions of the frontal lobes may give rise to all of the following EXCEPT

(A) ocular signs.
(B) UMN lesion signs.
(C) gait apraxia.
(D) hemianopias.
(E) sucking, groping, and grasping reflexes.

9. All of the following statements concerning the primary motor cortex are correct EXCEPT

(A) it is found in the paracentral lobule.
(B) it is located in the frontal lobe.
(C) it contains the giant cells of Betz.
(D) it corresponds to Brodmann's area 4.
(E) ablation results in a permanent flaccid paralysis.

10. All of the following statements concerning the frontal eye field are correct EXCEPT

(A) it is located in the middle frontal gyrus.
(B) it corresponds to Brodmann's area 8.
(C) ablation results in contralateral homonymous hemianopia.
(D) stimulation results in conjugate deviation of the eyes to the opposite side.
(E) destruction results in conjugate deviation of the eyes to the ipsilateral side.

11. Occlusion of the anterior cerebral artery may result in all of the following neurologic deficits EXCEPT

(A) an expressive aphasia.
(B) an UMN lesion.
(C) loss of pain and temperature sensation in the contralateral foot.
(D) infarction of the supplementary motor cortex.
(E) Babinski's sign.

Directions: Each group of items in this section consists of lettered options followed by a set of numbered items. For each item, select the **one** lettered option that is most closely associated with it. Each lettered option may be selected once, more than once, or not at all.

Questions 12–17

Match each of the areas described with the appropriate lettered area shown in the figure.

Questions 18–22

Match each of the areas described with the appropriate lettered area shown in the figure.

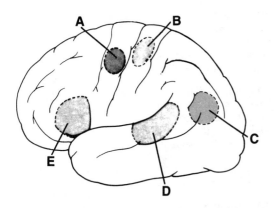

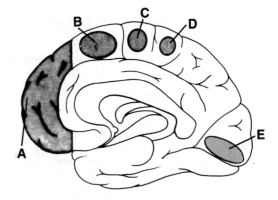

12. Broca's speech area

13. Wernicke's speech area

14. Lesion in this area results in contralateral astereognosis

15. Infarction in this area results in an UMN lesion

16. Lesion in this area results in a contralateral homonymous hemianopia

17. Lesion in this area results in finger agnosia, agraphia, and dyscalculia

18. Supplementary motor area

19. Lesion in this area results in paresthesias and numbness in the contralateral foot

20. Lesion in this area results in contralateral lower homonymous quadrantanopia

21. Lesion in this area results in a contralateral Babinski's sign

22. Lesion in this area results in loss of initiative and inappropriate social behavior

Answers and Explanations

1–E. Dressing apraxia is a symptom of the nondominant parietal lobe. A lesion of the dominant angular gyrus is known as Gerstmann's syndrome, which includes finger agnosia (autotopagnosia or somatotopagnosia), right-left confusion, agraphia, and dyscalculia. Alexia may be associated with Gerstmann's syndrome.

2–C. A nonfluent, expressive motor aphasia (Broca's aphasia) results from a lesion in the posterior inferior frontal gyrus (areas 44 and 45) of the dominant frontal lobe.

3–D. Broca's aphasia is frequently associated with an UMN lesion of the contralateral face and arm and occasionally of the leg. Broca's speech area lies just anterior to the motor strip; both Broca's speech area and the motor strip are irrigated by the superior division of the middle cerebral artery (prerolandic and rolandic arteries). Broca's aphasia is frequently associated with a "sympathetic apraxia," an apraxia of the nonparalyzed left hand.

4–E. Wernicke's speech area (included in Brodmann's area 22) is found in the posterior part of the superior temporal gyrus of the dominant hemisphere. Wernicke's speech area includes the planum temporale, which lies on the lower bank of the lateral sulcus.

5–C. In split-brain syndrome, the blindfolded patient with a dominant left hemisphere can correctly name an object placed in his right hand, but he cannot name an object placed in his left hand. The pathway from the nondominant hemisphere (via the corpus callosum) to the language center of the dominant hemisphere has been disconnected.

6–D. The six-layered neocortex represents 90% of the cortical mantle. It gives rise to the pyramidal tract, which arises from the premotor cortex (area 6); the motor cortex (area 4); and the primary sensory cortex (areas 3, 1, and 2). The giant cells of Betz are found in the fifth layer of the precentral gyrus and the anterior paracentral lobule (neocortex). The three-layered olfactory cortex is paleocortex; this cortex overlies the uncus of the parahippocampal gyrus.

7–E. The three-layered allocortex, the "other cortex," consists of archicortex (hippocampus and dentate gyrus) and paleocortex (olfactory cortex). It represents 10% of the cortical mantle. The visual cortex is a sensory neocortex; it contains densely packed granule cells and is called granular cortex or koniocortex.

8–D. Frontal lobe lesions may affect the frontal eye field, the motor cortex, and the premotor and prefrontal cortices (gait apraxia). Sucking, groping, and grasping reflexes are seen in frontal lobe lesions. Hemianopias result from lesions of the visual pathway. The visual pathway is not found in the frontal cortex.

9–E. The primary motor cortex, the motor strip (area 4), is located in the precentral gyrus and in the anterior part of the paracentral lobule, both of which are found in the frontal lobe. The giant motor cells of Betz are found in layer V of the motor cortex. Ablation of the motor strip initially results in flaccid paralysis, which becomes a spastic contralateral hemiparesis with Babinski's sign.

10–C. The frontal eye field (area 8) is located in the posterior part of the middle frontal gyrus. Stimulation results in conjugate deviation of the eyes to the opposite side. Destruction of this area results in conjugate deviation toward the side of the lesion. The frontal eye field projects via the tectobulbar tract to the contralateral lateral gaze center of the pons, located in the abducent nucleus (of CN VI).

11–A. Occlusion of the cortical branches of the anterior cerebral artery may result in infarction of the paracentral lobule and the supplementary motor cortex. A destructive lesion of the paracentral lobule would result in an UMN lesion affecting the contralateral foot and a sensory loss in the same foot. Occlusion of the ganglionic branches (medial striate arteries) could result in contralateral weakness of the face (involvement of the corticobulbar fibers). The anterior cerebral artery does not supply the inferior frontal gyrus, which contains Broca's speech area in the dominant hemisphere.

303

12–E. Broca's speech area (areas 44 and 45) is found in the posterior part of the inferior frontal gyrus of the dominant hemisphere, directly anterior to the premotor and motor cortices.

13–D. Wernicke's speech area is located in the posterior part of the superior temporal gyrus (part of Brodmann's area 22) of the dominant hemisphere. A lesion of this area results in a fluent sensory (receptive) aphasia.

14–B. A lesion of the left postcentral gyrus results in a right astereognosis (tactile agnosia), the inability to identify objects by touch. Lesions of the superior parietal lobule result in contralateral astereognosis and in sensory neglect.

15–A. A lesion in the precentral gyrus is an UMN lesion. The precentral gyrus (motor strip) gives rise to one-third of the pyramidal tract (corticospinal tract) fibers.

16–C. A deep lesion of the angular gyrus could involve the visual radiation, resulting in a contralateral homonymous hemianopia.

17–C. The dominant angular gyrus is the neurologic substrate of Gerstmann's syndrome, which consists of right-left confusion, finger agnosia, agraphia, and dyscalculia.

18–B. The supplementary motor cortex (area 6) lies on the medial aspect of the hemisphere, just anterior to the paracentral lobule.

19–D. A lesion in the posterior part of the paracentral lobule would result in loss of joint and position sense (astatognosia) and loss of tactile discrimination (astereognosis) in the contralateral foot.

20–E. A lesion of the superior bank of the calcarine sulcus (cuneus) would result in a contralateral lower homonymous quadrantanopia. A lesion destroying both cunei would produce a lower homonymous altitudinal hemianopia.

21–C. A lesion of the anterior part of the paracentral lobule results in a contralateral paresis of the foot muscles and in Babinski's sign (i.e., plantar reflex extensor or extensor toe sign).

22–A. Lesions of the prefrontal cortex may result in personality changes, with disorderly and inappropriate conduct and facetiousness and jocularity (witzelsucht). Lesions interrupt fibers that interconnect the dorsomedial nucleus and the prefrontal cortex (e.g., prefrontal lobotomy or leukotomy).

Comprehensive Examination

Directions: Each of the numbered items or incomplete statements in this section is followed by answers or by completions of the statement. Select the **one** lettered answer or completion that is **best** in each case.

1. The cuneus is separated from the lingual gyrus by the

(A) rhinal sulcus.
(B) calcarine sulcus.
(C) parieto-occipital sulcus.
(D) collateral sulcus.
(E) intraparietal sulcus.

2. Each of the following statements concerning the temporal lobe is true EXCEPT

(A) it contains the primary somatosensory cortex.
(B) it contains the primary auditory cortex.
(C) it contains Wernicke's speech area.
(D) it is separated from the frontal lobe by the lateral sulcus.
(E) it contains an auditory association cortex.

3. Each of the following statements concerning cerebral ventricles is true EXCEPT

(A) all ventricles contain choroid plexus.
(B) the frontal and occipital horns of the lateral ventricles lack choroid plexus.
(C) the body of the lateral ventricle contains the calcified glomus of the choroid plexus.
(D) the third and fourth ventricles are interconnected by the cerebral aqueduct.
(E) the fourth ventricle contains the foramina of Luschka and Magendie.

4. Each of the following circumventricular organs is highly vascularized with fenestrated capillaries EXCEPT the

(A) area postrema.
(B) pineal body.
(C) subcommissural organ.
(D) subfornical organ.
(E) median eminence of the tuber cinereum.

5. The middle cerebral artery irrigates each of the following structures or areas EXCEPT

(A) the paracentral lobule.
(B) the inferior parietal lobule.
(C) Broca's speech area.
(D) Wernicke's speech area.
(E) the primary auditory cortex.

6. Which sinus receives drainage from the greatest number of arachnoid granulations?

(A) Straight sinus
(B) Transverse sinus
(C) Sigmoid sinus
(D) Superior sagittal sinus
(E) Cavernous sinus

7. Each of the following statements concerning the cavernous sinus is true EXCEPT

(A) it surrounds the sella turcica.
(B) it receives blood from the ophthalmic veins.
(C) it contains fibers from the superior cervical ganglion.
(D) it contains the mandibular nerve.
(E) it contains cranial nerves III, IV, and VI.

8. The posterior cerebral artery supplies all of the following structures EXCEPT the

(A) parahippocampal gyrus.
(B) temporal pole.
(C) occipital lobe.
(D) midbrain.
(E) thalamus.

9. The neural crest gives rise to all of the following cells EXCEPT

(A) cells of the sympathetic trunk.
(B) cells of the suprarenal medulla.
(C) dorsal root ganglion cells.
(D) Schwann cells.
(E) ventral horn cells.

10. Which of the following statements concerning Rathke's pouch is true?

(A) It is a mesodermal diverticulum.
(B) It is derived from the neural tube.
(C) It gives rise to the adenohypophysis.
(D) It gives rise to the epiphysis.
(E) It gives rise to the neurohypophysis.

11. Which of the following statements concerning the lateral horn of the spinal cord is true?

(A) It contains preganglionic parasympathetic neurons.
(B) It gives rise to a spinocerebellar tract.
(C) It is present at all spinal cord levels.
(D) It gives rise to preganglionic sympathetic fibers.
(E) It is most prominent at sacral levels.

12. Which of the following statements concerning the nucleus dorsalis of Clarke is true?

(A) It is found in the ventral horn.
(B) It projects to the cerebellum.
(C) It is present at all spinal levels.
(D) It is most prominent at upper cervical levels.
(E) It is homologous to the cuneate nucleus of the medulla.

13. Each of the following statements concerning spinal cord nuclei is true EXCEPT

(A) the parasympathetic nucleus is located in the lateral horn.
(B) the intermediolateral nucleus extends from T1 to L3.
(C) the spinal accessory nucleus extends from C1 to C6.
(D) the phrenic nucleus extends from C3 to C6.
(E) the spinal border cells extend from L1 to S3.

14. Each of the following statements concerning the fasciculus cuneatus is true EXCEPT

(A) its neurons of origin are in the dorsal horn.
(B) its fibers project to a nucleus in the medulla.
(C) it contains input from the upper extremity.
(D) it mediates two-point tactile discrimination.
(E) its fibers do not decussate in the spinal cord.

15. Each of the following statements concerning the spinocerebellar tracts is true EXCEPT

(A) the dorsal spinocerebellar tract originates from the nucleus dorsalis of Clarke.
(B) the spinocerebellar tracts receive input from muscle spindles and Golgi tendon organs.
(C) the cuneocerebellar tract originates in the medulla.
(D) the ventral spinocerebellar tract originates from the spinal border cells of the ventral horns.
(E) the ventral spinocerebellar tract enters the cerebellum through the inferior cerebellar peduncle.

16. Each of the following statements concerning the lateral spinothalamic tract is true EXCEPT

(A) it mediates pain and temperature sensation.
(B) its second-order neurons are located in the dorsal horn.
(C) it decussates in the ventral white commissure.
(D) axons of its first-order neurons enter the dorsolateral tract of Lissauer.
(E) it projects to the ventral posteromedial (VPM) nucleus of the thalamus.

17. Each of the following statements concerning the pons is true EXCEPT

(A) it contains the nucleus that innervates the stapedius muscle.
(B) it contains the nucleus that innervates the tensor tympani muscle.
(C) it contains the mesencephalic nucleus.
(D) it contains a nucleus that innervates the parotid gland.
(E) it contains the center for lateral conjugate gaze.

18. In the brainstem, intra-axial fibers of the facial nerve are closely associated with all of the following structures EXCEPT the

(A) abducent nucleus.
(B) medial longitudinal fasciculus (MLF).
(C) medial lemniscus.
(D) spinal nucleus and tract of CN V.
(E) middle cerebellar peduncle.

19. Which of the following groups of cranial nerves is closely related to the corticospinal tract?

(A) CN III, CN IV, and CN V
(B) CN III, CN V, and CN VII
(C) CN III, CN VI, and CN VIII
(D) CN III, CN VI, and CN XII
(E) CN III, CN IX, and CN X

20. All of the following structures are present in the cavernous sinus or its lateral wall EXCEPT

(A) the ophthalmic nerve.
(B) the maxillary nerve.
(C) the mandibular nerve.
(D) cranial nerves III, IV, and VI.
(E) postganglionic sympathetic fibers.

21. The mandibular nerve innervates all of the following structures EXCEPT the

(A) mucosa of the anterior two-thirds of the tongue.
(B) posterior belly of the digastric muscle.
(C) tensor tympani muscle.
(D) external auditory meatus.
(E) muscles of mastication.

22. Each of the following statements concerning the ventral trigeminothalamic tract is true EXCEPT

(A) it mediates pain and temperature sensation from the head.
(B) it receives input from cranial nerves VII, IX, and X.
(C) second-order neurons are found in the caudal spinal trigeminal nucleus.
(D) it is a crossed pathway.
(E) decussation of pain fibers occurs in the pons.

23. Each of the following structures is part of the auditory pathway EXCEPT the

(A) spiral ganglion.
(B) cochlear nuclei.
(C) trapezoid body.
(D) inferior olivary nucleus.
(E) nucleus of the inferior colliculus.

24. The primary auditory cortex is located in

(A) the frontal operculum.
(B) the postcentral gyrus.
(C) the superior parietal lobule.
(D) the inferior parietal lobule.
(E) the transverse temporal gyri.

25. Each of the following statements concerning vestibular nuclei is true EXCEPT

(A) they receive input from semicircular ducts.
(B) they receive input from the saccule and utricle.
(C) they receive input from the spiral ganglion.
(D) they project to cranial nerves III, IV, and VI.
(E) they have reciprocal connections with the flocculonodular lobe.

26. Each of the following statements concerning the MLF is true EXCEPT

(A) it contains ascending and descending fibers.
(B) it contains vestibular fibers that project to all ocular motor nuclei.
(C) it is very close to the internal genu of CN VII.
(D) it is very close to the motor nucleus of CN V.
(E) it extends from the spinal cord to the midbrain.

27. Each of the following statements concerning the vestibular nerve is true EXCEPT

(A) it consists of the central processes of bipolar neurons.
(B) it traverses the internal auditory meatus.
(C) it projects direct fibers to the cerebellar cortex.
(D) it enters the brainstem at the pontomedullary junction.
(E) it does not contain efferent fibers.

28. Transection of the facial nerve between the geniculate ganglion and the chorda tympani results in the loss of all of the following EXCEPT

(A) taste sensation from the anterior two-thirds of the tongue.
(B) innervation of the lacrimal gland.
(C) innervation of the sublingual and submandibular glands.
(D) the corneal reflex.
(E) the ability to wrinkle the brow on the affected side.

29. Each of the following statements concerning the nucleus ambiguus is true EXCEPT

(A) it contains preganglionic parasympathetic neurons that innervate the heart.
(B) it innervates the musculature of the larynx and pharynx.
(C) it is located near the hypoglossal nucleus.
(D) it is located near the spinal trigeminal nucleus and tract.
(E) it sends SVE fibers to cranial nerves IX, X, and XI.

30. Each of the following statements concerning Purkinje cells is true EXCEPT

(A) they project to the cerebellar nuclei.
(B) they project to the thalamus.
(C) they project to the vestibular nuclei.
(D) they are inhibited by basket cells.
(E) their neurotransmitter is GABA.

31. Each of the following statements concerning the cerebellar peduncles is true EXCEPT

(A) the superior cerebellar peduncle is the major efferent pathway from the cerebellum.
(B) the middle cerebellar peduncle attaches the cerebellum to the midbrain.
(C) the inferior cerebellar peduncle includes the juxtarestiform body.
(D) the ventral spinocerebellar tract is found in the superior cerebellar peduncle.
(E) the neocortex influences the cerebellum via the middle cerebellar peduncle.

32. The neocerebellum projects to the motor cortex via the

(A) anterior thalamic nucleus.
(B) ventral anterior nucleus.
(C) ventral lateral nucleus.
(D) lateral dorsal nucleus.
(E) lateral posterior nucleus.

33. The dentatothalamic tract decussates in the

(A) diencephalon.
(B) rostral midbrain.
(C) caudal midbrain.
(D) rostral pons.
(E) caudal pons.

34. Each of the following statements concerning the retina is true EXCEPT

(A) it is of diencephalic origin.
(B) the fovea centralis contains rods and cones.
(C) the optic disk is the blind spot.
(D) the macula lutea surrounds the fovea centralis.
(E) the retina has a dual blood supply.

35. A pituitary tumor is most frequently associated with

(A) a homonymous hemianopia.
(B) a homonymous quadrantanopia.
(C) a bitemporal hemianopia.
(D) a binasal hemianopia.
(E) an altitudinal hemianopia.

36. Resection of the anterior portion of the left temporal lobe is most frequently associated with a

(A) left homonymous hemianopia.
(B) right upper homonymous quadrantanopia.
(C) right lower homonymous quadrantanopia.
(D) left upper homonymous quadrantanopia.
(E) left lower homonymous quadrantanopia.

37. Each of the following statements concerning transection of the left optic tract is true EXCEPT

(A) the direct pupillary light reflex is unaffected.
(B) the consensual pupillary light reflex is unaffected.
(C) it causes ganglion cell degeneration in the right nasal hemiretina.
(D) it causes cell degeneration in the right lateral geniculate body.
(E) it causes a right homonymous hemianopia.

38. Each of the following statements concerning ocular motility is true EXCEPT

(A) the frontal eye field is located in the inferior frontal gyrus.
(B) the occipital eye field is located in areas 18 and 19.
(C) the subcortical center for vertical conjugate gaze is located at the junction of the midbrain–diencephalon.
(D) the subcortical center for lateral conjugate gaze is located in the abducent nucleus.
(E) stimulation of the frontal eye field causes contralateral deviation of the eyes.

39. Each of the following statements concerning autonomic innervation of the eye is true EXCEPT

(A) stimulation of the intermediolateral cell column at T1 causes ipsilateral mydriasis.
(B) transection of the cervical sympathetic trunk causes ptosis and miosis.
(C) stimulation of the Edinger-Westphal nucleus causes miosis and ptosis.
(D) destruction of the ciliary ganglion interrupts both sympathetic and parasympathetic postganglionic fibers en route to the globe.
(E) destruction of the superior cervical ganglion causes ipsilateral Horner's syndrome.

40. Parasympathetic stimulation causes all of the following reactions EXCEPT

(A) profuse watery secretion of the salivary glands.
(B) constriction of the lumina of the bronchial tubes.
(C) ejaculation.
(D) increased gastrointestinal motility.
(E) penile erection.

41. Horner's syndrome can result from all of the following lesions EXCEPT

(A) hemisection of the spinal cord at C7.
(B) occlusion of the posterior inferior cerebellar artery.
(C) an aneurysm of the cavernous sinus.
(D) a tumor of the apex of the lung.
(E) a tumor of the base of the pons.

42. Each of the following statements concerning olfactory receptor cells is true EXCEPT

(A) they are first-order neurons in the olfactory pathway.
(B) they are unmyelinated bipolar neurons with central processes that form the first cranial nerve.
(C) they synapse with mitral cells in the olfactory bulb.
(D) they are incapable of regeneration.
(E) they enter the skull via the lamina cribrosa of the ethmoid bone.

43. Each of the following structures is a part of the gustatory pathway EXCEPT

(A) cranial nerves VII, IX, and X.
(B) the solitary tract and nucleus.
(C) the parabrachial nucleus.
(D) the ventral posterolateral (VPL) nucleus.
(E) area 43 of the parietal lobe.

Directions: Each group of items in this section consists of lettered options followed by a set of numbered items. For each item, select the **one** lettered option that is most closely associated with it. Each lettered option may be selected once, more than once, or not at all.

Questions 44–50

Match each of the following structures with the appropriate part of the brain.
(A) Diencephalon
(B) Medulla
(C) Midbrain
(D) Pons
(E) Telencephalon

44. Cerebral aqueduct

45. Cranial nerves III and IV

46. Caudate nucleus

47. Optic chiasma

48. Olive and pyramid

49. Pineal gland

50. Cranial nerves IX, X, XI, and XII

Questions 51–55

Match each of the following descriptions with the most appropriate type of cell.
(A) Astrocytes
(B) Ependymal cells
(C) Microglial cells
(D) Oligodendrocytes
(E) Schwann cells

51. Are derived from the neural crest

52. May myelinate numerous axons

53. Have filaments that contain glial fibrillary acidic protein

54. Myelinate only one internode

55. Arise from monocytes

Questions 56–60

Match each of the following symptoms with the appropriate lettered lesion (shaded area) in the diagram of a cross-section of the spinal cord.

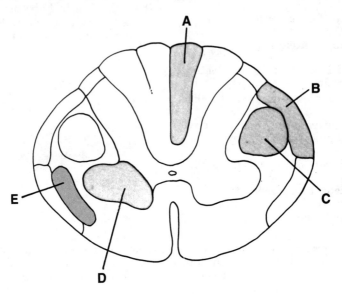

56. Ipsilateral leg dystaxia

57. Ipsilateral flaccid paralysis

58. Contralateral loss of pain and temperature sensation one segment below the lesion

59. Exaggerated muscle stretch reflexes below the lesion

60. Loss of two-point tactile discrimination in the ipsilateral foot

Questions 61–66

Match each of the following neurologic conditions with the appropriate lettered lesion (shaded area) shown on one of the two cross-sections of the brainstem.

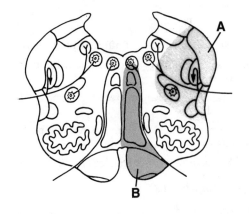

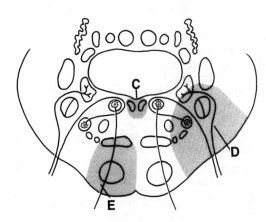

61. Medial rectus palsy on attempted lateral gaze

62. Lateral rectus paralysis; contralateral spastic hemiparesis

63. Occlusion of the posterior inferior cerebellar artery

64. Loss of the corneal reflex; contralateral loss of pain and temperature sensation from the body and extremities

65. Hemiatrophy of the tongue; contralateral hemiparesis; contralateral loss of vibration sensation

66. Hoarseness; Horner's syndrome; singultus

Questions 67–72

Match each of the following descriptions with the appropriate nucleus.
(A) Anterior thalamic nucleus
(B) Centromedian nucleus
(C) Ventral lateral nucleus
(D) Ventral posteromedial nucleus
(E) Mediodorsal nucleus

67. Receives input from the dentate nucleus

68. Receives input of taste sensation from the parabrachial nucleus

69. Receives input of pain and temperature sensation from the face

70. Receives the mamillothalamic tract

71. Projects to the putamen

72. Has reciprocal connections with the prefrontal cortex

Questions 73–78

Match each description with the most appropriate hypothalamic nucleus.
(A) Anterior nucleus
(B) Arcuate nucleus
(C) Mamillary nucleus
(D) Paraventricular nucleus
(E) Suprachiasmatic nucleus

73. Receives input from the hippocampal formation

74. Destruction results in hyperthermia

75. Receives input from the retina

76. Projects to the neurohypophysis

77. Regulates the activity of the adenohypophysis

78. Regulates water balance

Questions 79–83

Match each description with the most appropriate nucleus.
(A) Caudate nucleus
(B) Globus pallidus
(C) Centromedian nucleus
(D) Substantia nigra
(E) Subthalamic nucleus

79. Destruction causes contralateral hemiballism

80. Receives dopaminergic input from the midbrain

81. Gives rise to the ansa lenticularis and the lenticular fasciculus

82. Destruction causes hypokinetic-rigid syndrome

83. A loss of cells in this griseum causes greatly dilated lateral ventricles

Questions 84–90

Match each of the following nuclei or cells with the appropriate neurotransmitter.
(A) Acetylcholine
(B) Dopamine
(C) GABA
(D) Norepinephrine
(E) Serotonin

84. Raphe nuclei

85. Purkinje cells

86. Nucleus basalis of Meynert

87. Motor cranial nerve nuclei

88. Pars compacta of the substantia nigra

89. Locus ceruleus

90. Globus pallidus

Questions 91–95

Match each description below with the appropriate neurotransmitter.
(A) Glutamate
(B) Glycine
(C) β-Endorphin
(D) Enkephalin
(E) Substance P

91. Neurotransmitter of afferent pain fibers

92. Major inhibitory neurotransmitter of the spinal cord

93. Major neurotransmitter of the corticostriatal pathway

94. Located almost exclusively in the hypothalamus

95. Helps inhibit input from afferent pain fibers

Questions 96–102

Match each of the following neurologic deficits with the most likely site of the responsible lesion.
(A) Left frontal lobe
(B) Left parietal lobe
(C) Right parietal lobe
(D) Left temporal lobe
(E) Right occipital lobe

96. Left upper quadrantanopia

97. Muscle weakness and clumsiness in the right hand; slow effortful speech

98. Inability to identify a key placed in the left hand with the eyes closed

99. Denial of hemiparesis; patient ignores stimuli from one side of the body

100. Poor comprehension of speech; patient is unaware of the deficit

101. Patient is unable to identify fingers touched by examiner when eyes are closed; is unable to perform simple calculations

102. Babinski's sign and ankle clonus

Questions 103–107

Match each structure below with the appropriate lettered structure shown in the MRI axial section of the brain.

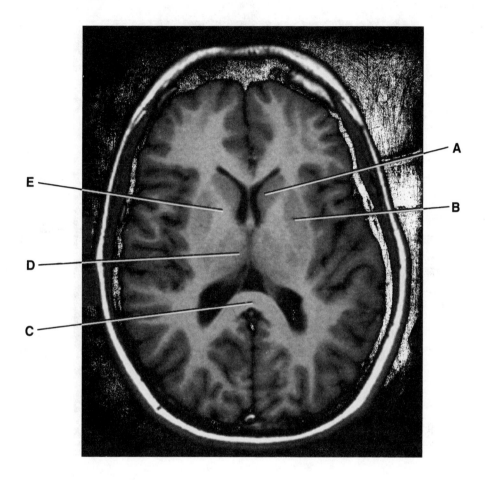

103. Thalamus
104. Internal capsule
105. Putamen
106. Caudate nucleus
107. Splenium

Questions 108–112

Match each structure below with the appropriate lettered structure shown in the MRI axial section of the brain.

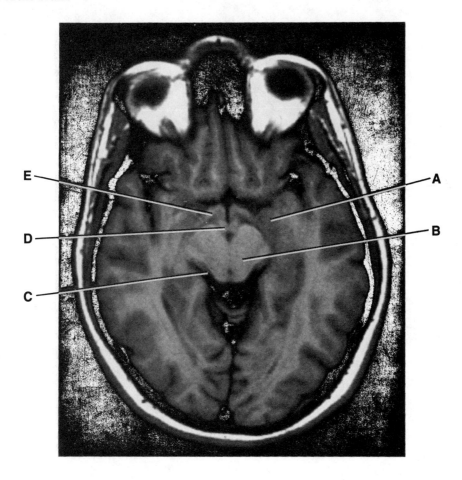

108. Medial geniculate body

109. Mesencephalon

110. Mamillary body

111. Optic tract

112. Amygdala

Questions 113–117

Match each structure below with the appropriate lettered structure shown in the MRI midsagittal section of the brain.

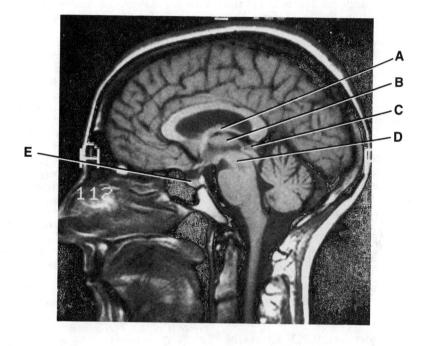

113. Pineal gland
114. Hypophysis
115. Mesencephalon
116. Thalamus
117. Fornix

Answers and Explanations

1–B. The calcarine sulcus separates the cuneus from the lingual gyrus. The banks of the calcarine sulcus contain the visual cortex.

2–A. The primary somatosensory cortex (areas 3, 1, and 2) is located in the postcentral gyrus (sensory strip) of the parietal lobe.

3–C. The trigone of the lateral ventricles contains the calcified glomera of the choroid plexus. These calcifications are visible in radiographs and CT images.

4–C. The subcommissural organ lies in the roof of the cerebral aqueduct near the posterior commissure. All circumventricular organs except the subcommissural organ have fenestrated capillaries and, thus, lack a blood–brain barrier.

5-A. The anterior cerebral artery irrigates the paracentral lobule, which lies on the medial surface of the hemisphere.

6–D. The superior sagittal sinus receives drainage from the greatest number of arachnoid granulations.

7–D. The mandibular nerve (CN V-3) exits the skull through the foramen ovale; it is not found in the cavernous sinus.

8–B. The temporal pole is supplied by the anterior temporal artery, which is a branch of the middle cerebral artery.

9–E. Ventral horn neurons develop in the basal plate of the mantle layer of the neural tube.

10–C. Rathke's pouch is an ectodermal outpocketing of the stomodeum anterior to the buccopharyngeal membrane and gives rise to the adenohypophysis (pars distalis, pars tuberalis, and pars intermedia).

11–D. The lateral horn (T1–L3) gives rise to preganglionic sympathetic fibers.

12–B. The nucleus dorsalis of Clarke (C8–L3) gives rise to the dorsal spinocerebellar tract, which ascends and enters the cerebellum through the inferior cerebellar peduncle.

13–A. The parasympathetic nucleus of the spinal cord is located in the ventral horn (Rexed lamina VII) at sacral levels S2–S4.

14–A. The neurons of origin (i.e., first-order neurons) of the gracile fasciculus are found in the dorsal root ganglia from T6–S5. Second-order neurons are located in the nucleus gracilis of the medulla. Third-order neurons are located in the contralateral ventral posterolateral nucleus of the thalamus.

15–E. The ventral spinocerebellar tract enters the cerebellum through the superior cerebellar peduncle. The dorsal spinocerebellar and the cuneocerebellar tracts enter the cerebellum through the inferior cerebellar peduncle.

16–E. The lateral spinothalamic tract projects to the ventral posterolateral (VPL) nucleus of the thalamus. The VPM receives pain fibers via the trigeminal system (i.e., via the ventral trigeminothalamic tract).

17–D. The parotid gland receives parasympathetic innervation from the glossopharyngeal nerve (CN IX). The inferior salivatory nucleus of CN IX is found in the medulla; it projects preganglionic fibers via the lesser petrosal nerve (CN IX) to the otic ganglion. The otic ganglion projects postganglionic fibers to the parotid gland.

18–C. The intra-axial fibers of the facial nerve are closely associated with the abducent nucleus, the MLF, the spinal trigeminal tract and nucleus, and the middle cerebellar peduncle. Lesions involving the facial nerve within the pons frequently include these associated structures. The medial lemniscus lies more distant (medial) to the intra-axial fibers of the facial nerve.

19–D. In the midbrain, the pyramidal tract lies in the basis pedunculi; oculomotor fibers of CN III pass through the medial part of the basis pedunculi. In the pons, the pyramidal tract lies in the base of the pons; abducent fibers of CN VI pass through the lateral part of the pyramidal fasciculi. In the medulla, the pyramidal tracts form the medullary pyramids; hypoglossal fibers of CN XII lie just lateral to the pyramids.

20–C. The mandibular nerve (CN V-3) is not located in the cavernous sinus. The cavernous sinus includes cranial nerves III, IV, VI, V-1, V-2, postganglionic sympathetic fibers, and the internal carotid artery.

21–B. The mandibular nerve (CN V-3) innervates the anterior belly of the digastric muscle. The facial nerve (CN VII) innervates the posterior belly of the digastric muscle.

22–E. The ventral trigeminothalamic tract mediates pain and temperature sensation. The second-order neurons mediating pain are located in the caudal third of the spinal trigeminal nucleus. Decussation of these fibers occurs in the medulla. Fibers that mediate the corneal reflex decussate at a higher level. Thus, trigeminal tractotomies at lower medullary levels (e.g., foramen magnum) may spare the corneal reflex fibers while abolishing pain sensation from the face.

23–D. The inferior olivary nucleus is a cerebellar relay nucleus located in the medulla; it is not part of the auditory system. The superior olivary nucleus, however, has an important role in the auditory pathway. It receives input from the cochlear nuclei and projects to, and forms, the lateral lemniscus.

24–E. The primary auditory cortex (i.e., areas 41 and 42) is located in the transverse temporal gyri of Heschl, a part of the superior temporal gyrus.

25–C. The vestibular nuclei receive input from the vestibular ganglion, which is found in the base of the internal auditory meatus. The spiral ganglion innervates the cochlear organ of Corti and gives rise to the cochlear nerve (CN VIII).

26–D. The MLF extends from the spinal cord to the rostral midbrain. It contains ascending vestibular fibers to the oculomotor nuclei of cranial nerves III, IV, and VI; abducent fibers (i.e., fibers from the lateral gaze center of the pons) to the contralateral oculomotor complex (medial rectus subnucleus); and descending vestibulospinal fibers. The MLF is a paramidline structure that lies distant to the motor nucleus of the trigeminal nerve (CN V).

27–E. The vestibular nerve contains efferent fibers that arise from neurons in the superior and medial vestibular nuclei. These inhibitory fibers innervate the hair cells of the cristae ampullares and the maculae of the utricle and saccule.

28–B. Transection of the facial nerve (CN VII) between the geniculate ganglion and the chorda tympani spares the GVE fibers from the superior salivatory nucleus that synapse in the pterygopalatine ganglion and innervate the lacrimal gland. These preganglionic lacrimal fibers are located in the major petrosal nerve (CN VII).

29–C. The nucleus ambiguus of cranial nerves IX, X, and XI is located in the lateral medulla, midway on a line connecting the hypoglossal nucleus and the postolivary sulcus; it is not near the hypoglossal nucleus of CN XII. The nucleus ambiguus is supplied by the posterior inferior cerebellar artery; the hypoglossal nucleus is supplied by the ventral spinal artery, a branch of the vertebral artery.

30–B. Purkinje cells project only to the vestibular and cerebellar nuclei. One of the cerebellar nuclei is the dentate nucleus, which projects to the contralateral ventral lateral nucleus of the thalamus, which projects to the motor cortex (area 4 of the precentral gyrus).

31–B. The superior cerebellar peduncle connects the cerebellum to the pons and midbrain. The middle cerebellar peduncle connects the cerebellum to the pons. The neocortex influences the cerebellum via the middle cerebellar peduncle. The inferior cerebellar peduncle connects the cerebellum to the medulla.

32–C. The neocerebellum (the posterior lobe minus the vermis and the paravermis) sends input to the motor cortex through the ventral lateral nucleus of the thalamus. The pathway is the neocerebellar cortex, dentate nucleus, contralateral ventral lateral nucleus of the thalamus, and motor cortex (area 4).

33–C. The dentatothalamic tract decussates in the caudal midbrain tegmentum at the level of the inferior colliculus. This massive decussation of the superior cerebellar peduncles is diagnostic of this level.

34–B. The fovea centralis of the retina is the site of highest visual acuity; it contains only cones. The retina has a dual blood supply. The choriocapillaris perfuses the outer layers of the retina, including the outer plexiform layer. The central retinal artery supplies the remaining inner layers of the retina.

35–C. Pituitary tumors frequently compress the decussating fibers of the optic chiasm and produce a bitemporal hemianopia. Nasal fibers decussate and temporal fibers remain ipsilateral.

36–B. Resection of the anterior portion of the temporal lobe transects the fibers of the loop of Meyer and results in a contralateral upper homonymous quadrantanopia. Inferior retinal quadrants are represented in the inferior banks of the calcarine sulcus. The loop of Meyer is located approximately 4 cm posterior to the temporal pole and projects to the inferior bank of the calcarine sulcus.

37–D. Transection of the optic tract results in transsynaptic (transneuronal) degeneration of cells in the ipsilateral lateral geniculate body. The optic tract contains pupillary and visual fibers from the contralateral nasal hemiretina and from the ipsilateral temporal hemiretina. Pupillary fibers from both eyes are present in the optic tract; therefore, interruption of one optic tract does not abolish pupillary light reflexes.

38–A. The frontal eye field is found in the middle frontal gyrus (area 8). Destruction of a frontal eye field results in a deviation of the eyes toward the side of the lesion.

39–C. The Edinger-Westphal nucleus contains preganglionic parasympathetic neurons that innervate the sphincter muscle of the iris and the ciliary muscle. Stimulation of this nucleus causes a constricted (miotic) pupil but does not cause ptosis. Severe ptosis results from damage to the superior division of the oculomotor nerve, which innervates the superior levator palpebrae. Slight ptosis results from sympathetic paralysis of Müller's superior tarsal muscle (smooth muscle) in Horner's syndrome.

40–C. Although erection is caused by parasympathetic stimulation, ejaculation is the result of sympathetic stimulation. Sacral somatic motoneurons also have a role in ejaculation: They evoke spasmodic contractions of the bulbocavernosus and ischiocavernosus muscles.

41–E. Horner's syndrome results when sympathetic input to the eye, at any level, is interrupted. Descending sympathetic pathways to the ciliospinal center of the thoracic cord (T1–T2) are located in the lateral tegmentum of the brainstem and in the lateral funiculus of the spinal cord. Horner's syndrome is seen in PICA, AICA, and Brown-Séquard syndromes; it is frequently associated with lung (Pancoast tumor) and neck tumors that encroach upon the sympathetic trunk and cervical sympathetic ganglia. Disease of the neck and cavernous sinus may also cause Horner's syndrome.

42–D. Olfactory receptor cells are located in the olfactory mucosa of the superior nasal conchae and opposing septum. These cells have a lifespan of 1 month and are capable of regeneration.

43–D. The gustatory (taste) pathway (SVA) is taste buds of the tongue; cranial nerves VII, IX, and X; solitary tract and nucleus; central tegmental tract; parabrachial nucleus of the pons; ventral posteromedial nucleus of the thalamus; and primary olfactory cortex (area 43).

44–C. The cerebral aqueduct is located in the midbrain (mesencephalon). It interconnects the third and fourth ventricles.

45–C. The tegmentum of the midbrain contains the nuclei of the oculomotor nerve (CN III) and the trochlear nerve (CN IV). The midbrain also contains the mesencephalic nucleus of the trigeminal nerve (CN V).

46–E. The caudate nucleus, a basal ganglion, is located in the white matter of the telencephalon. It forms the lateral wall of the frontal horn of the lateral ventricle.

47–A. The optic chiasm is located in the diencephalon. It lies between the anterior commissure and the infundibulum of the pituitary gland (hypophysis).

48–B. The olive and the pyramid are prominent structures on the surface of the medulla. The olive contains the inferior olivary nucleus; the pyramid contains the corticospinal tract.

49–A. The pineal gland (epiphysis cerebri) is part of the epithalamus, which is a subdivision of the diencephalon.

50–B. Cranial nerves IX, X, XI, and XII are located in the medulla.

51–E. Schwann cells of the peripheral nervous system are neural crest derivatives.

52–D. Oligodendrocytes of the central nervous system may myelinate numerous axons. Schwann cells myelinate only one internode.

53–A. The filaments of astrocytes contain glial fibrillary acidic protein (GFAP), a marker for astrocytes.

54–E. Schwann cells myelinate only one internode.

55–C. Microglial cells arise from monocytes.

56–B. Interruption of the dorsal spinocerebellar tract results in ipsilateral leg dystaxia (i.e., incoordination). The cerebellum is deprived of its muscle spindle input from the lower extremity.

57–D. Destruction of ventral horn cells (LMNs) results in an ipsilateral flaccid paralysis (a LMN lesion), with muscle atrophy and loss of muscle stretch reflexes (areflexia).

58–E. Interruption of the lateral spinothalamic tract results in a contralateral loss of pain and temperature sensation one segment below the lesion. The decussation occurs in the ventral white commissure in the spinal cord.

59–C. Interruption of the lateral corticospinal tract results in an ipsilateral UMN lesion, which is characterized by exaggerated muscle stretch reflexes (hyperreflexia), spastic paresis, muscle weakness, a loss or diminution of superficial reflexes (i.e., abdominal and cremaster reflexes), and Babinski's sign. The deficits are below the lesion on the same side. The lateral corticospinal tract decussates in the caudal medulla.

60–A. A lesion of the gracile fasciculus results in a loss of two-point tactile discrimination in the ipsilateral foot. The dorsal column–medial lemniscus pathway decussates in the caudal medulla.

61–C. This lesion includes the two MLFs. The patient has MLF syndrome and will have a medial rectus palsy on attempted lateral gaze to either side. Convergence remains intact.

62–E. This lesion includes three major structures: the medial lemniscus, corticospinal fibers, and exiting abducent root fibers (CN VI) traversing the corticospinal fibers. Interruption of the abducent fibers causes an ipsilateral lateral rectus paralysis with medial strabismus. Damage to the uncrossed corticospinal fibers results in contralateral spastic hemiparesis.

63–A. Occlusion of the posterior inferior cerebellar artery (PICA) infarcts the lateral zone of the medulla, causing PICA syndrome. The major structures involved are the inferior cerebellar peduncle, spinal trigeminal tract and nucleus, spinal lemniscus, the nucleus ambiguus, and exiting vagal fibers of CN X.

64–D. This lesion includes the facial motor nucleus of CN VII and its intra-axial fibers, thus, accounting for the loss of the corneal reflex (efferent limb). The spinal trigeminal tract and nucleus and the spinal lemniscus also are damaged by this lesion. Damage to the spinal trigeminal tract and nucleus causes an ipsilateral facial anesthesia, including loss of the corneal reflex (afferent limb). Damage to the spinal lemniscus (lateral spinothalamic tract) causes a contralateral loss of pain and temperature sensation from the body and extremities.

65–B. This lesion damages the hypoglossal nucleus of CN X and exiting root fibers, the medial lemniscus, and the corticospinal tract. Damage to the hypoglossal nerve results in an ipsilateral flaccid paralysis of the tongue, a LMN lesion. Damage to the medial lemniscus results in a contralateral loss of tactile discrimination and vibration sensation. Damage to the corticospinal (pyramid) tracts results in a contralateral spastic hemiparesis. This symptom complex is known as medial medullary syndrome.

66–A. Lateral medullary syndrome (PICA syndrome) usually includes hoarseness, Horner's syndrome, and singultus (hiccups). Damage to the nucleus ambiguus causes a flaccid paralysis of the muscles of the larynx with hoarseness (dysphonia and dysarthria). Interruption of descending autonomic fibers to the ciliospinal center at T1 causes sympathetic paralysis of the eye (Horner's syndrome). The anatomic causes of singultus are not clear.

67–C. The ventral lateral nucleus receives input from the dentate nucleus of the cerebellum and projects to the motor cortex (area 4). The VPL nucleus also receives input from the dentate nucleus and projects to the motor cortex.

68–D. The VPM nucleus receives input of taste sensation from the medial parabrachial nucleus of the pons and projects this input to the gustatory cortex of the parietal operculum (area 43).

69–D. The VPM nucleus receives GSA input from the face, including pain and temperature sensation. It also receives SVA (taste sensation) input from the tongue and epiglottis.

70–A. The anterior thalamic nucleus receives input from the mamillary nucleus via the mamillothalamic tract and direct input from the hippocampal formation via the fornix. The anterior nucleus projects, via the anterior limb of the internal capsule, to the cingulate gyrus (areas 23, 24, and 32).

71–B. The centromedian nucleus, the largest of the intralaminar nuclei, projects to the putamen and to the motor cortex. The centromedian nucleus receives input from the globus pallidus and the motor cortex (area 4).

72–E. The mediodorsal nucleus of the thalamus, or the dorsomedial nucleus, has reciprocal connections with the prefrontal cortex (areas 9–12).

73–C. The mamillary nucleus receives input from the hippocampal formation (i.e., subiculum) via the fornix.

74–A. The anterior nucleus of the hypothalamus helps prevent a rise in body temperature by activating processes that favor heat loss (e.g., vasodilation of cutaneous blood vessels, sweating). Lesions of this nucleus result in hyperthermia (hyperpyrexia).

75–E. The suprachiasmatic nucleus receives direct input from the retina; it plays a role in the maintenance of circadian rhythms.

76–D. The neurons of the paraventricular and supraoptic nuclei of the hypothalamus produce ADH (vasopressin) and oxytocin. These peptides are transported via the supraopticohypophyseal tract to the neurohypophysis. Lesions of these nuclei or their hypophyseal tract result in diabetes insipidus.

77–B. The neurons of the arcuate nucleus (infundibular nucleus) produce hypothalamic-releasing and release-inhibiting hormones, which are conveyed to the adenohypophysis through the hypophyseal portal system. These hormones regulate the production of adenohypophyseal hormones and their release into the systemic circulation.

78–D. The paraventricular and supraoptic nuclei produce ADH, which helps regulate water balance in the body.

79–E. Hemiballism results from circumscript lesions of the subthalamic nucleus.

80–A. The caudate nucleus and the putamen (caudatoputamen) receive dopaminergic input from the pars compacta of the substantia nigra, the nigrostriatal tract.

81–B. Neurons of the globus pallidus give rise to the ansa lenticularis and the lenticular fasciculus, two pathways that project to the ventral anterior, ventral lateral, and centromedian nuclei of the thalamus.

82–D. Destruction or degeneration of the substantia nigra results in parkinsonism (hypokinetic-rigid syndrome).

83–A. In Huntington's chorea, there is a lossof neurons in the striatum. Cell loss in the head of the caudate nucleus causes dilation of the frontal horn of the lateral ventricle (hydrocephalus ex vacuo), which is visible on CT and MRI studies.

84–E. Serotonin (5-HT) is produced by neurons located in the raphe nuclei. This paramidline column of cells extends from the caudal medulla to the rostral midbrain.

85–C. Purkinje neurons are GABA-ergic. GABA-ergic neurons are also found in the striatum, globus pallidus, and in the pars reticularis of the substantia nigra.

86–A. The nucleus basalis of Meynert contains cholinergic neurons, which project to the entire neocortex. This griseum is a ventral forebrain nucleus found embedded in the substantia innominata (located ventral to the globus pallidus). This nucleus degenerates in Alzheimer's disease.

87–A. Acetylcholine is the neurotransmitter of motor cranial nerves (GSE, SVE, and GVE) and anterior horn cells of the spinal cord.

88–B. Neurons of the pars compacta of the substantia nigra contain dopamine. Dopamine also is present in the ventral tegmental area of the midbrain, the superior colliculus, and the arcuate nucleus of the hypothalamus.

89–D. The locus ceruleus is the largest assemblage of noradrenergic (norepinephrinergic) neurons in the entire brain. It is located in the lateral pontine and midbrain tegmenta. Locus ceruleus neurons project to the entire neocortex and cerebellar cortex.

90–C. The globus pallidus contains GABA-ergic neurons that project to the thalamus and subthalamic nucleus.

91–E. Substance P is contained in dorsal root ganglion cells and is the neurotransmitter of afferent pain fibers. Substance P also is produced by striatal neurons, which project to the globus pallidus and substantia nigra.

92–B. Glycine is the major inhibitory neurotransmitter of the spinal cord. The Renshaw interneurons of the spinal cord are glycinergic.

93–A. Glutamate is the major excitatory neurotransmitter of the brain; neocortical glutamatergic neurons project to the caudate nucleus and the putamen (striatum).

94–C. β-Endorphinergic neurons are located almost exclusively in the hypothalamus (arcuate and premamillary nuclei).

95–D. Enkephalinergic neurons in the dorsal horn of the spinal cord presynaptically inhibit the dorsal root ganglion cells that mediate pain impulses.

96–E. A lesion of the lingual gyrus of the right occipital lobe can cause a left upper homonymous quadrantanopia. Lower retinal quadrants are represented in the lower banks of the calcarine sulcus.

97–A. A lesion of Broca's speech area (areas 44 and 45) and the adjacent motor cortex of the precentral gyrus (area 4) can cause Broca's expressive aphasia and an UMN lesion involving the hand area of the motor strip. This territory is supplied by the superior division of the middle cerebral artery (prerolandic and rolandic arteries).

98–C. A parietal lesion in the left postcentral gyrus (areas 3, 1, and 2) or in the left superior parietal lobule (areas 5 and 7) can cause astereognosis, the deficit in which a patient with eyes closed cannot identify a familiar object placed in the right hand. This territory is supplied by the superior division of the middle cerebral artery (the rolandic and anterior parietal arteries). The dorsal aspect of the superior parietal lobule on the convex surface is also supplied by the anterior cerebral artery.

99–C. Characteristic signs of damage to the nondominant hemisphere include hemineglect, topographic memory loss, denial of deficit (anosognosia), and construction and dressing apraxia. A lesion in the right inferior parietal lobule could account for these deficits. This territory is supplied by the inferior division of the middle cerebral artery (posterior parietal and angular arteries).

100–D. Wernicke's receptive aphasia is characterized by poor comprehension of speech, unawareness of the deficit, and difficulty finding the correct words to express a thought. Wernicke's speech area is found in the posterior part of the left superior temporal gyrus (area 22). This territory is supplied by the inferior division of the middle cerebral artery (posterior temporal branches).

101–B. Gerstmann's syndrome includes left-right confusion, finger agnosia, dysgraphia, and dyscalculia. This syndrome results from a lesion of the left angular gyrus of the inferior parietal lobule. This territory is supplied by branches from the inferior division of the middle cerebral artery (angular and posterior parietal arteries).

102–A. A lesion of the anterior paracentral lobule results in an UMN lesion (spastic paresis) involving the contralateral foot. Ankle clonus, exaggerated muscle stretch reflexes, and Babinski's sign are common.

103–D. The thalamus.

104–E. The anterior limb of the internal capsule.

105–B. The putamen.

106–A. The head of the caudate nucleus.

107–C. The splenium of the corpus callosum.

108–C. The medial geniculate body.

109–B. The mesencephalon.

110–D. The mamillary body.

111–E. The optic tract.

112–A. The amygdala (amygdaloid nuclear complex).

113–C. The pineal gland (epiphysis).

114–E. The hypophysis (pituitary gland).

115–D. The mesencephalon (midbrain).

116–B. The thalamus.

117–A. The fornix.

Suggested Readings

Adams RD, Victor M. (1989) *Principles of Neurology*, 4th ed. McGraw-Hill, New York.

Barr ML, Kiernan JA. (1988) *The Human Nervous System*, 5th ed. JB Lippincott, Philadelphia.

Carpenter MB. (1991) *Core Text of Neuroanatomy*, 4th ed. Williams & Wilkins, Baltimore.

Clemente CD. (1985) *Gray's Anatomy*, 30th American ed. Lea & Febiger, Malvern, Pa.

Cooper JR, Bloom FE, Roth RH. (1986) *The Biochemical Basis of Neuropharmacology*, 5th ed. Oxford University Press, New York.

Fix JD. (1987) *Atlas of the Human Brain and Spinal Cord*. Aspen, Gaithersburg, Md.

Moore KL. (1988) *The Developing Human*, 4th ed. WB Saunders, Philadelphia.

Noback CR, Strominger NL, Demarest RJ. (1991) *The Human Nervous System*, 4th ed. Lea & Febiger, Malvern, Pa.

Williams PL, et al. (1989) *Gray's Anatomy*, 37th ed. Churchill Livingstone, New York.

Index

Note: Page numbers in italics denote illustrations, those followed by t denote tables, those followed by Q denote questions, and those followed by E denote explanations.